DATE DUE

HIGHSMITH #45115

The Letters of
Sigmund Freud and Otto Rank

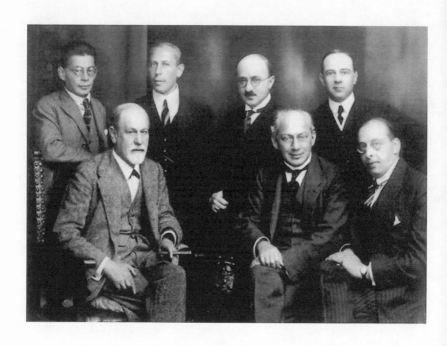

The Letters of
Sigmund Otto
Freud & Rank

Inside Psychoanalysis

Edited by

E. James Lieberman, M.D.

Robert Kramer, Ph.D.

Letters translated by

Gregory C. Richter

THE JOHNS HOPKINS UNIVERSITY PRESS

Baltimore

Published by arrangement with the Estate of Otto Rank and The Trustees of
Columbia University in the City of New York.

For the Sigmund Freud Letters
© A. W. Freud et al. (2012)

The Johns Hopkins University Press
2715 North Charles Street
Baltimore, Maryland 21218-4363
www.press.jhu.edu

Library of Congress Cataloging-in-Publication Data
Freud, Sigmund, 1856–1939.
[Correspondence. English. Selections]
The letters of Sigmund Freud and Otto Rank : inside psychoanalysis /
edited by E. James Lieberman and Robert Kramer ;
letters translated by Gregory C. Richter.
p. ; cm.
Includes bibliographical references and index.
ISBN-13: 978-1-4214-0354-0 (hardcover : alk. paper)
ISBN-10: 1-4214-0354-4 (hardcover : alk. paper)
1. Freud, Sigmund, 1856–1939—Correspondence. 2. Rank, Otto,
1884–1939—Correspondence. 3. Psychoanalysts—Austria—Correspondence.
4. Psychoanalysis. I. Lieberman, E. James, 1934– II. Kramer, Robert, 1953– III. Title.
[DNLM: 1. Freud, Sigmund, 1856–1939. 2. Rank, Otto, 1884–1939. 3. Psychoanalytic
Theory—Collected Correspondence. 4. History, 19th Century. 5. History, 20th Century.
6. Psychoanalysis—history. WM 460]
BF173.F85A4 2012
150.19′52092—dc23
[B]   2011016274
A catalog record for this book is available from the British Library.

Frontispiece: The Committee, 1922. *Seated:* Freud, Ferenczi, Sachs; *standing:* Rank, Abraham,
Eitingon, Jones. Guiding the movement from 1913, members in each location sent letters
to the other locations: Vienna, Budapest, Berlin, London. All were physicians except Rank
and Sachs; all were Jewish except Jones. Courtesy of the estate of A. W. Freud et al., by
arrangement with Paterson Marsh Ltd., London

*Special discounts are available for bulk purchases of this book. For more information,
please contact Special Sales at 410-516-6936 or specialsales@press.jhu.edu.*

The Johns Hopkins University Press uses environmentally friendly book materials, including recycled text paper that is composed of at least 30 percent
post-consumer waste, whenever possible.

Contents

Preface

Newly available unpublished letters shed light on the remarkable professional and personal relationship between Sigmund Freud and his youngest colleague, Otto Rank. The two lived near each other in Vienna during the formative years of psychoanalysis, from 1906 to 1926. This volume presents some two hundred fifty letters (most written when one or both men were away from home) within a narrative that provides historical and psychoanalytic context for general readers as well as specialists. The letters add a missing piece to the biographies of these men and to the history of an idea that held sway for much of the last century in Western—and global—thought and culture. The psychoanalytic movement had, and still has, an impact beyond psychology, psychiatry, and anthropology—in literature, philosophy, art, religion, entertainment, marketing, and politics.

Sigmund Freud wrote about twenty thousand letters in his lifetime of 83 years (1856–1939) and received just as many himself.[1] He kept a log of mail sent and received from hundreds of correspondents. Freud spent most evenings writing thoughtful, often elegant, letters by hand (his angular *Frakturschrift* can be read today only by specialists). A superb speaker and writer in his native language, he learned Latin and Greek, Italian, some Hebrew, enough Spanish to read Cervantes, enough French to work with Charcot and translate a book on hypnosis, and enough English—his favorite—to translate John Stuart Mill's *On Liberty* and to analyze British and American patients. He corresponded in fluent English with Ernest Jones, whose German was limited.

Rank, 28 years younger than his mentor, wrote in modern script. Trained as a locksmith, he enjoyed technology; he fixed things, typed, drove a car, and used a camera. He loved music, unlike Freud, who was described by his son Martin as unmusical. According to Martin, Freud hated bicycles but provided his children with "good new models. This did not prevent him from expressing his opinion whenever he had the chance." Freud did not object to cars or airplanes, and he enjoyed his first flight at age 75.[2]

Freud's family lived in an apartment (also his office) on Berggasse (Hill Street) from 1891 to 1938. He often worked 16 hours a day, beginning at 8 A.M. and ending between midnight and 3 A.M., with evening hours devoted to correspondence, reading, and writing. His wife, Martha, entertained often, mostly upper-middle-class Jewish friends, Freud's colleagues, and some patients. Rank routinely dined there before the Wednesday meetings of the psychoanalytic group. Martha had, besides her unmarried sister, Minna Bernays, five helpers: a maid (Paula Fichtl, who also received Freud's patients), a cook, a governess for the older children and a nanny for the younger, and a charwoman. Punctuality was important, "something then unknown in leisurely Vienna. There was never any waiting for meals: at the stroke of one [main meal] everybody in the household was seated at the long dining-room table and at the same moment one door opened to let the maid enter with the soup while another door opened to allow my father to walk in from his study to take his place at the head of the table facing my mother at the other end."[3]

As secretary of the Vienna Psychoanalytic Society, Rank kept the *Minutes*. Later he headed the *Verlag* (publishing house) and coauthored the Vienna *Rundbriefe* (circular letters) to Committee members in Budapest, Berlin, and London. Freud, about 5' 7", had his hair and beard trimmed daily at the barber's, posed for portraits, and imagined his bust on display at the University of Vienna. Rank, a few inches shorter and rather homely, nevertheless had three attractive women in his life: his two wives and Anaïs Nin.

The Freud-Rank letters do more than fill a gap in the history of psychoanalytic theory, practice, and organization. They dramatically reveal the interplay of personality and profession, theory and practice. From a father-son and teacher-pupil beginning, the two men become colleagues. The letters provide access to their work, family, travels, humor, anger, pathos, friends and rivals, sickness and health. This mentorship is insufficiently appreciated because of its ending, with Rank excommunicated from the organizations and texts of psychoanalysis during its heyday. The mentorship brings to mind that of Plato and Aristotle (well known to our principals), where the best pupil became a formidable critic.

One of the most influential thinkers of the twentieth century, Freud is the subject of more biographies than anyone can digest. The most influential is *The Life and Work of Sigmund Freud*, by Ernest Jones, in three large volumes (1953, 1955, 1957), with at least 14 printings, a one-volume abridgment, and many translations. Jones knew both Freud and Rank for 30 years and had access to Freud letters only published in full after 1990. Jones's partisan view of rivals Ferenczi and Rank becomes clear in our volume, which helps balance the record.

Freud's papers reside in the Library of Congress in Washington, D.C. Some items have only recently been opened to researchers, and some remain closed for years, even decades. Rank's papers, including originals of Freud's letters and some manuscripts, are at Columbia University, open to scholars. Most of Rank's letters to Freud came to Dr. Judith Dupont in Paris from the late Michael Balint, student and friend of Sándor Ferenczi. We assume that Freud gave the Rank letters to Ferenczi.

Freud's published letters, besides an early anthology to 90 different recipients, include extensive correspondence with Carl Jung, Karl Abraham, Ernest Jones, Sándor Ferenczi, Max Eitingon, and family members. There are smaller published exchanges with Eduard Silberstein, Wilhelm Fliess, James Jackson Putnam, Lou Andreas-Salomé, Ludwig Binswanger, Hilda Doolittle, Georg Groddeck, Oskar Pfister, Eduardo Weiss, Arnold Zweig, and others. Unpublished Freud letters include those with A. A. Brill and Ruth Brunswick, among many others. There are six major Freud correspondences published since 2000: the unabridged letters with Abraham; the letters with Ferenczi (3 vols.); the letters with Eitingon (2 vols.); the Committee *Rundbriefe* (4 vols.); travel letters to his family (*Reisebreife*, 1895–1923), and letters to his children (2010; 680 pages!). The last four collections—eight volumes—have not been translated into English. We rely on these primary sources, grateful for the labors of our predecessors and colleagues, especially Ernst Falzeder, the preeminent Freud scholar.

Rather than publish this collection in the conventional catalog format, we placed letters of minor significance—which would interrupt but not add to the narrative—in a chronological appendix (A). Letters of medium and major importance appear in full in the text. Along with some high drama and deep thoughts, these tell of everyday work, the business of editing and publishing, colleagues and rivals, health, friends, travel, and the weather. A volume of record for scholars, this book is meant to be a readable text for non-specialists interested in ideas and their history.

In personal correspondence Freud was prolific, eloquent, and amazingly frank for one who knew his letters would be saved for posterity. The Freud-Rank collection is small compared to Freud's correspondence with other Committee members such as Ferenczi: 1,240 letters, half of them from Freud. The Jones and Abraham volumes are about half that size, the Eitingon collection two-thirds the size. There are, in addition, four volumes of *Rundbriefe,* the circular letters sent from each station—Vienna, Berlin, Budapest, London—to the other three. These, written for the group, are generally more formal, less personal, than the one-to-one letters.

Freud and Rank had quite different ideas about biographical access. At 29, in 1885, Freud wrote to Martha, his future wife, that he had destroyed all papers and letters except hers and those of family, to frustrate future biographers. He hoped to bury his letters to Wilhelm Fliess, but they were saved by Princess Marie Bonaparte. Rank kept letters from Freud, and many Rundbriefe—but little other correspondence, professional or personal. He wrote a diary from age 17 to age 21 and copied the original pencil version carefully in ink; he preserved the diaries, along with notes and drafts of articles and books. Unlike Freud, he published only one case history, and there are no patient records—if indeed he maintained any.

The drama of Freud's professional and personal relationships is well known from published primary sources—except, until now, the one with his closest ally. Jessie Taft, Rank's American friend, translator, and first biographer, described his reticence: "Whatever he had to say came out freely in his books but always impersonally. In the 13 years of my association with him he never discussed with me his relation to Freud or others on the 'Committee' except once in answer to something I had said about their attachment to Freud, when he replied, 'and I was in deepest of all'; and once painfully about Ferenczi, whom he had met in the railroad station in New York in 1926, 'He was my best friend, and he refused to speak to me.' "[4]

The letters tell how Rank, with Freud's support, evolves from a reticent disciple into an intellectual and administrative force in psychoanalysis. Close and warm colleagues for twenty years, Freud and Rank come alive through these letters, their collegial—indeed, loving—relationship ultimately strained to the breaking point: unforeseen, unwanted, inevitable.

NOTE TO THE READER: In the pages of this book, where the date, sender, and recipient of a letter are evident, the letters are not cited in the notes. Notes indicate the sender with an asterisk before the initials: *F-Fer or F-*Fer. The notes use the letter dates and numbers given in the primary sources (not page numbers, which vary in different editions). As mentioned above, the minor Freud-Rank letters (sometimes quoted in part) appear in full in appendix C. "[...]" indicates an illegible word or illegible words in a letter, usually no more than a sentence. Rarely, a paragraph or a page is missing, and the omission is so indicated.

There are gaps in the collection; missing letters are sometimes noted. There are only two from Freud in 1916, then none until 1921. There is only one from Rank between 1918 and 1921. Correspondents often abbreviate psychoanalysis: Pa, Psa, P/A, or Ψ. Some but not all names, places, and texts mentioned in letters are annotated.

The Letters of
Sigmund Freud and Otto Rank

≈ ≈

Introduction

Born Otto Rosenfeld in 1884, Rank adopted his surname from a sympathetic character in Henrik Ibsen's *A Doll's House*. He surely knew that 1884 also marked the publication of his favorite play, Ibsen's *Wild Duck*, and his favorite book, Twain's *Huckleberry Finn*, from whom in later years he took his American nickname, Huck. The second son in a working-class Jewish family, with a loving mother and an abusive, alcoholic father, Otto was relegated to trade school due to financial constraints, while Paul Rosenfeld became a lawyer. Locksmith by training, poet, psychologist, and philosopher by nature, Rank savored plays and concerts from the free or cheap seats in Viennese theaters, read voraciously, and kept a diary from age 17 to 21. In 1905, at 21, having read Freud's *Interpretation of Dreams*, he wrote a critical reanalysis of one of Freud's own dreams and *Der Künstler,* an essay on the sexual psychology of the artist. Alfred Adler, Rank's doctor and an early Freudian, brought the young man to Freud's attention. It is generally assumed that Freud was impressed by the "Artist" manuscript, but it may have been the audacious dream analysis, the carefully copied diary, or all three.

In his analysis of Freud's Frau Doni dream (see App. B), Rank expounds on the mention of Freud's "poetic" eldest son: "F's son cannot become a great poet because he protected him through puberty from all real harm. But on the other hand, from the psychological riches and keen insight of the father, from his half-poetic, half-scientific talents (studies-stories), his perception of people and relationships, it could well be possible! And that would be interesting (the first case of its kind!)."

In his diary (*Tagebuch* [manuscript], 1905), Rank reacts to Freud's *Interpretation of Dreams*: "A medically proven artist!" He was intrigued with Freud's

1

ability to make scientific sense out of dream-work and the unconscious. He greatly admired Darwin—and Schopenhauer, Nietzsche, Shakespeare, Beethoven, Wagner, and others. Rank wanted to understand the artist without diminishing the irrational, a source of creativity. From his diary:

> The most beautiful thing in an artist's life is that which he cannot work out. An artist, whose creative work would be his life! The peak! If the whole man, whole life, is not contained in every moment of life as the sea in its drops, then life makes no sense! What does nature make of the myriad lost days, hours, lives? How much advantage the least of the living has over the greatest of the dead!
>
> Instinct is the unconscious of animals. Religion is the synthesis of poetry and philosophy. Art is life's dream interpretation. Artists know the rules of art, but a work of art cannot be created by following them. Does the hysteric know the rules by which his illness is formed? Perhaps not entirely, for then he would be the doctor.[1]

The adolescent Rank writes of coming close to suicide at one point and rejecting it. "Afterwards there grew in me the greatest lust for life and courage toward death." Living became a conscious choice, a willing rebirth. Rank was a religious skeptic, though not a militant atheist like Freud. The diary includes "Ten Commandments," one of which states, "Thou shalt not give birth reluctantly." Two decades later, in *The Trauma of Birth*, Rank writes that "Socrates himself likened his dialectic therapy of drawing forth thoughts to *the practice of midwifery* as he practices it in imitation of his mother, who was a midwife." He saw Socrates as the "primal father of the analytic technique, which found in Plato its worthy theorist" (181–82).

Freud hired Rank as secretary of his Wednesday Psychological Society in 1906, stipulating that he finish academic high school (*Gymnasium*) and go on to the University. Rank was 28 years younger than his mentor and three years older than Mathilde, the first of Freud's six children: three daughters and three sons. The youngest, Anna, knew Rank from age 10. The only one of Freud's children to follow in his footsteps, she worked closely with both men from age 23 (1919). For two decades Rank and "Professor" steered the psychoanalytic movement from a smoky room at Berggasse 19 to an intellectual, social, and cultural force in much of the world for most of a century. Rank said he might write a history of psychoanalysis one day, but, along with unfinished projects on humor, women, and Judaism, he left that undone at his death at 55, in 1939, a month after Freud died in London, at 83.

Their partnership coincided with historic movements in science, the arts, philosophy, and politics. The year 1905 brought Albert Einstein's theory of relativity, along with Freud's *Three Essays on the Theory of Sexuality*. Soon after came Henri Bergson's *Creative Evolution* and William James's *Pragmatism*. Bergson moved from initial scientific positivism to favor intuition and interior personal experience—in the spirit of Henri Matisse's remark, "Exactitude is not truth." With the relativity concept came attention to inseparable relationships—space-time, energy-matter—and awareness of the influence of the observer on the observed. The history of psychoanalysis shows some parallels, with the notion of transference (Freud) and the discovery of new aspects of therapeutic influence (Ferenczi and Rank).

In 1914 Freud, like many intellectuals, lost his initial patriotic enthusiasm as the massacre of World War I went on. His sons and his virtual sons, Rank and Ferenczi, were drafted. Rank returned in 1918 from army service in Krakow newly married. Postwar Vienna, former capital of the Austro-Hungarian Empire, was a head without a body, a palatial city with bread lines. Psychoanalysis gained adherents from medicine and the arts, drawing patients, trainees, and money from abroad, so Freud's project flourished. Rank and Freud took up where they left off, but Rank was no longer just an apprentice and a scholar. Allied with Ferenczi in "active therapy" and pioneering a new theory on the early mother-child relationship, Rank, who coined and emphasized the term *pre-Oedipal,* ran afoul of conservative colleagues Abraham and Jones. In 1923, Ferenczi and Rank modified Freud's medical-authoritarian model in pursuit of more effective therapy at the same time Freud published his *Ego and Id*—literally *The I and the It* (*Das Ich und Das Es*), and Martin Buber defined the I-Thou relationship (*Ich und Du*). That year a fraternal battle erupted in the Committee after Freud's diagnosis of oral cancer.

We present the story of the Freud-Rank bond, its development and denouement, as much as possible in the words of the participants. Important questions are clarified if not answered: Can there be a science of the irrational? Is psychoanalysis an art form, a science, or both? Can the therapeutic relation be standardized, codified, measured, or is it existential, ineffable, beyond psychology?

Chapter 1

The Vienna Psychoanalytic Society

1906–1910

The basis for your complaint seems to me to lie in the oppression of your imagination by your intellect. . . . You are ashamed or frightened of the momentary, passing madness found in every true creator, the longer or shorter duration of which distinguishes the thinking artist from the dreamer. You complain of your unfruitfulness because you spurn too soon and sift too fine.
—Schiller to C. G. Körner, 1788

During their first four years together, Freud, with Rank's help, published the second edition of *The Interpretation of Dreams* (1909) and presided over the first two international psychoanalytic congresses. The *Jahrbuch* (Yearbook) was established in 1909 with Carl Jung as editor. Rank published two books, worked on two more, and emerged as second only to Freud in the pantheon of psychoanalytic writers. A summary of their early years sets the stage for the correspondence, which becomes significant in 1911.

1906. Freud, then 50, introduced Rank, 22, as secretary of the Wednesday Psychological Society, precursor of the Vienna Psychoanalytic Society (VPS). About a dozen physicians and intellectuals had met weekly at Berggasse 19, Freud's home and office, since 1902—holding about 25 meetings annually, with a long summer break. By 1906 Freud had written five books and 70 journal articles. During the day he treated patients, devoting evening hours to correspondence with an enlarging circle, which included English sexologist Havelock Ellis and Swiss psychiatrist Carl Jung. Rank soon became the youngest member of the VPS on the basis of three presentations that became his third and largest book, *The Incest Motif in Literature and Legend* (1912). His VPS *Minutes* include précis of each formal presentation along with members' lively dialog, eventually filling four volumes. Freud must have read and approved these minutes.

Rank endured and parried criticism in the meetings; Wilhelm Stekel, for example, said he was diligent but lacking maturity and too beholden to Freud. While Freud's devotees took *The Interpretation of Dreams* and *Three Essays on Sexuality* as scripture, not all members bowed to the Professor. In October, Alfred Adler ventured his own theory of organ inferiority and overcompensation, while Stekel argued that neurosis derives from psychological causes, not heredity and sexual frustration. He said that modern man is "haunted by anxiety. Due to a superabundance of hygienic restrictions, meant to preserve his life, he does not live at all; it is precisely his anxiety that makes him ill."[1] Freud recalled his own work with Josef Breuer before 1896: "In curing neuroses one takes hold of the floating part of the patient's libido and transfers it to one's own person. The translation of the unconscious material into consciousness is performed with the help of the transference. The cure, therefore, is effected by means of a conscious love. . . . The patient, like the child, believes only one whom he loves."[2] At year's end Freud complained to Jung that his own supporters sometimes made him feel like a crank or fanatic.[3]

1907. On New Years Day Freud mentioned Rank to his Swiss correspondent, Carl Jung: "I know of only one who might be regarded as your equal in understanding, and of none who is able and willing to do so much for the cause as you."[4] In the spring, psychiatrists Carl Jung, Ludwig Binswanger, and Max Eitingon visited the society for their first meeting with Freud, Adler, and Rank. Jung thought Alfred Adler's organ-inferiority theory was "brilliant." To his visitors Freud disparaged the Viennese group. That upset Binswanger but not Jung, who knew how much Freud preferred his non-Jewish supporters. When Karl Abraham broached visiting from Berlin, Freud wondered whether this German psychiatrist was Jewish. He was, and he knew Jung well, having worked three years at the Burghölzli clinic in Zurich.

In May, Fritz Wittels presented a paper on why women should not be medically trained. Some members disputed his thesis, but most agreed that medical education might be harmful and that women physicians should never touch men's genitals. Rank elaborated Freud's idea that medical education is a less neurotic path than philosophy and religion to resolve childhood curiosity about sex, birth, and "where did I come from?"

Rank published his monograph, *The Artist: Toward a Sexual Psychology*. Its epigraph from Shakespeare (in English) reflects the twentieth-century artist's concern about self-consciousness: "Is it possible, he should know what he is, and be that he is?" (*All's Well That Ends Well*). Rank elaborated a grand theory in dense prose. The artist transforms repressed sexual impulses into a socially acceptable product that gratifies, even heals, the admiring audience. If art is insufficient, the audience needs and gets a prophet or savior who delivers it from sin by suffering and atoning for it. This idealized creative figure provides a therapeutic cure for the masses as the artist does for the cultured few. The neurotic must be cured individually: "He is the complete egotist, his opposite is the prophet who suffers for the people, and the artist stands between the two."[5]

Freud sent *The Artist* to Jung, who replied with criticism of Rank's fealty to Freud's sexual theory: "The public that Herr Rank writes for won't understand it at all. . . . In reading him I have more than once had to think of Schelling and Hegel. But your theory is pure empiricism and should be presented empirically too."[6] Freud answered: "I feel sure Rank will not get very far. His writing is positively autoerotic; he is utterly lacking in pedagogic tact. Besides, as you observe, he has not overcome the influence of his previous intellectual fare and wallows in abstractions that one cannot get one's teeth into. But he is more independent of me than might appear; he is an able man, very young and, what is especially estimable in one so young, thoroughly honest."[7]

Probably due to his academic work Rank did not present a paper during the VPS year beginning in October, but he was active in discussions, duly recorded in his minutes. Rank took issue with Freud's dualistic libido theory, preferring the monism of Schopenhauer's will as the source of both desire and suffering and that of the Greek philosophers: desire resembles that which fosters growth in plants, from which other drives differentiate.[8]

1908. On March 4, Rank quoted Friedrich Schiller (epigraph, above) on the conflict between intellect and emotion. Freud added the passage, thanking Otto Rank for unearthing it, to the second edition of *The Interpretation of Dreams*, stating that analysis requires turning unwilled, often threatening, thoughts into voluntary ones, as poets do.[9] In that session Rank used Adler's theory to analyze Schiller's *William Tell*, which portrays a blind archer. Since Schiller himself had eye problems, the overcompensation thesis could apply. Several members attacked Rank, while Adler and Freud were supportive:

"Rank's interpretation is a particularly beautiful mythological confirmation of Adler's principle and secure as are few interpretations." On April 1, Nietzsche's *Genealogy of Morals* was the topic. Rank said Nietzsche "explored not the external world, as did other philosophers, but himself . . . reversing the earlier transfer from within onto the external world." Freud said his own attempt to read Nietzsche was "smothered by an excess of interest. . . . I can assure you that Nietzsche's ideas have had no influence whatsoever on my own work." Freud drew a clear line between science and art: poets had flashes of insight that he had to reach gradually with methodical theory and research.

The first International Psychoanalytical Association (IPA) Congress brought 42 people to Salzburg on Easter Sunday, where Freud displayed his spellbinding oratory. The attendees, mainly Austrian, included two women and some important outsiders: Jung, Ferenczi, Jones, Abraham and A. A. Brill, the Hungarian-American psychiatrist who first translated Freud into English. On Monday morning Freud spoke without notes for three hours about the "Rat Man" and was pressed to continue, which he did for another two hours after lunch. Rank presented the Schiller quotation. Elated by the event and enamored with Jung, Freud chose the tall, handsome Protestant minister's son to be editor of the new *Yearbook* (*Jahrbuch*). This offended the Viennese, whose jealousy and distrust of the Swiss psychiatrist were no secret. Freud overruled them, explaining that they had to keep psychoanalysis from being dismissed as a Jewish affair. Freud nominated Rank as reporter for the *Yearbook,* telling Jung, "You know from his *Artist* how well he can formulate my ideas."[10]

Relations between Abraham and Jung had been strained; in a letter of October 11 Freud pleaded with his Berlin colleague to extend himself to "the more alien" Aryan. He also calls Abraham's attention to Rank's work on the myth of the birth of the hero. Meanwhile Rank entered the University of Vienna, majoring in philosophy and German. Freud, a neurologist himself, confident of medical support from physicians like Adler, Ferenczi, Jones, and Jung, counseled Rank to pursue the Ph.D. rather than an M.D. He opposed medical education for his own three sons, also.

1909. The *Minutes* reveal Rank's independent, emboldened voice. In February he presented and analyzed the story "Cursed to Stand," from Grimm. Therein a boy who refuses an order is cursed by his father to stand in one spot forever; after some years, he dies. Rank said, "In this case of hysterical paralysis the motivation—that is, the stubborn boy's resistance to his father's order—is clearly expressed." Freud called it the prototype of passive resistance.

The next month Alfred Adler spoke on Karl Marx. Freud, receptive, outlined a theory of human progress: "The enlargement of consciousness is what enables mankind to cope with life in the face of the steady process of repression." And vice versa: each process is a condition for the other. Freud praised Rank's work on the incest motif in literature for examples of how poetry reflects repression and called Rank's *Artist* "the first introduction of psychology into historical studies." At the end of March, discussing poets and psychology, Rank restated his conviction, "when the unconscious is made conscious, art ceases to exist." Freud ended the session with praise for Henrik Ibsen, who, he said, made issues clear while concealing himself. Both Freud and Rank held that historical progress led to the decline of literary art. In Rank's favorite play, Ibsen's *Wild Duck*, the father, Ekdal, is self-absorbed and insensitive, like Rank's. Such a man, says the budding analyst, can be neither helped nor hurt by interpretation: he is impervious.

In April, Rank delivered "The Psychology of Lying," based on observations of real people, not literature. He linked pathological lying, which is compulsive and clumsy, to some kind of sexual secret, usually masturbation, while compulsive truthfulness relates to self-control of masturbation. Rank proposed a "masturbatory character," listing, as indicators, cleanliness, defiance, avarice, collecting, frugality, punctuality, secrecy, and shyness. Freud called this useless speculation but gave Rank credit for having "touched very intelligently on a series of most interesting problems." Freud considered Emile Zola to be a "truth fanatic" but doubted that he fit Rank's thesis. Rank said that his ideas had not been refuted, and he thanked the three members who supported him and Professor Freud for "affirmation of my main point—the fanaticism for truth."

Rank's *Myth of the Birth of the Hero* would soon be out. Freud contributed several paragraphs on "The Family Romance"—the common, grandiose fantasy of children that they were adopted from royal families by their current parents. Rank inscribed Freud's copy as co-parent, not son or student.

To the father of this book
In gratitude from—the Mother[11]

In September, Freud, Jung, and Ferenczi sailed to the United States for a conference at Clark University. Freud gave five talks in German to a mostly nonmedical audience; the published lectures became an introduction to psychoanalysis. Newspapers in Boston and New York interviewed Freud, reporting with enthusiasm about a radical departure from asylum psychiatry, speculative neurology, hypnosis, and quackery. Psychologist-philosopher (and M.D.) William James was amicably skeptical, while Boston neurologist James Jackson Putnam became Freud's first important American supporter. British psychiatrist Ernest Jones met his future colleagues there and soon wrote Freud that he was using Rank's *Hero* book for a study of Hamlet.[12]

In the fall session of the VPS Freud spoke of weaning in relation to traumatic anxiety. A footnote is added to *The Interpretation of Dreams* (2nd ed., 1909), saying that "birth is the first experience of anxiety." Another session was devoted to Nietzsche, whose autobiographical *Ecce Homo* (*Behold the Man*) had just appeared, posthumously. To members who diagnosed that philosopher as neurotic, Rank replied that neurotic elements were ubiquitous in normal and exceptional people. Freud thought the book's mastery of form supported its validity. He praised Nietzsche's introspection but faulted him for transforming "is" to "ought," so that moral-theological matters trump science. Though fascinated by Nietzsche's brilliant insights, Freud again explained that he couldn't read past page one of the opus "partly because of the resemblance of his intuitive ideas to our laborious investigations, and partly because of the wealth of ideas."[13]

1910. The first mention of Rank's involvement in clinical work occurs in January: he analyzes a young woman friend's dream.[14] Some of this material found its way into *The Interpretation of Dreams* (3rd ed., 1911), and Freud called it "perhaps the best example of a dream interpretation." Jones called it "delightful."[15] At the second IPA Congress in Nuremburg, in March, a storm hit. Ferenczi, by arrangement with Freud, nominated Jung to be IPA president for life! The Viennese—20 of the 80 attendees—banded together in protest. A distraught Freud scolded them, arguing that a psychiatrist and a Gentile must lead the movement. But Freud had to reduce the term to only two years. Even loyalist Jones (a non-Jewish psychiatrist) concluded that Freud's wishful thinking made him a poor judge of character; the Viennese protesters foresaw Jung's defection. To assuage the VPS, Freud stepped down as its president, allowing Adler to take over. In April a medical group in Hamburg proposed to boycott clinics where psychoanalysis was practiced. Freud expressed his anger to Ferenczi: "There they make the argument that I wanted to deflect by moving [the presidency] to Zurich, namely that Viennese sensuality cannot be found elsewhere! You can still read between the lines that we Viennese are not only pigs but also Jews."[16]

Writing Freud from Toronto (June 19, 1910) Jones was introspective: "The originality-complex is not strong with me; my ambition is rather to know, to be 'behind the scenes' and 'in the know,' rather than *to find out*. . . . Any talent I may have lies rather in the direction of being able to see perhaps quickly what others point out. . . . To me work is like a woman bearing a child; to men like you, I suppose it is more like the male fertilization. That is crudely expressed, but I think you will understand what I mean." (Freud did not address this specifically in reply.)

The VPS, now too large for Freud's home, began to meet in a rented room. Dues were raised to about $15. Probably Freud tapped a wealthy contributor for Rank's salary of $200, the rent, and a new publication: *Zentralblatt für Psychoanalyse*, co-edited by Stekel, Adler, and Freud, which would supplement Jung's *Yearbook*.

Rank and Hitschmann were working on Freud's *Neurosenlehre* (*Collected Papers*) and read chapters aloud to Professor, who wrote "it will be quite usable . . . the first textbook of P/a."[17] In 1902, Freud's academic title was raised from the lowest, adjunct, to "Professor Extraordinary"—still minimal, without a chair, like "clinical professor": one who is in practice, teaches occasionally, has no university office, no salary, just the title and library privileges. Anti-Semitism may have denied him earlier or higher academic recognition. In any case, he taught little but prized the title, which everyone used. The VPS grew; any qualified applicant could join except current patients of members. Hanns Sachs, a lawyer, became a member; soon he, Freud, and Rank were meeting for a weekly dinner at Freud's home, followed by a brisk walk on the Ringstrasse. Freud cited Rank as a good reason for Jung to include non-physicians in the Swiss group.[18]

At year's end Freud complained to Jung that Adler was departing from the path of psychoanalysis by deemphasizing sexual themes.

≈ Chapter 2 ≈

Alfred Adler Departs

1911

The psychoanalytic movement began to splinter as it grew. Early in 1911, Alfred Adler took three Vienna Psychoanalytic Society sessions to present and defend his ideas, which Freud considered a departure from psychoanalysis. Adler argued that the therapeutic value of transference resides in rebellion against the therapist, not as a love-bond that fosters continuing treatment. He praised Freud but elaborated his own theory of organ inferiority and masculine protest. Freud considered it a major deviation—"acutely observed ego-psychology"—but it was, with its lessened emphasis on sex, reactionary, superficial, unscientific, and dangerous.[1]

Freud wrote to Jones: "We had a series of Adler-debates and as the incompatibility of his views with our ΨA came out clearly, he resigned his leadership, though he was not obliged or suggested to do so. . . . Adler's views were clever but wrong," his motives and behavior must stem from neurosis, and he has "a morbid sensibility." And, "I am glad you like Rank's work ['A Dream That Interprets Itself']. He is growing rapidly in sharpness and good forms and keeps his honest character unharmed. I gave him some help in this paper but he wanted very little. I am of intention to use his force broadly in my next works and to make him a partner in the coming edition of *Traumdeutung*."[2]

Ten days later, March 8, Jones replied, "Rank seems to be grandly active in his work. You must be proud of him as a disciple." Rank updated the bibliography and proofread *The Interpretation of Dreams* for the second and third editions (1909 and 1911). He would contribute two chapters, with his name appearing below Freud's on the title page in the fourth through the seventh editions (1914–22).

Freud wrote Jung about Adler, making clear that ego-psychology was out of bounds, a false triumph of rationality over instinct: "I must avenge the offended goddess Libido. . . . I would never have expected a psychoanalyst to be so taken in by the ego [*das Ich:* the I]. In reality the ego is like the clown in the circus [canoe], who is always putting in his oar to make the audience think that whatever happens is his doing."[3] Freud wrote Ferenczi, "there is only one of the Viennese who has a scientific future, and that is little Rank, who has held on very valiantly alongside me."[4] In April, Rank traveled to Greece for two weeks on a university excursion, paid for by Freud as thanks for editorial work. A grateful Rank left Freud the draft of his doctoral thesis, a psychoanalytic monograph on *Lohengrin.*

In all their letters Freud and Rank use the formal *Sie* (you); Freud used *du* only with family and a couple of others. His young associates eventually came to use the *du* form with one another.

Athens ¶April 20, 1911

Esteemed Professor:

Just a half hour before my leaving Athens your friendly lines were forwarded to me and I must answer in great haste, in pencil, so this letter can go ashore and arrive in Vienna before I do.

We've had almost constantly beautiful weather, but were somewhat rushed, which I really regretted today in the National Museum, where you were on Sept. 5, 1904 according to a note in your Baedeker's Guide. I can't possibly describe right now all my impressions of this magnificent world—hoping to have the chance to do so in Vienna.

Concerning the proofs, I worried some, since nothing came until today. Now that they're here all is well, with our long sea voyage ahead of us.

Your comments on Lohengrin *are brilliant. I was mostly concerned with collecting material, trying to put it together as much as possible. What attracted me were the correspondences, which fit almost without exception. I'd appreciate further hints from you in person regarding its overall balance.*

My apologies for writing in haste: the gangway can be lifted any moment, but before leaving these glories I felt compelled, esteemed Professor, to express my heartfelt, sincere thanks for your great kindness, which made this experience possible.

With best regards to your dear wife, and greetings to your daughter [Anna] and sons, I am your devoted Rank

Back home for the early May meeting of the Vienna Psychoanalytic Society, Rank found himself on the spot when Paul Federn spoke of libido in a broad sense, "as Rank has done." Freud's *libido* meant strictly "the urging of the sexual instincts." He criticized Jung but not Rank for broadening the concept to include "every kind of psychic tension." Adler's supporters kept pressing Rank, who hedged: "It's true that I took the libido concept broadly, but I consider the things to which I extended it as sexual. Thus one could take my statement as an unjustified extension of Freud's concept just as much as being an enrichment of it."[5]

That spring, Rank and Sachs proposed a new nonmedical psychoanalytic journal, *Imago*, for psychoanalytic papers on literature, mythology, and philosophy. In June, Freud announced he would no longer serve with Adler as co-editor of *Zentralblatt*. Adler got a lawyer, set some conditions that Freud ridiculed, and resigned from the VPS with three others. Seven Adlerians remained, declaring that his resignation had been provoked.[6] In July Rank wrote from his vacation.

Maria-Wörth [Carinthia], Villa Belvedere ¶July 17, 1911

Esteemed Professor!

At last I have put things in order and rested enough to write at leisure. The trip was indescribably beautiful, and though I ventured two days in Naples, tempted by its proximity and reassuring news, Rome impressed me most. I enjoyed all the worthy sights, and the last day was in Tivoli, where I recovered from the tiring Roman study. Not completely, though, for I was in Hadrian's Villa, one of the most beautiful things I've ever seen. I'm very proud that at the Forum, without a guide, I could identify nearly every stone, for which I thank my previous study-sojourn in Greece. I stayed as briefly as possible in Naples proper, just to be in the museum and at one scenic outlook, spending the rest of the time in Pompeii and Sorrento. I'd have disobeyed your order not to buy antiquities had not the price of the marvelous artifacts excavated at Pompeii exceeded my travel fund. On the trip out I stopped in Florence, where I beheld an unforgettable sunset from the Piazza di Michelangelo; on the return spent a night in Genoa (saw the leaning tower of Pisa en route) and had a day in Milan. Alas, I was half an hour too late to see "The Last Supper" by Leonardo da Vinci. Attempts to bribe were fruitless, as keys and guides are not in the house, but in the convent. That's the one dark spot in the annals of this otherwise extremely successful voyage, and I can't thank you often enough or warmly enough for making it possible.

Of our Austria I've heard nothing the whole trip, first getting some news now. Dr.

Bach sent a membership application with a statement declaring his wish to withdraw; he joins the protest of those gentlemen who see in the proceedings against A[dler] an infringement of scholarly freedom.

Dr. Maday of Innsbruck asked for information about what's recently happened so he can express his own opinion. Dr. Sachs reports that he and his project were cordially received in Zurich. Maeder wrote a detailed letter assuring me of his warmest sympathy for the project. From correspondence between Stekel and Bergmann, Dr. Sachs and I have the impression that Stekel is working against our plan, which he seems to have represented to Bergmann as his own.

Yesterday I visited Dr. Steiner, who is here in Velden. Jones wrote that after a six-month break he is again working on Nightmare.

With the very best wishes for your recovery, and
with most respectful greetings, I am your grateful, Rank

P.S. Dr. Tausk sent me a ms. about suicide by Drosnés in Odessa. I don't know what I should do with it. Please let me know.

On July 13, Jones announced that he would leave Toronto for London. His common-law wife, Loe, "a chronic invalid," suffered from pyelonephritis, had almost constant pain, and was dependent on morphine. A native of the Netherlands, "she is away from her friends and relatives, and cordially detests the Canadian people, as I do myself. She has made big sacrifices for me in the past in many ways, although she does not believe in my work and is very fearful about the dangers of it to my reputation." Jones had told Freud in an earlier letter (June 28, 1910), "I have always been conscious of sexual attraction to patients; my wife [Loe] was a patient of mine." Now Jones would not subject Loe to another year in Toronto in hopes of getting a professional appointment—one had already been denied because of opponents who thought him "dangerous." His only choice was "to return with her to London or to separate, which is unthinkable."

Freud praised Jones and commiserated (Aug. 9), then reported on Adler: "I have ripened the crisis. It is the revolt of an abnormal individual driven mad by ambition. . . . I hope we will lose a great many others of little or no use who are ready to follow him." On August 31, Jones reported that a professorship had been granted after all: the chancellor, whose daughter he had successfully treated, weighed in, among others.

Mark Twain would become Rank's favorite author, Huck Finn his "twin." He tells here how it all started.

Maria-Wörth ¶July 25, 1911

Esteemed Professor!

Many thanks for your kind letter [missing]. As to the ambitious plan you read accurately from my unconscious, I'd like to realize it only for Rome, and hope to once more. Also I'd like to study more and enjoy longer some parts of Florence and Naples, not getting over-sated; only in Rome do I feel that could never happen. Here, by the way, where all goes well, there is plenty of opportunity to recover from the stress of travel and get strength for the winter; already I feel quite refreshed and fear I'm getting lazy.

A sketch of my daily inactivity will make that fear credible to you. Up at 7, breakfast at 8, then I take part in the children's English lesson. Then I usually row over to the post office to see whether I got anything, which almost every day is the case. Then I swim (yesterday the water was 21 degrees [70 F]) and sunbathe till noon. Lunch at 1, then, until tea, a lesson in Latin and Greek, my real activity. And now the decision whether I do some work or loaf the rest of the day—mostly the case. Evenings we usually have a concert, or the children's American governess reads us Huckleberry Finn *in an awful Nigger-dialect. Today the children are away and so I hope I can use it to work.*

Otherwise I have no special plans besides my wish to assemble and sort material accumulated over the course of the year. Corrections for Lohengrin go slowly; I hope to finish before the Congress. As you see from the enclosure, I got the invitations from Jung and already sent them out. Also Drosnés ms. sent to Stekel.

May I inquire about the "magical"?

Somewhere in the Worcester [Clark University] Lectures is a note citing your Sexual Theory *with the wrong title and year. Presumably they'll catch the error.*

I've come to an understanding with Stekel and got over my initial irritation at his presumptuous written comments: no wonder, given these temperatures. After the last (July) issue, which is quite "eropsychic," I understand his resistance. Deuticke [publisher] would be ideal for us in every way, and always hovered quietly in our thoughts. After your comments we do have reason to be hopeful and are glad to know the matter is safely in your hands.

Adler's letter to Jung indicates that he'll stubbornly carry on "the old fight with his teacher." In his last article on syphilophobia he revealed that phobias are for security and therefore did not even think of the nice simile of the border fortification. Thus he cites Stekel, using Leuthold's lines:

Like Goethe I'm gold?

Then you are just brass—

like Lessing. Behold:

Not diamond but glass.[7]

He's also trying to recruit allies by quotes with praise (Philipp Frey), which was never his way before.

Maday would like to know what happened in the Society so he can express his own opinion; I'll send him the bare facts on a card. Maybe Sachs will stop off here during his return trip.

> *Best wishes for your recovery. Yours with grateful respect, Rank*

Maria-Wörth, August 7, 1911

Esteemed Herr Professor!

Time flies incredibly fast here, and, doing nothing, I make no headway; it's worthwhile, for once, just to live in the day.

News flows meagerly. Dr. Sachs has happily returned to Vienna from his successful mission, and until further notice leaves the whole business to me, which I have to present at the Congress in his place—at least with private courting of coworkers and subscribers. I hope to be in Weimar a day before the Congress and get further instructions from you about this; I do hope your personal involvement in this will render my task superfluous.

Jones wrote that he won't go back to America after the Congress, but will stay in London and try to get your psychology into the hard skulls of the English. He's again working on Nightmare, *the first part of which he hopes to bring along to Weimar. He laments that* Zentralblatt *is not run internationally enough to have articles in other world languages, saying the many difficulties of translation have kept him and many of his countrymen from submitting their works more often. In this context, after a comment from you, I felt it appropriate to recommend that he contact* Eros und Psyche. *Hitschmann wrote me, among other things, that he had met Friedjung, who was at a Tuesday evening meeting at the home of A., but was apparently so appalled at the shady wheeling and dealing of Grüner and comrades that he swore never to return. He also writes that Franz Servaes tore Abraham's "Segantini" [article] to shreds in the* Frankfurter Zeitung, *and the next day "a Frankfurt physician poured manure on Stekel."*

Maday of Innsbruck will be in Vienna in a few days, and I asked him to look up Dr. Sachs. The young musician I once introduced to you sent me from Paris some interesting essays on musical production, the psychology of music, and Bruckner's emotional life in particular; I believe he could also contribute lots of fine articles for us.

The new interpretation of the calf [leg] impressed Jones very much, and he con-

gratulated me for it, which praise I dutifully pass on to you. Hopefully "Psychoanaly-
sis" has now been completed. This time Deuticke is so slow that I'm afraid I'll be leav-
ing here without finishing Lohengrin. In any case, the book is getting bigger than I
expected. Nor is there any sign thus far of the Jahrbuch. Jung wrote me that in early
August one more issue of the Korrespondenzblatt will appear, and after September
1 the complete Congress program will be available. Since I may be in the Dolomites
then, I'll have to leave Dr. Sachs in charge of distribution. Unfortunately, I probably
can visit only the Ampezzo Valley. Otherwise from Bolzano I'd have taken the liberty
to visit you and your family, to whom I extend my best greetings.

I've again been doing some work on "The Nudity Theme," which promises to be
very fruitful. In this article I've poked a psychological wasps' nest and don't know my
way in or out. I hope it goes better soon.

I hope you've had a good cure in Karlsbad and thoroughly recuperated at Kloben-
stein am Ritten [Collalbo sul Renon, Italy].

Respectful greetings. Gratefully yours, Rank

In the next letter, Rank explains his behavior psychoanalytically: the unconscious having its way in determining behavior.

Maria-Wörth, August 27, 1911

Esteemed Herr Professor!

Many thanks for your kind letter [missing]. Lacking outside events or inner ex-
periences worth reporting, I wouldn't have answered except that time, which gets me
to do everything, presses me on, and my departure from here fast approaches.

The Dolomites tour did not work out; although in a way disappointed, I have a
welcome opportunity to complete several projects. I await the last 11(!) proof sheets of
Lohengrin. Only now can I see what a huge piece of work I must have done, finishing
in one month; in light of this I decided to do nothing more here except loaf. But since
this tendency resided in my unconscious the whole summer, expressing itself unre-
strained in corresponding symptoms, I'm inclined to interpret my new resolve as a
"rationalization" of the unconscious tendency. Fortunately, my article on the theme of
nudity in literature and legend, intended for Eros und Psyche, is nearly finished and
will not be harmed by this new resolve. Material and topic were not infrequently fine,
furthermore self-organizing in surprising and, to me, unexpected relationships. At
several points, however, if the material didn't organize itself, I couldn't fully master it.
I don't attribute the fault to my inability, although I feel I'd have done better in Vienna
with less rest and more work. Perhaps I'll talk about this in the VPS. In any case, may I

take the liberty of asking your advice about this, for I know that you always see at first glance where I have failed, and how it can be helped.

I am getting along with Sachs really well, and if he shows me just the positive side of his brother complex, we'll be fine.

Jones wrote that he's leaving on September 10. So I won't be able to answer him again.

I wrote Abraham today about the hotel in Weimar, and I told him the plan for the new project.

From Vienna I hear only from Sachs and Hitschmann from time to time. Hitschmann wrote that in the most recent edition of Jugend *there's a poem about Segantini [Italian artist]. One could become more popular in Germany only if the Kaiser personally had the "cause" presented to him.*[8]

Hopefully your plans during this hot summer will ripen enough so that Eros und Psyche *can present a fine fruit to readers.*

Before mid-September (11/12) I go via Salzburg to Munich; I want to study the Glyptothek [museum], and will come to Weimar on the 20th. From there I'd like to go to Berlin for two or three days, where I need to read some things in the library that can be found only in Berlin.

> *Best regards to your honored family and you. With grateful respect, Rank*

Maria-Wörth, Villa Belvedere to Klobenstein [Collalbo] ¶August 30, 1911

Hochverehrter [Highly Esteemed] Herr Professor

Jung wrote today that due to the low count of announced presentations, the program will be delayed. He encourages me to volunteer a presentation since there is only one from Vienna so far. I'm wholly unprepared right now, and would gladly yield to older and, especially, foreign colleagues, though I don't want to leave Congress overseers or our group in the lurch. Please release me from this psychological conflict through an imperative, which I'll follow obediently.

Do you think the nudity theme would be appropriate? In any case, I'd first have to work out a few basic types by omitting all secondary information. Is there still enough time? Or do you think a few nice bladder dreams with rain and water symbolism more appropriate?

> *Meanwhile, cordial thanks from your grateful Rank*

The Third International Psychoanalytical Association Congress took place in Weimar, September 21–22, without the Adlerians. Rank reviewed some of the presentations in *Zentralblatt* no. 2. His paper, "Nudity in Literature and

Legend," was singled out for mention in the local press—prurient interest. As a result, journalists were unwelcome at future psychoanalytic meetings.[9]

On October 11, the VPS expelled members of Adler's "Society for Free Psychoanalytic Investigation," stating the two groups were incompatible. Freud wrote Abraham: "I've completed the purge of the society and sent Adler's seven followers packing . . . with the single exception of Rank, I have no one here in whom I can take complete pleasure."[10]

After a long silence Rank led one of a series of discussions on masturbation in December. He spoke of guilt that arises from within the individual and is not just a result of social disapproval. Freud praised Rank for "the most correct statements about it up to now," supporting more emphasis on this inner sense of guilt.[11] Rank's Ph.D. thesis, *Die Lohengrinsage* (1911), was published, in addition to articles, reviews, and translations in the *Yearbook*. His paper on narcissism was cited by Havelock Ellis, an originator of the concept, as an important influence on Freud. "Rank's study evidently impressed Freud, who in 1914 accepted and emphasized Rank's view, stating positively that there is a primary narcissism in every individual, the libidinal complement to the egoism of the instinct of self-preservation."[12]

The founders of depth psychology—Freud, Adler, Jung, and Rank—never met together after the Nuremberg Congress of 1910. The Weimar Congress of 1911 took place without the Adlerians.

Jones attended the Weimar IPA Congress and wrote Freud a long, enthusiastic letter from Toronto on October 17 (including praise for Rank's "beautiful" *Lohengrin* monograph). "I found my wife distinctly better. Adolf Meyer had done her much good by talking to her very reasonably about my work." She was optimistic, even amenable to treatment when she learned that Freud thought it could help. She stipulated that she would "do anything so long as she wasn't expected to believe something she couldn't believe (i.e., have ideas forced upon her against her will)." She preferred analysis with Freud above anyone, which Jones thought would not be possible; they would await Freud's judgment. Jones reported a "disagreeable dream, which after a difficult analysis showed the wish that she might die instead of getting better. I felt greatly relieved after having it out with myself, and ever since have been freer and happier than for years."

In November Freud was 55½, the age at which Rank died (in 1939).

≈ Chapter 3 ≈

Judging Jung

1912–1913

Freud used a charming illustration provided by Rank in the revision of *The Psychopathology of Everyday Life* (German edition, 1912). An insecure young man misspoke when addressing a young woman on the street, saying *begleitdigen* instead of *begleiten*, "accompany"—a slip of the tongue. The slip combines the intended word with *beleidigen*, "insult." Interpretation: the man expected that the woman would be insulted by his underlying carnal motive. Freud used the example in lectures, pointing out that the man— doubtless Rank himself—was timid and had little chance with the lady.[1]

On January 19, Rank responded to Oskar Pfister's request for a gift suggestion for Freud. From his own experience he knows how hard it is to find something for a man who is a "giver of gifts in the best sense of the word, who barely understands and cannot enjoy the fact that someone needs to give him something. This is his nature. I don't mean to say he wouldn't be pleased by a little gift (though he takes most pleasure—as I've often seen—in the things he gives to himself)." Rank had brought Freud a pair of antique vases from Greece: "the first and only time in my life I allowed myself such a thing, the double joy in seeing he was very pleased." Having said that, Rank noted that Freud had a substantial collection of museum-quality antiques, that it's hard to find something genuine, and that it would be expensive. So he suggests a book, for "the most beautiful private library I know." Rank offered to help with the choice, if only in a negative way. For the price of a modest antique one can get "a sumptuous volume," in which case, "I would with greatest pleasure consult with our publisher who knows well the Professor's tastes and the library."[2]

Regarding *Imago,* the new cultural journal, Freud wrote Jones (Feb. 24): "It brings the excellent chance into existence of being directed by two bright and honest boys like Rank and Sachs, who besides stand in excellent relations to each other." He also mentions that *Taboo* is half-written and "all finished in thought."

In late July Freud alerted Ferenczi to a growing schism with Jung, who, after a disturbing five-week silence, wrote that keeping his distance "will guard against any imitation of Adler's disloyalty." Freud senses that the Swiss (Jung, Riklin, Maeder) are leaning toward "symbolism instead of reality" and "doubting the influence of infantile complexes," while invoking racial difference as an explanation. That Jung accepts "tendencies," neglecting deeper probing of patients' experiences, means he has taken "the path for traveling salesmen." He adds, "Jung must now be in a florid neurosis. However this turns out, my intention of amalgamating Jews and goyim in the service of ΨA seems now to have gone awry. They are separating like oil and water."[3]

Ferenczi was glad that Freud had "finally given up the frantic effort to appoint a personal successor." He wrote that Jung's "declaration of war saddened but did not surprise me.... [The Swiss] are all a bunch of anti-Semites." Ferenczi found an advantage in being Jewish: "You must always keep an eye on Jones."[4]

In brief letters of August 11 and 18 Freud invites Rank to join him and Ferenczi on a visit to England in September, hosted by Jones (see App. A). Freud would pay Rank's expenses as a reward for his "latest excellent book," *Das Inzest-Motiv in Dichtung und Sage (The Incest Motif in Literature and Legend).* This huge—685 pages—cross-cultural study is dedicated, "To my revered teacher, Professor Dr. Sigmund Freud, in gratitude."

Prof. Dr. Freud Karersee ¶Aug. 22, 1912

Lieber Herr Rank,

I am very happy with your decision [to go to England]. Ferenczi, who just today praised your book highly, also looks forward to your company. We plan to depart September 8 from Caldonazzo in Valsugana [Italy], probably to make Munich our first stop and there you can join us. Of course you'll get precise details in good time.

Imago no. 3 is in my hands and so far as I was not involved, pleased me very well. Please make sure I can complete proofreading for the second section before we travel. We stay here another 8 days, then my address is: Hotel Seehof, San Cristoforo, Valsugana, Tirol.

You must deal directly with Löwenfeld. I respect the sense of obligation you and Dr. Sachs have in the decision.

With Zurich, most regrettable is the certainty that togetherness of Jews and anti-Semites, whom I hoped to unite on the foundations of psa., miscarried. Otherwise, I'm not too upset. Jung's behavior toward me—not his opinion about the libido—has damaged our close relationship a lot, but things shouldn't come to a split as with Adler, given many solemn assurances. But who knows? Anyway, it's time we worked more closely together, and the London trip will help. Also try to suppress all in Vienna that raises expectations of a civil war. I could not admit that this is getting to me person-ally. C'est la vie. We'll survive these difficulties too, if we don't let them drive us crazy.

We're having a wonderful stay here en famille, *enhanced by Sophie's bridegroom [Max Halberstadt]. Unfortunately the weather is inconsistent and often too cold, so the boys have nothing to do. The old bones feel it, though.*

> *I greet you warmly and hope you won't fail [academically] in autumn due to your very sensible choice of the pleasure principle. Yours, Freud*

The next letter expressed uncertainty about the trip, which was canceled.

Prof. Dr. Freud Karersee ¶August 25, 1912

Lieber Herr Rank,

Thank me no more! You've no idea how much pleasure I take from your accepting my proposal.

Sadly I have to tell you today that the trip has become uncertain. Not giving up yet, I must prepare you for the possibility, and ask that you keep the secret. My eldest daughter [Mathilde] who has caused us so much worry, has become ill again. What will come of this is still unclear. Perhaps things will be in order again in 2 weeks, departure time, but that's the condition for my leaving the house. Otherwise, I'll come to Vienna ahead of schedule, and incognito.

Naturally, I'll keep you apprised of all changes in our chances. I'd be very sorry to give up the trip, which would serve to forge a closer relation between you and Ferenczi, but human aims are powerless.

Given this situation, I don't want to become interested in anything else. I got the article in the Frankfurter Allgemeine Zeitung; *it left me cold, like everything from that quarter. It's all malicious nonsense. Let's keep working; a book like yours on incest, or a creation such as* Imago, *are more important than all the newspaper articles and "scholarly" discussions of literature.*

Cordial greetings. Please await further news from me. Yours, Freud

On September 7, Freud told Jones: "I bade Rank prepare for a sojourn at London and I had to disappoint him as well as you owing to the illness of the eldest daughter." He further asked Jones to assure his wife that "not seeing her at London" was his "greatest regret."

Prof. Dr. Freud S. Cristof ¶September 13, 1912

Lieber Herr Rank

I was quite ill for some time, but now I feel energetic, so on Sunday the 15th I'm going to Rome. I've sent you the last corrections for Imago, *and ask you to take care of the page proofs. Should you wish to send anything back to me, my address is: Roma, ferma in poste. (For Italy, one must always print the F in Latin script. Otherwise the letters will be lost, as the Italians do not recognize our F.)*

I hope you're approaching the end of your study for examinations. At least the cancellation of the trip to London was good in that respect. More idiotic jealous comments from Stekel against Imago. *It is difficult, but one must not take him seriously.*

Cordial greetings to you and Dr. Sachs from your Freud

From London (Sept. 18), Jones told Freud about a talk he had with Mrs. Jung, who, recently analyzed, "seems to take a fairly objective view of her husband's failings." As for a permanent presidency, "We cannot have a monarchy unless one man is strong enough to be king, and willing. Perhaps the best solution after all would be a yearly changing President . . . with a strong central committee of about six who would conduct the campaign, organize the forces, and formulate the plans."

In November Rank, at 28, passed his final exam for the Ph.D., after which Freud addressed him as "Herr Doktor." Stekel left the Vienna Psychoanalytic Society but kept control of the *Zentralblatt* (Central journal). In response the VPS planned a new journal, the *Zeitschrift* (Chronicle).

After the Wednesday night meetings, Freud took Rank and Sachs on a vigorous walk through Vienna's quiet streets. They surely discussed Ferenczi's analysis of Jung: "He identifies confession [to priest] with psychoanalysis and evidently doesn't know that the confession of sins is the lesser task of Ψa therapy: the greater one is *demolition of the father imago*, which is completely absent in confession. Evidently Jung never wanted (and was not able) to let himself be demolished by a patient. So he has *never* analyzed, but to his patients has always been the *savior* who suns himself in his Godlike nature!"[5]

Loe Kann, Jones's common-law wife, came for analysis with Freud in November. Freud sent progress reports to Jones and Ferenczi: ". . . doing very well and has given up the first half of her dose of morphine without difficulty."[6]

Jung bridled at Freud's attempts to control him. "I've done more to promote psychoanalysis than Rank, Stekel, Adler, etc., put together."[7] He berated Freud for treating pupils like patients: "You produce slavish sons or impudent puppies"—Rank and Ferenczi on the one hand, Adler and Stekel on the other.[8] Freud strategized with Rank, Sachs, and Ferenczi about Jung: "He is obviously disposed to provoke me so that the responsibility for the break will fall to me and he can say that I can't tolerate analysis. . . . He is behaving like a florid fool and the brutal fellow that he is. The master who analyzed him could only have been Fräulein Moltzer, and he is so foolish as to be proud of this work of a woman with whom he is having an affair."[9] (Maria Moltzer was a nurse who became an analytical psychologist. In 1909 Jung disclosed to Freud an affair with a patient, Sabina Spielrein, who later became a psychiatrist and analyst.) In the same letter Freud told Ferenczi that Rank "is day by day becoming more indispensable."

Rebutting Jung, Freud wrote that he himself was criticized for allowing his followers too much latitude. "It is a convention among us analysts that none of us needs be ashamed of his own bit of neurosis. But one who, behaving abnormally, keeps shouting that he's normal gives cause to suspect he lacks insight into his illness." With this Freud severed the personal relationship, saying that the emotional tie has long been only a thin thread.[10]

Freud announced the *Internationale Zeitschrift für ärtzliche Psychoanalyse* (International Journal of Medical Psychoanalysis), edited by Ferenczi and Rank (to replace Stekel's *Zentralblatt*). Rank would handle relations with the VPS and the publisher, Heller. In December Freud wrote, "The [Balkan] war mood dominates our daily life; it hasn't affected my practice yet, but it could turn out that I have three sons on the battlefield at the same time."[11]

Lou Andreas-Salomé, writer, friend of Nietzsche and Rainer Maria Rilke, attended VPS sessions through the academic year as well as Freud's Saturday lectures. She had attended the Weimar Congress and met Karl Abraham, who praised her grasp of Freud's work. She kept a diary and corresponded with Freud from Göttingen, Germany, where she practiced analysis. Concerned about Freud's troubles with Jung and with Victor Tausk, a brilliant, provocative newcomer to the VPS, Lou wrote in her diary (Feb. 12, 1913):

I understand very well that men of intelligence and ability like Otto Rank, who is a son and nothing but a son, represent for Freud something far more to be desired. He says of Rank: "Why is it that there can't be six such charming men in our group instead of only one?" Even in his wish for a half-dozen the individuality of the man referred to is put in some doubt. And yet just this serves to reassure Freud in the face of threatening "ambivalence." During one evening's discussion, when Rank lectured on regicide, Freud wrote the following note to me on a piece of paper: "R disposes of the negative aspect of his filial love by means of this interest in the psychology of regicide; that is why he is so devoted."

Internationale Zeitschrift für Ärtzliche Psychoanalyse ¶Feb 11, 1913
Lieber, verehrter Professor!

I take the liberty of sending Zentralblatt *for your examination, and ask you to bring it please Wednesday evening so I may report on the contents. It seems we must be prepared to face determined competition, which we need not fear so long as the contributions are so weak and deluded, blind. Nevertheless, the question—raised by Ferenczi today in a letter to me, too—is whether we should report critically on* Zentralblatt *(to the extent that the articles, though polemical, are of psa. interest, I think they should be included in the bibliography). I'd favor that just in exceptional cases, of course leaving the decision to you; on the other hand, I'd say it's time to critically rip up Adler's approach, pull out by its roots this whole fruitless and false system of opposition. If Jung or Reitler can't or won't do this, Tausk would be the next logical choice; bait is now being thrown to him (in the critique on the onanism debate). I might be willing to do this, as soon as I have gotten some more done. Yesterday I began work for Löwenfeld.*

Yesterday, as before, I got a package from Bergmann with Zentralblatt *copies, which I didn't accept, so they went back. I let him know, with instructions to turn to Jung with any questions. I also wrote Jung that sending out* Zentralblatt *through Bergmann to all members—again, it seems—would create great confusion, and asked him to reach an agreement with Bergmann if need be.*

Frau Dr. Stöcker (Berlin), who wrote about editorial matters, apologizes for her support for Stekel (bound by the name! [stecken, "stick fast"]), whose presentation appears in Neue Generation, *saying that she wishes to be "informed [...] only of research as such." I responded that she need not justify herself to us, that we accept her impartiality, but there are limits that can, in other perspectives, be breached even by psa. research, which she advocates.*

From Jung I got a very flattering card (re his criticism), in which he is encouraged to refute a new opponent (Stärring?) who has come out in Specht's journal.[12]

[...] Greetings. Rank

By early summer Freud finished *Totem and Taboo,* in which he applies psychoanalysis to society and history, based on the primordial, fatal rivalry between father and sons. Rank and Sachs had just published their book, *The Significance of Psychoanalysis for the Mental Sciences* [Humanities]. In June a celebratory dinner for *Totem* took place in Vienna with Freud, Rank, Sachs, Ferenczi, and Jones. Jones suggested that they, with Karl Abraham, form a committee to guide and guard the psychoanalytic movement.

≈ Chapter 4 ≈

The Committee

1913–1914

Jones, Ferenczi, Rank, Sachs, and Abraham joined with Freud in May 1913 to launch the Committee, which Freud insisted be kept secret. Ferenczi wished each of the five to be analyzed by Freud, as he would later be, but that was impractical. Freud gave each member an antique engraved stone to be mounted in a ring, and expressed his gratitude and relief: "I was so uneasy about what the human rabble would make out of it [psychoanalysis] when I was no longer alive.... Since [the Committee was formed] I've felt more lighthearted and carefree about how long my life will last."[1]

Jones presented Freud with personal rather than ideological problems. Freud discussed Loe Kann's analysis with him, her de facto husband. Freud said her dependence on morphine has lessened but her sexual anesthesia was less tractable. To the dismay of all concerned, Jones, traveling in Europe, renewed an old affair with Loe's maid, Lina. He remorsefully apologized to Freud, admitting "a repressed spirit of hostility against my dear wife as punishment for her anesthesia."[2] Loe relapsed on morphine and threatened to abandon Freud as well as Jones. To keep the analysis going, Freud accepted her wish to be free of commitment to Jones. "I could not go on in the role of your friend," he wrote Jones, "as long as I am to act as her physician."[3]

Jones hoped to reconcile with Loe. He apologized to her but not abjectly, as he had done the first time, writing that "no woman can altogether demand this in her heart from a man, in spite of friend Adler." He refers to the theory of masculine protest, which in women presses for social and sexual equality with men. Thinking it unmanly to beg, Jones projected on all women his anti-Adlerian wish to be firm, real guilt notwithstanding.[4] Freud wrote Abraham: "Jones is off today for two months' analysis with Ferenczi. I enjoy the thought that your marriage shows that Ψa does not necessarily lead to divorce."[5]

Ferenczi had hoped to spend June in Vienna for analysis with Freud and a diet cure. Freud demurred, saying even six weeks would be too little, and expressed concern about exposing "one of my indispensable helpers to the danger of personal estrangement brought about by the analysis. I don't yet know how Jones will bear finding out that his wife, as a consequence of the analysis, no longer wants to remain his wife." The next sentence contains a slip. "Should it turn on the fact that women are more intelligent than we and are justified in subjecting us to our! their will?"[6]

Perhaps "our will" mixes the male sexual drive with Loe's indignant resistance. She is intelligent and sexually alienated. When a man's sexual need overrides his good judgment, the intelligent, sensitive woman finds him less attractive. Jones thought Loe's anesthesia could excuse his philandering, but that only exacerbated the anesthesia. Loe's outrage at Jones's behavior with Lina is justified, though she was unduly hopeful, if not masochistic, to keep Lina after the first episode. By justifying a weaker apology Jones kept his pride but increased Loe's distrust and sealed his fate. This case pits two different men's presumptions about the "weaker sex" against two very different women.

Freud, hoping to save the relationship, remained calm with Jones, as he had a few years before in the case of Jung's tryst with patient Sabina Spielrein. Freud confessed then to being tempted himself, and minimized the damage of such experiences: "No lasting harm is done. They help us develop the thick skin we need and to dominate 'counter-transference' which is after all a permanent problem for us. . . . They are a blessing in disguise."[7]

Freud sometimes analyzed both members of a couple (in tandem). Although he sent Jones to Ferenczi for analysis, there would still be boundary and transference problems. In 1895 Freud defined transference—the displacement of feelings from early relationships onto the analyst—and emphasized its importance. He said little about counter-transference—the analyst's own unconscious projected onto the patient—a concept that grew in importance later on.[8] Axel Hoffer commented about the early years of psychoanalysis: "The implications of the fact that the analyst was a lover or a relative were insufficiently taken into account; the magnitude of the unanalyzable difficulties created by such blurring of personal and professional relationships was only superficially recognized."[9]

Jones began analysis with Ferenczi in Budapest just as Loe ended the relationship. Jones reported to Freud that Ferenczi was "very tactful and kind, and I am sure we shall get some good work done, which I both want and need." He asked about Rank, who had not been well.[10] Freud replied: "Rank is all right. I had to tremble at the idea of his getting disabled for a longer time as he is—in every department of the work—the indispensable helpmate and a most intelligent companion. If anyone of us is getting rich it will be his duty to provide for him in a satisfying way." Freud said the tension between him and Jones about Loe "will pass away when you see my part more clearly. I had to work against my own interest." Anglophile Freud assumed the Jones house in London would be a regular accommodation for him: "One of my earliest wish-fancies."[11]

Ferenczi also had problems with women. A bachelor approaching 40, he was romantically involved with Gizella Palos, 48, whom he had analyzed. He began analyzing her daughter, Elma, in 1911 and fell in love with her. He asked Freud to take over the analysis, in part to find if Elma's love for him was real, not just transference. Freud soon returned the patient to Ferenczi, who was trying to decide which woman to marry. Freud claimed to be neutral but favored Gizella. Elma dropped Ferenczi for an American suitor. Freud took Ferenczi into analysis for three short periods between 1914 and 1916. Rank probably knew about these interlocking triangles.[12]

During Freud's vacation, Rank reported an exchange with Victor Tausk, lawyer-turned-psychiatrist and member of the Vienna Psychoanalytic Society since 1909. Five years Rank's senior, Tausk became close to Lou.

Wien ¶July 19, 1913

Lieber und verehrter Herr Professor!

I hope you're comfortable in Marienbad, experiencing better weather than we are here, so you can, at least for a while, relax from your strenuous literary activities. Otherwise, I have no doubt that this summer will yet provide the opportunity to complete the technical article.

The July issue of Zeitschrift *has been printed, to be distributed in the next few days. Meanwhile I'm putting the Sept. issue together, which goes to the printer next week, along with an index and instructions to Ferenczi who'll now have to become familiar with editorial problems and irritations, too. Dr. van Emden still hasn't decided to let us do the work for September; I said the deadline is Monday.*

I got Dr. Tausk to delete for now the theoretical part of his discussion of childhood dreams, and publish the dreams alone (with just a brief note on their theoretical interest). In this context, apparently to compensate for failing with you, he revealed to me part of his narcissism theory (I almost said, of his narcissism). He claims that in narc., erogenous libido energies are not, as in the normal, also expended in object love (as an example, he noted anal eroticism, which connects with the external object through [...]) but always remains bound to, reacting upon, him. I do not know whether that is quite comprehensible, but if not, my brief manner of expression is at fault, for I believe I understood Tausk quite well. He then discusses two more mechanisms of ego-differentiation: the supposition of emotions in another person, and the imitation in one's own ego of another's expressions; both of these are to be subsumed under identification.

I also spoke with van Emden about establishing local groups in the Netherlands, and advised him to proceed since it seems he is being too cautious here [...] as well.

Jahrbuch V:1 must have appeared already, as Pfister sent an offprint. I still haven't seen the issue, though, which really should be read before the Congress. In the literature otherwise there is not much [...]. In the July issue of L'Encéphale, Hesnard completes his presentation with a criticism that I haven't read yet.

With me till now things have been topsy-turvy, but start to shape up better. I've ordered the most important furniture, which won't be ready before [...]. In my old apartment I'm beginning [...] am dealing with whatever comes up.

By the time Sachs returns (27th or 28th) I hope to have everything arranged more or less, and by then my brother will be in Vienna to take over my private affairs. It's a relief that I must go then, as my old apartment will be cleared out and the new one not ready. All indications are that, given this weather and other things, I'll go to Paris; reports from Sachs don't scare me off fulfilling this long-held wish. Anyway, there's nowhere else I'd like to go, and whenever I think about where I should go, the answer "comes to mind": Paris. It would flout the basic rule of psychoanalysis if I forsook the thought.

Jones is resigned: the nice plan won't be a reality this year. His wife returned from Budapest yesterday; I'll visit her today.

Many thanks also for kindly sending me Totem and Taboo. I couldn't get an offprint from Heller, and want to take the book along on the trip so at last I can enjoy you as an actual reader. Next week we'll return the favor with the brochure by Löwenfeld. I'd be much obliged, Herr Professor, if you'd kindly give me the address of Herr von Redlich, to whom I'd also like to send a copy.

Please give my best regards to your dear family as I unfortunately had no time to bid them farewell. With best wishes for summer, and cordial greetings. Your grateful and devoted, Rank

Prof. Dr. Freud Marienbad, July 23, 1913

Lieber Herr Rank,

Many thanks for the news. I hope I won't disappoint your interest in my literary accomplishments during vacation. At the moment the idea is beyond imagining.

Marienbad must be a glorious place in the summer. Right now we are freezing and rained on. The forests are very refreshing. I'm in very cheerful company. We endure the injustice together.

On Paris I congratulate you. Pity that you should be so alone in that city of millions.

Herr von Redlich is staying in Grand Hotel Ott——. Literary news comes from England (Brit. Med. J. *July 5, Forsyth, and a* Leader *[weekly magazine]). Judging from letters I get, interest in* ΨA *must be very lively. The* Jahrbuch *has come out. When you pass by Deuticke, please remind them to send it here. Eitingon was here Monday, with Abraham's mandate that I speak at the Congress. I said that would depend on the decision whether to have discussion or not. Abraham will look into it.*

If you see van Emden, try to put some pressure on him. You know he is a cunctator [procrastinator].

Cordial greetings, and wishing you a wonderful vacation, interrupted as it was by the events you mentioned. Yours, Freud

Internationale Zeitschrift für Ärtzliche Psychoanalyse ¶July 24, 1913
[Names/addresses of Freud, Ferenczi, Rank, and publisher, Hugo Heller]
Lieber, verehrter Herr Professor!

Many thanks for your kind letter, which gladdens me to learn you don't dwell on work, and do bear the bad summer with humor; perhaps the second half will be all the more beautiful.

I've heard about the English movement from Frau Loe, who is kind enough to keep me posted; I'm coming to appreciate her more and more. She's a great person, with not a trace of neurosis.

I'm also very glad for Jones, coming to London at just the right time; sorry that Eder is so unreliable, as we need a really dependable person there. I believe he'll have a small circle of people around him.

The Zeitschrift *(July issue) goes out today, and the ms. for September is already at the printer: enclosed the table of contents as sent to Ferenczi, Sachs, Heller and the publisher. For contents, arrangement or scope, if there's anything unsuitable, please let me or Ferenczi know; further, when Ferenczi reads the final draft in San Martino you'll have the last review. Having your contribution here by August 15 would be good. Please send the ms. directly to Heller (registered). I'll give instructions for forwarding. Yesterday I got an article by Morton Prince on [...], with a very nice accompanying letter. I sent him an equally cordial letter accepting the article with thanks, immediately sent it to Budapest so that Jones can evaluate it. Emden can't make up his mind to go through with publication. He has already read portions of the* Jahrbuch. *Deuticke hasn't sent it to me and today I urged him to send me both copies; nothing is in Jung's article other than what is in* Transformations.

The Zentralblatt *came a few days ago: really genuine Stekel. Psa. ever more recedes while the Stekel spirit moves to the front. He's made so many non-analytic contributions, like some in our camp (Rorschach, Kaplan, [...], etc.). Adler still has a "top" position in the journal. [...] His elaborately worked out "tabular" response to Maeder's letter shows how right was our decision not to include these [...] formulations in our journal. Furtmüller discusses some issues of* Imago *(and your first three concurring opinions) in the usual way. Stekel scorned Ferenczi's article on the sense of reality and [Maxim] Steiner's book [1913; preface by Freud]. On the last page, Stekel takes a tone of familiarity with his [...] and declares that the journal won't die with this volume. "On the contrary! There will be no change in our approach....As always, our basic principle will be strict self-criticism and full objectivity!" I thought to send the journal, but will only if you send a card requesting it, in which case please send it back to Dr. Sachs.*

Sachs arrives Sunday the 27th, and we meet on Monday to discuss all details. I'll be free then if I've taken care of all my private business. I plan to travel as soon as possible, latest the 1st, and hope you won't take offense if I don't find free time to write to you—other than important things.

In any case, if it should seem that I am "residence unknown" my new address in Vienna will be valid.

With cordial greeting and best wishes, your grateful Rank

Marienbad ¶July 25, 1913

Lieber Herr Doktor

You won't be angry if I "thank" you for Stekel! That his journal is not going to its rest is surely disappointing, but we shall bear it. Though perhaps it will go on spouting lies until the end. Jahrb. & Zeitschr. received. Many thanks. Once more: good wishes for vacation.   *Your Freud.—My greetings to Paris!*

On August 5 Ferenczi wrote Freud that Jones had left. "I miss him *very much*. We have become intimate friends; I grew to love and treasure him. . . . Let's hope he'll succeed in mastering his neurotic tendencies from now on, but I won't venture to make a *definite* prognosis on this."

Middelkerke [Belgium] Hotel du Kursaal ¶August 17, 1913

Lieber Herr Professor,

I'm finally here on the Belgian coast, vis-à-vis Jones, settled for a while and getting myself and my thoughts in order.

In the Berner [Swiss] Oberland, gaining strength for Paris, I had marvelous weather and was so charmed that I almost wished to go no further. Yet Paris drew me on, and compensated richly for the mountains. As a city it falls well short of the unique impression Rome made on me, but the Louvre is such a storehouse of magnificent objects that again it was just exhaustion that got me away. I hope to recover here in a few days.

Then I must think about my presentation for the Congress; the form concerns me more than the content. Jung wrote in early August asking me to send an abstract of my Munich paper to be printed with the program. I explained that the paper doesn't exist, and he shouldn't delay printing the program. I got an extremely nice letter from Riklin—like old times—saying that preparations for the Congress will be done by month's end—along with other misinformation.

I heard from Sachs that everything is going well with Imago and that the issue will appear on time. (It may already have appeared.) However, I've heard nothing about Zeitschrift.

In London things seems to have erupted again. In the Neue Freie Presse v. 13:8 that I happened to come across here, I noticed a report that in London [Seventeenth International Congress of Medicine, Aug. 7–12] Janet criticized the Viennese school— it's already distinctly known as a scientific society—but there were also defenders. I asked Jones for a report. Have you heard anything? Nor have I had any news from

Ghent. If you know anyone who was there, I'll ask for a report. I thought Emden was going, but at a Press evening of the 14th I saw his name on the list of guests taking the cure in Abbadia [Italy][...]. Isn't he there?

I heard from Sachs that both Joneses left for London as planned; I'll write them today.

I'd so appreciate it, esteemed Professor, if you'd kindly let me know how you envision my Congress paper, i.e. whether (as planned) I present on the function of dreams addressing Maeder's approach peripherally, or whether my comments should go more in the direction of a response. I think I'm right in interpreting Jung's request for an abstract in the first sense.

I'd also be glad to receive your personal news—whether you enjoyed Marienbad this year, and if you've been having good weather lately.

The location of the Munich Congress we'll learn only from the programs, which hopefully will be mailed out soon.

Cordial greetings to you and Ferenczi. Regards to your family....R

At the London meeting mentioned by Rank, both Pierre Janet and Carl Jung proclaimed their respective contributions to psychoanalysis and their differences with Freud. Janet said Freud's use of "free" association was influenced by suggestion from the analyst, and he criticized his dream recording and analytic tools. Like Jung, he denied that sexuality was "the essential and unique cause" of neuroses. Ernest Jones, the only Committee member there, boasted that he "put an end to his [Janet's] pretensions of having founded psychoanalysis and then seeing it spoiled by Freud." Rank sent disappointing reports from the *Neue Freie Presse* to Jones, who explained that reporters had not attended the session but used handouts from Janet and Jung.[13]

The Fourth Congress of the International Psychoanalytical Association took place in Munich, September 7–8. Jung presided, and stood for reelection after two years in office. Freud supported this, still hoping to unite Jews and anti-Semites in the cause. Alphonse Maeder said that scientific differences between Swiss and Viennese reflected differences between Aryans and Jews. Freud stood fast: There can be no Aryan or Jewish science, notwithstanding differences in outlook on life. Jung was elected with 52 ballots "for," but the Viennese expressed displeasure, with 22 abstentions.[14] After the meeting Freud went to Rome for 17 "delicious" days with his wife's sister, Minna: Jones reports this and four similar trips beginning in 1903, but asserts Freud's unbroken fidelity to Martha.[15]

Internationale Zeitschrift für Ärtzliche Psychoanalyse Wien ¶September 20, 1913
Lieber und verehrter Herr Professor!

First, many thanks for your kind congratulations, which came a bit early only in the sense that due to sloppy work of various parties making deliveries, I'm still far from feeling my current abode is home.

Hearing of your good mood and your appetite for work makes me very happy. I was sure you couldn't resist Rome's charms, and by the first day you'd have shaken off the shabby and unpleasant Munich Congress. Knowing you won't settle for the results makes me twice as glad.

I'll have your work published at the end of the month—of course with citations, all of which I recognize [...]. I've received some material for the next issue too. Ferenczi sent the Weimar [...] paper on homosexuality [...] urgent printing (I'm not sure it's good that he injects himself so often as editor), and Abraham wants to submit his Congress paper (light phobia) to our Zeitschrift—*in installments apparently. The September issue—somewhat smaller than planned—will come out in the next few weeks. Jones' name is on the title page and the inside cover.*

You probably know that Jones is in the midst of establishing the local group in London with [...] twelve members (including some in India and Scotland). He sent a business letter to Heller which we have to discuss later.

My assistance is of course at your disposal. That you so value my work is a great honor and flattering, though undeserved.

I attended some sessions of the Congress on Medical Psychology, meeting here yesterday and today, though I thoroughly regret it now. (Once again, you were right.) I've never heard anything so pitiful as the discussion on repression. The speakers (by the way very [...]) were helplessly muttering stupid things (Hattingberg too), and the few who knew anything (e.g. Bleuler) kept silent. Adler [...] is as far from all psycho-analysis as ever. Fortunately he's completely outside. Stekel fancifully peers into every facet with huge exaggerations and hairsplitting formulations (moreover got strong objections from almost everyone). I call his approach, his style, Balkan psychology.

Last evening I had the pleasure of being with your family. We talked a lot about the summer, and I had to recount the main events of Munich.

Please remember me to your sister-in-law with best regards.
Enjoy your days in Rome! In cordial devotion Your, Rank

Freud met with Rank every Friday evening to prepare the fourth edition of *The Interpretation of Dreams.* He wrote Ferenczi, "Reading through all that jumble is a harsh punishment." A month later the task claimed "every free hour. . . . I wouldn't be able to get started without Rank."[16] Rank's published output already surpassed that of his peers. He would soon become the first and only coauthor listed on the title page of *The Interpretation of Dreams* (4th ed. 1914), to which he contributed the chapters "Dreams and Creative Writing" and "Dreams and Myths."[17]

After the Munich Congress in September Freud wrote, "Since being taken in by Jung my confidence in my political judgment has greatly declined," expressing a stronger dependence on the opinions of the Committee.[18]

In April 1914, Jung resigned as International Psychoanalytical Association president and editor of the *Yearbook*. Karl Abraham became interim president when Freud suggested this to the presidents of the six European branches: Berlin, Budapest, London, Munich, Vienna, and Zurich. He expected to hold on to three of the four American groups after the schism: New York, founded by Brill (M.D.s only); the American, founded by Jones; and the Boston, founded by J. J. Putnam and I. Coriat. The Washington-Baltimore, founded by W. A. White, was doubtful because the group around White and his colleague Smith Ely Jelliffe accepted Jung's desexualized libido concept.[19]

Rank's *Myth of the Birth of the Hero*, translated by F. Robbins and S. E. Jelliffe, was published in their prestigious American *Journal of Nervous and Mental Disease* in 1914, and in monograph form—reprinted for decades, despite the publication of a much enlarged second German edition in 1922 (1st English ed., 2004).

Freud, Ferenczi, and Rank met in Budapest to witness Loe Kann's marriage to Herbert Jones, an American, in June, one of only two weddings Freud ever attended outside his immediate family. Reviewing his correspondence with Freud, Jones says much of it "was taken up with reports of a treatment he was conducting of a very difficult case, with a mixture of mental and organic symptoms, in a lady who stood in a personal relationship to myself."[20]

The planned fall meeting of the IPA in Dresden would be canceled due to the outbreak of World War I in August. Within the psychoanalytic movement stability endured for most of the decade ahead, although from 1914 to 1918 the Committee included members on both sides of that Great War.

≈ Chapter 5 ≈

War

1914

*The truth is that they [Jung and Adler] have picked out a few cultural overtones
from the symphony of life and have once more failed to hear the
mighty and primordial melody of the instincts.*
—Freud, *History of the Psychoanalytic Movement*

Freud's first grandchild was born to Sophie, 21, his fifth child, in March. That spring Freud turned 58, Rank 30, just before *History* was published. Freud's *Interpretation of Dreams,* 4th edition, appeared with Otto Rank as contributing author. Rank had, since 1912, published many articles, including "Homosexuality and Paranoia," "Masturbation and Character Formation," "Nudity in Literature and Poetry," "Multiple Meanings of Dreams during Awakening," and "The Double," prompted by the 1913 silent film *The Student from Prague* and a theme he developed later in a book.

Freud wrote Jones about Loe's marriage. The ex-husband was gracious toward the new couple but showed resentment toward Loe. He praised Freud's *History,* calling one sentence "magnificent" (epigraph, above).[1] Jones was nervous about Jung's upcoming presentations in London. Freud reassured him: Jung now "concedes that his 'constructive psychology' is *no science* and lands in unveiled adherence to [Henri] Bergson. So you see he has found another Jew for his father complex. I am no more jealous."[2]

A major review of *Totem and Taboo* came from Carl Furtmüller, a former Vienna Psychoanalytic Society member who left in the purge of Adlerians. He wrote that Freud ignores critics, misuses Darwin, and presumes confir-

mation of the Oedipus hypothesis in totemism. Granting Freud's wit, as-
tuteness, and poetic spirit, Furtmüller chides "the free play of fantasy" and
metapsychology in lieu of scientific logic: "The Oedipus complex of the psychoanalyst has become the original sin of the human race."[3]

From new quarters closer to Freud, Rank reports on June 6 that the May
issue of *Zeitschrift* is out and encloses the contents of the July issue. He asked
Abraham, Ferenczi, and Jones to vote on the location of the fall Congress
(Dresden—canceled by the war). On June 12 he reports that the April *Imago*
is out and the June issue will appear soon. He's working with E. Régis and
A. Hesnard on the first psychoanalytic textbook in French.

Wien, Grünangergasse 3 ¶June 25, 1914

Lieber Herr Professor!

*Yesterday I also wanted to ask you whether you'd be so kind as to speak with Heller
concerning the publication of my writings on mythology. Yesterday I found him in
a very [...] mood, which had not been the case for some time. I spoke about this with
Sachs. He believes there won't be any problems with Bergmann, or that they will be
easily resolved.*

The contents of the book would be:

*Introduction (the chapter from "Grenzfragen" [Boundary Questions]) in expanded
form.*

Folktales of brothers

Folk-psychological parallels to infantile sexual theories

Belated obedience as a theme in legend (Manneken Pis)

Nudity

Griselda

The Matron of Ephesus

The Double[4]

*Perhaps one of the themes I am considering working on next: fire, Parsifal, Samson.
I'd estimate the size (without the possible new work) at 15–16 bound sheets.*

*It would be very nice to know before the start of the vacation whether this is going to
work out, since my work during the vacation will partly depend on that.*

Many thanks for your kind efforts. Your devoted Rank

*P.S. During the double holiday I'll be at the Rax and surrounding mountains. On
Tuesday [...]*

"Fire" refers to a discussion among Freud, Ferenczi, and Rank in April. Afterwards Freud wrote, "There is nothing at all left for me on the acquisition of fire. Cultural history is mute on the subject. But I'm very curious as to what kind of serious things both of you will come up with."[5]

Wien, Grünangergasse 3 ¶June 26, 1914

Lieber Herr Professor!

Many thanks for your kind letter and your generous efforts with Heller, which will doubtless lead to the desired success.

I gladly promise to leave mythology behind then; I merely wished to do so gradually, without a sudden break. Perhaps Sachs—though overwhelmed with assignments too—will take over Samson himself. The discussion of fire, if anything becomes of it, will go somewhat beyond the narrow confines of mythology, so that only Parsifal, a topic I've been planning to address for two or three years, will remain. I hope to get to Parsifal during the summer.

I'm very sorry my tour conflicts with your kind invitation; I regret that I can't enjoy both simultaneously. But it was some comfort to me that your express letter came before the invitation, thus anticipating the regrettable need for me to decline. For several weeks I've been scheduled to participate, and see no other possibility of preparing for the tour of the Dolomites. With activities like that, bad weather is as rare as good clothing, so the chances of my coming to see you on Sunday are quite slim. If something unexpectedly comes up, I'll permit myself to contact you by phone by 9:00 a.m. Saturday. Otherwise, please excuse me this time and convey my regrets to your family and guests....R

On June 28 Archduke Franz Ferdinand, heir to the Austro-Hungarian throne, and his wife were assassinated in Sarajevo by a Bosnian supporter of an independent Greater Serbia. Freud, while concerned, underestimated the sequel, and allowed Anna to leave for a two-month stay in England. During July Austria bombarded Belgrade; when Russia mobilized to counterattack, Germany declared war on Russia and France and invaded Belgium, which brought Britain in against the Central Powers. Freud, like many, expected a short war, a brief storm that would clear the air. At the outset, when 100 German scientists were asked to petition against the war, only four accepted, among them Albert Einstein.[6]

Freud wrote to Frau Lou Andreas-Salomé, "Rank with his usual kindness has taken over the mass distribution of the offprint [of *History*]."[7] The

Committee hoped this "bombshell" would provoke the Jungians to leave the International Psychoanalytical Association. That came to pass after earlier rumors of the split were found to be false.

Wien I Grünangergasse 3 ¶July 9, 1914

Lieber Herr Professor,

Congratulations on Bleuler's reaction [favorable to History*]! Sachs knows about it, and I hope to deliver it to Ferenczi in person. I'll be available on Saturday, and Sachs agrees.*

Abraham writes that he'll send out the circulars on the 12th. On July 3 he gave a paper on partner selection and exogamy for Ärztliche Gesellschaft für Sexualwissenschaft [Medical Sexology Society] in Berlin, which I immediately ordered for Imago. In the discussion, I. Bloch confirmed the incest complex based on his own experience.

Jones wrote to Sachs that due to your article, [M. D.] Eder [British analyst] has completely turned to Jung. Today I received a letter from him (Eder) without a word about it. He promises to work "further" on translating my work, though he hasn't even begun.

[Karl] Landauer reported that you received his ms; I hope to get it from you on Saturday. From the ethnologist Wilhelm Löwenthal he learned that Wundt and Weule (Leipzig) have spoken more favorably of the folk-psychological value of P/A. The latter assigns a number of analytical papers in his ethnology seminar.

Tausk sent in an announcement of his lectures for Fall from [...] newspapers. Yesterday the discussion group at the "Landtmann" shrunk to five, counting two guests (van Emden and Sokolnicka).

Correspondence with L, Jung, and Maeder on the dream problem for the Jahrbuch. A publication with a presumptuous foreword has appeared. The first reference is Hitschmann, and I'm 2nd. Disgusting how these people puff up with empty phrases. Adler's and Stekel's Zschr. came out, without notable content. The best thing in Stekel's publication now is the Varia, which attracts fine poets and [...] to confirm your points of view.

Sachs shared this with me from Bernstein's collection of Yiddish proverbs: "Wos ejner wolt gern gehat, dus cholojm't sich ihm in bett" [Whatever someone really wants, he dreams of in bed].

After my last inquiries with Deuticke, it still seems that several copies of ID will arrive this week.

Working with Jekels is a cross to bear; I proofread parts of his work in ms. after he discussed it with me. Now Sachs has proofread the galleys, and I'll look at them once more before they go to the printer. One would really need to revamp the whole work, or better yet, the author.

At the moment I'm somewhat unfit for work, or not in the mood, which adds up to the same thing. Sachs is probably going on vacation next Wednesday (July 15); I won't be able to go until the end of the month. In the meantime, I hope I'll develop more of an urge to travel.

Looking forward to seeing you. Cordial greetings. . . . R

Loe and her husband, Herbert, relocated to London at the same time Ernest returned there with Lina, Loe's former maid and companion. According to Loe, who socialized with the Freud family and Rank, Ernest had a romantic interest in Anna. Freud's distress about Anna in London moved Rank to sympathetic anger.

Internationale Zeitschrift für Ärtzliche Psychoanalyse Wien ¶July 16, 1914
Lieber Herr Professor!

Many thanks for your kind missive, and for Pfister's letter [he will side with Freud, not Jung] which I'll forward to Abraham.

At least Pfister is an honest and decent person, which can hardly be said of the others as they do not even have a sufficient sense of honor to acknowledge the [...] which is now clear. Hopefully we'll be rid of them soon.

Jekels, who now visits daily at the same morning hour with analytical punctuality—evidently substituting me for his son, who has sent no word for three weeks—told me about a letter from Federn saying that after your article you should not be surprised at the defections and enmity—as if that were not the situation before. He plans to leave for New York August 1.

There's nothing new here. Saison morte—dog days. Sachs left yesterday, as did [Herbert] Jones with his whole family. I brought them to the station myself, you can rely [...] on that. Their address in London is London NW [...] Road, West Hampstead, c/o Detiel.

Loe just told me about Ernest's new problems, and the problems he's caused you. It's really too bad that analysts, with so few exceptions—almost none—lack insight into their personal, private affairs. The fact that they're all neurotics excuses this only to some degree, for most people are neurotics, but analysts should surely be healthier or at least enlightened neurotics who'd rather suffer than inflict suffering on those around them. Loe worries about Ernest, and I must say that I do too. If one path of revenge is cut off he'll look for another. But he's very good-natured and maybe will handle the situation.

The mailing of copies of ID I can arrange to be done by Deuticke: Five copies be sent directly from there [...] and I'll have the other five sent to you. I hope you'll find this method acceptable, and that you won't mind if I take the liberty of keeping one copy for our Society library. So you'll find ten copies here. I'll reimburse Deuticke's expenses since Ollie [Oliver Freud] gave me the funds for that.

Today or tomorrow I hope to be able to visit your sister-in-law [Minna]—if my lumbago lets up, which has plagued me for a few days.

I'm so glad that you're already feeling well [...] recovery. Best regards [...]. [Rank]

[P.S.] This week I'll send you one copy of the July issue of the Zeitschrift, as well as the correspondence that came in the meantime.

Internationale Zeitschrift für Ärtzliche Psychoanalyse Wien ¶July 19, 1914
Lieber Herr Professor!

Finally I can congratulate you—and myself; hopefully all will go now as wished.

So far no news from Abraham. I'd like to pose the following question (which I'll put to Abr. forthwith): Shall we announce the resignation in the next issue of the Zeitschr.? Under the heading "On the psa. movement," or in an "extra edition" of the Korr. blatt? But then it would also be good to be able to announce at the same time [...]. As you've observed from the Korr. the September issue of the Zschr is so far along that it can be out in 14 days. We'll be able to inform all members a month before the Congress. I'll ask Abraham if he wants to publish the Congress program in that issue. I'll inquire now, since I'd like to get that done before I leave. Maybe I'll just have to stay here a few more days till the situation is clear.

In looking over the book by Régis and Hesnard, please think about whether anything would be appropriate for a supplementary issue, or whether they should be approached about such a publication. My letter does not seem to have reached Hesnard in Bordeaux. I'd like to suggest that Régis be invited. I'll send Abraham's communication to [...] today.

I'm glad that Zschr. can count on contributions from you again. It really needs them, at least as much as Pa. Review, which finally has its well-deserved [...].

I heard today from Loe that Jones and family had arrived at the Hague after a terrible 27-hour journey (hot at night too), and that they are very comfortable there.

Your sister-in-law, whom I visited on Thursday, looks very well, and feels greatly

energized out of doors, but is understandably uncomfortable with the tempo of the [...].
She thinks she will also have to stay [...] next week.

  I had an encounter with Wittels in the vestibule; he was embarrassed, and I didn't
find the encounter exactly pleasant either. I certainly like him much less now than
before. Just let those Sadger [Wittels's uncle] family traits show through the cultural
veneer!

  You've probably received the issue and the proofs. Suggestions for improvement
(sent to Jekels) will be thankfully appreciated. Your devoted, Rank

  [P.S.] Today I received from Sokolnicka a [dream] of transference and resistance,
from Munich. Of course it concerns you, and applies to me [...] as your Double who
has stayed behind in Vienna. I'll respond to the dream as analytically as possible.

Viennese psychologist Theodore Reik, four years Rank's junior, was in analysis with Abraham, in Berlin, depressed, and looking for work. Abraham wrote Freud that Reik was comparing himself with Rank, who got a stipend for his work. Freud replied, "He is a good chap, intelligent and modest. But he can't really compare himself with Rank. It's true the Association has done a great deal for Rank. But R. would not have gone under if none of us had bothered about him. He'd have found others; I know of few people who can make themselves so generally loved and deserving. Also, Rank was there earlier. Perhaps Reik has a sibling rivalry complex in this respect."[8]

Anna, 18, arrived in London accompanied by her godmother on July 16, the same day her father wrote her, on a tip from Loe, "Dr. Jones has a serious intention of wooing you." Freud also wrote Jones thanking him "for your kindness with my little daughter. . . . She is the most gifted and accomplished of my children and a valuable character besides." He cautioned Jones, who was twice Anna's age: "She does not claim to be treated as a woman, being still far away from sexual longings and rather refusing man." Father and daughter have a pact, he wrote: she won't consider marriage "or the preliminaries" for another few years. Freud put it bluntly to Ferenczi, "I don't want to lose the child to a clear act of revenge," and "Loe will keep watch like a dragon." Loe, 32, and Anna had become close. Ernest's revenge would be against both Loe and Freud, for her leaving him.[9]

Celebrating the Jungians' resignation was premature, Rank wrote Freud on July 21, saying he had no word from Ferenczi and Sachs. He has travel plans, including Dalmatia (Croatia). The next two days Rank wrote postcards; one says he'll bring Minna some reading matter and then leave. A day later he writes that Heller would like to publish a German edition of the new *La Psychoanalyse*: perhaps Rank would translate and edit it. Not having seen the finished book, Rank asks Freud's opinion.

> *Internationale Zeitschrift für Ärtzliche Psychoanalyse* Wien ¶July 26, 1914
> *Lieber Herr Professor!*
>
> *Many thanks, above all, for "my portion" of ID which, as always, given your generosity is more than deserved. [Rank's name appears on title page.]*
>
> *Many thanks moreover for the news for Heller. [Librairie] Alcan wrote: not a single copy [La Psychoanalyse] left! I had Heller send me one, and began reading from the end, as is my wont. Just in reference list III after a cursory look I found about 30 errors. That was enough.*
>
> *Abraham also told me about the resignation of the Swiss members. The only question left is what they'll put in print: apparently a "sufficient" answer to our temporary note. [...]: as droll as your comparison to warfare is, this is no longer amusing. Here everything stands under the impression and [...] of a crisis.*
>
> *I don't know for sure if and when I'll be able to get away with special travel restrictions officially in effect on Tuesday, and unofficially, already today with colossal movements of troops. I'm glad Fräulein Bernays left today just before the deadline. I had the pleasure of being useful at the train station. I reserved a half-compartment. All right [in English].*
>
> *In any case, I'll try going this week to the Tirol, otherwise to Germany. Dalmatia is of course impossible now. Hopefully you'll arrive safely in Seis [Siusi, Italy], where I hope to see you.*
>
> *Again, cordial thanks for everything, and for the congratulations & good luck wish, so needed now, and which are most cordially returned by your devoted R*

The next day Rank wrote Miss Bernays, pleased that she'd arrived safely in Italy. "From Privy Councillor [Martin] Freud, whom I just visited, I learned that south and west railroads are open until further notice and will remain so for the duration of the war. . . . Prof. Freud will be able to get to Seis easily." He acknowledges the possibility of disruptions affecting the family of Herr Priv. Coun., delayed in Marienbad. He signs, "Yours, Dr. Rank."

Neutral Italy allowed both travel and a channel for letters to and from Jones, now in a country at war with Austria. Rank left Vienna on July 29, and relates his experience to Freud after a fortnight.

Dr. Otto Rank Semmering am ¶August 12, 1914

Lieber Herr Professor!

I just received your letter of August 2 [missing] this evening and I hope mine will still reach you in Karlsbad.

I left Vienna just 14 days ago, and will describe my adventure briefly. Since it was impossible to travel via the Glockner [Road] into the Puster Valley due to persistent poor weather, I went to Innichen, which had its first day of glorious weather. Nevertheless, I felt a bit uneasy. Drei Zinnen to Cortina. There, due to the news, I decided with heavy heart to break off my trip. Since I'd sent my baggage ahead to Bolzano, I had to get there immediately. Luckily I caught the last bus, and made the eleven-hour trip along that glorious route. At the Bolzano train station I was told that only two trains were running, with no assurance about routes reopening. The next day at [...]:25 p.m. I bought a ticket to Vienna and rode all night. I wanted to have breakfast in Mürzzuschlag, but could only get a newspaper, which I thank for this stay in Semmering. It said some local transport will continue. So I got off, and spent a wonderful week here. The weather is perfect, the town empty except for a few Hungarians I can't converse with, and it's quite cheap. I spend whole days in the forest, where cyclamen, strawberries, and wild animals abound. I thought of how busy you'd be here, collecting things. I plan to stay here a few more days, until the 15th, then return to Vienna, since there's no peace anywhere. As for the military, so far I've been spared.

I'm sorry this letter is so narcissistic, but vacations are of course a narcissistic period, and besides I got no mail here until today, and really had nothing to report. Among the messages today is a letter from Ferenczi, who won't go to London after all, and from Jones, who asks about everything, and reports that your daughter is having a good time in London.

I hope you and your wife are well rested, and that Miss Bernays is completely well again. I suppose none of your sons must go.

Please write me next in Vienna: given the current post, a letter might not reach me here.

I hope to hear good things from you soon. Best wishes in the meantime.

Cordially, your devoted R

[postcard] Pension Hirschvogel *Internationale Zeitschrift für Ärtzliche Psychoanalyse* Semmering, en route to Vienna ¶Aug. 13, 1914

Verehrter Herr Professor,

After receiving your letter [missing] I wrote you yesterday in Karlsbad but just learned from Sachs that you're in Vienna. On the way back from Tirol I stayed here

a while but will be home again in the next few days and hope to find you well rested.
Best regards to your family and cordial greetings from your grateful Rank

On August 25 Freud wrote Abraham, "Rank, as cheerful as ever, has, as we're all for the moment incapable of scientific work, found himself work arranging and cataloguing my library." Anna returned August 26 via Gibraltar and Italy with the Austrian ambassador, arranged by Herbert and Loe Jones.[10] A week later Freud acknowledged to Abraham that the war would go on, the early German victories upon which he hung his hopes were not enough. But he could focus on work: "Rank, with whom I spend a great deal of time . . . will be writing to you about [scientific matters]." Martin and Ernst Freud signed up to serve in the army, leaving Oliver at home. Ferenczi was called for army duty as a physician. The Wednesday Vienna Psychoanalytic Society meetings were reduced to twice monthly.[11]

In late November Freud reported progress to Ferenczi: his own *Theory of Sexuality* (3rd ed.), a long case history and some important theoretical ideas. "Rank will probably avoid being mustered in and then will be able to do his p/a work on the epic," that is, essays on Homer and on the folk epic, intended to qualify him as university lecturer (*Habilitation*). "Sachs was freed today [mustered out due to nearsightedness]," Freud wrote Ferenczi on December 2: "next we expect to hear the same about Rank, who is defending himself *against* the fatherland like a lion." Two weeks later Freud is elated: "Rank has delightfully solved the problem of Homer with the aid of a p/a presupposition. We were very amused by it, almost as much fun as the investigation of fire on Brioni." To Abraham he wrote about Rank's insight, "I want to see him, you, and Ferenczi as university lecturers in order to enable p/a theory to survive the bad times ahead."[12]

A postcard from Rank to Jones, December 24, had to be sent through van Emden in neutral Holland. Rank mentions papers and editing, ending with: "Subjectively I feel quite badly, and would like to come to you earlier than you expect, if I could." Jones wrote in his Freud biography that the war interfered with Rank's plan to be analyzed by him in London, and this is the evidence.[13] Since Rank had little respect for Jones as a person and analyst, he probably sought to avoid military service while improving his English. Rank could act the part of patient even if his heart was not in it. Freud must have known of and approved the fruitless plan.

≈ Chapter 6 ≈

Limbo

1915–1916

The unworthiness of human beings, even of analysts, has always made a deep
impression on me, but why should analyzed people be altogether better than others?
Analysis makes for unity, *but not necessarily for* goodness. *I do not agree with*
Socrates and Putnam that all our faults arise from confusion and ignorance.
—Freud to James Jackson Putnam, June 7, 1915

The bond between Freud and Rank grew stronger during the war. They probably spent more time together in 1914–15 than ever before or after. Freud's clinical practice was reduced. Travel was limited. Activities of the International Psychoanalytical Association and Vienna Psychoanalytic Society slowed, as did correspondence for the Committee. A delayed volume 4 of *Imago* and 3 of *Zeitschrift* appeared in 1915, using articles by Freud that in better circumstances would have made a book. The first English translation of *The Interpretation of Dreams* (3rd ed.), by A. A. Brill, was published in New York. Freud enjoyed most of the summer away from Vienna. Karl Abraham was on military assignment in East Prussia, where he spent the rest of the war, joined by his family. Ferenczi was stationed west of Budapest, closer to Vienna. Jones had a busy psychoanalytic practice in London.

In January 1915 the VPS met every other week, "quietly and not very productively. Rank and Reik alone seem to be working hard."[1] In February Freud addressed his B'nai B'rith Lodge on the emotional aspects of war. As a youth he took military figures as heroes and himself as a conquistador, but now he spoke with ironic sorrow and cynicism:

Consideration for the dead, who no longer need it, is dearer to us than the truth, and certainly, for most of us, is dearer also than consideration for the living.... Life is impoverished, it loses in interest, when the highest stake in the game of living, life itself, may not be risked.... We cannot maintain our former attitude toward death, and have not yet discovered a new one.... Our mortification and our grievous disillusionment regarding the uncivilized behavior of our world-compatriots in this war are shown to be unjustified. They were based on an illusion to which we had abandoned ourselves. In reality our fellow-citizens have not sunk so low as we feared, because they had never risen so high as we believed.[2]

"The eight months of the war weigh upon us like a bad dream," Freud wrote in April. Martha set off for Hamburg for a few weeks, leaving Freud with Anna and Minna. Ration cards were issued. Anna was "developing charmingly, more gratifyingly than any of the other six children," he wrote, but "the situation with bread promises to escalate to a real calamity." Oskar Pfister visited from Switzerland with Freud, Rank, and Sachs: "He is a good fellow and will stay with us [not with Jung]."[3]

On July 8 Ferenczi tells of the loss of 41 officers and a thousand men killed or taken prisoner; "we mostly mourn the death of a cavalry captain we all loved." Freud replied, on July 10, "If this war lasts another year, which is probable, no one would be left who participated in its beginning." In the same letter he reports a "prophetic dream" about the death of his sons. Martin was grazed by a Russian bullet; Freud, considering telepathy, later asked about the time of the incident, but Martin couldn't remember.

On July 12, to Ferenczi, Freud outlines a parallel between specific mental illnesses and stages of human evolution, for example, anxiety is linked with privations in the Ice Age, as is hysteria: "When they had learned that propagation was now the enemy of preservation and had to be restricted they became—still lacking the faculty of speech—hysterical." He builds this phylogenetic theory with examples leading to the totem thesis and says, "Your priority in the above is evident." From vacation in Karlsbad, July 20, Freud writes, "Rank has unified all business in his hands. It would be very nice if you could find the means to support him on a number of points." A week later Freud encouraged Ferenczi to work on treatment of traumatic neuroses due to war—"the brain-crippled."[4]

Freud finished all but one of twelve papers on metapsychology before his vacation. Rank urged him "to get the book to press in the fall." This was a difficult time, but they could not expect better options right after the war. Rank "will attempt to keep the machine running."[5] Of Freud's output, Jones wrote later, "Such a furor of activity would be hard to equal in the history of scientific production."[6] Freud kept only the first five of 12 essays, those on instincts, repression, the unconscious, dream theory, and melancholia. Reflecting on this later, he called metapsychology "a method of approach according to which every mental process is considered in relation to three coordinates, which I described as *dynamic, topographical,* and *economic* respectively; and this seemed to me to represent the furthest goal that psychology could attain. The attempt remained no more than a torso.... I broke off wisely perhaps, since the time for theoretical predications of this kind had not yet come."[7]

On July 8 Freud wrote to J. J. Putnam, Harvard neurologist, Boston Brahmin, and supporter of psychoanalysis, whose new book, *Human Motives,* had just arrived. Putnam met Freud in 1909 at Clark University and at Weimar, 1911, with Rank, who translated one of his papers into German. Putnam, a Unitarian, explains in the book that psychoanalysis is a human science compatible with religion and philosophy. His optimistic emphasis on human spirit and will, to which Freud objected—but Rank may have liked—made psychoanalysis more palatable in the United States. Freud's letter, courteous, challenging, and revealing, shows his characteristic ability to mix humility and hubris.

I cannot see the connection between our ideas of perfection having a psychological reality and the belief that they have a material existence....I have no fear of God at all. If we were ever to meet I should have more reproaches to make to him than he could to me. I would ask him why he hadn't endowed me with better intellectual equipment, and he couldn't complain that I have failed to make the best use of my so-called freedom....I consider myself a very moral human being...when it comes to a sense of justice and consideration for others; to dislike of making others suffer or taking advantage of them, I can measure myself with the best people I have known. I have never done anything mean or malicious, nor felt any temptation to do so, hence am not at all proud of it. I am taking the notion of morality in its social, not its sexual, sense. Sexual morality as defined by society, to the extreme in America, seems to me quite contemptible. I advocate a far freer sexual life, though I myself have made very little use of such freedom. Only to the extent that I believed I myself was limiting the allowable in this realm....If knowledge of the human soul is still so incomplete that my poor mental faculties have managed to produce such ample discoveries, it is evidently premature to declare oneself for or against such assumptions as yours.

Freud forgot or dismissed his harshness with the Adlerians and Stekel and his betrayal of Wilhelm Fliess in 1902, for which, when caught, he hedged his apology.[8]

Imago [letterhead] ¶August 2, 1915

Lieber Herr Professor!

As you may already have heard from Sachs, Heller is creating difficulties. From a discussion with him today I had the impression that this is once again just a (hopefully temporary) problem, for which Heller, beside his subjective motives, can also adduce a convincing rationalization this time. Specifically, Heller claims that as of today he hasn't been paid by any local group for the Zeitschrift *subscription. Given the current situation, this understandably doesn't have an encouraging effect on him. This time I'd agree with his complaints, though the form of his resistance makes itself felt very unpleasantly: the printing of the current fourth issue is at a standstill. I promised him today—since despite two admonitions he supposedly has no response from local groups—that I'll contact Abraham (also Ferenczi) and have those in arrears urgently admonished. Whether this will help is another question, as uncertain as Heller's future behavior, which incidentally strikes me as strongly influenced by his upcoming medical examination for the military.*

Today I checked the addresses in your mailbox, and in the evening I spent some time with your son [Oliver]. I learned that your eldest is doing well, despite his adventure, and heard also of the change in Ernst's life.

Nothing new with me. My brother will probably be sent to fight soon. Sachs is hoping that the delay in his call-up will be extended.

Best wishes. Yours, Rank

In August Ferenczi was posted to Györ for six weeks to evaluate recruits: "testing the poor 43–50-year-olds for their fitness for war." On the way he stopped in Vienna, where he saw Rank for a few hours: "He was sweet, as always, and—even in the new situation—in a good mood—something that I couldn't say about myself," he told Freud (Aug. 24).

Imago ¶September 3, 1915

Lieber Herr Professor

Many thanks for your two postcards [missing] and the proof-corrections. Meanwhile Issue No. 3 has appeared and No. 4 (index will follow shortly) is as good as guaranteed. It now seems that No. 2 of Imago *will see the light of day now, so things are progressing again. Things are going well with me, as before. Objectively, my condition is good. Eitingon was here on a brief trip. Of course you already know about Sachs' fate. What do you hear from your sons, and are you and your family well? Hopefully the weather has become civilized again, too. My brother remains where he is for the time being.*

That someone should ask about The Artist *strikes me like something from a distant, vanished world, so the comparison with the votive image is correct.*

Shall I simply delete the last footnote about animals in Tausk's article?

With best regards to you and your family. Respectfully yours, Rank

Freud visited his daughter Sophie and grandson Ernst in September; he watched the 1½ year old invent a *fort/da* ("there/here") game, later described in *Beyond the Pleasure Principle*. In October Freud visited Ferenczi, who was preoccupied with the decision to let Frau Gizella go in favor of Elma. Back in Vienna, Freud writes him that "the war is becoming unbearable" (Oct. 17). He gave his first introductory lectures (Oct. 23 and 30) to an audience of about 70, including Rank, Sachs, and daughters Anna and Mathilde. At Rank's urging Freud published them promptly, noting to Ferenczi: "I want to make it impossible for me to lecture on this 'Introduction to P/A' again . . . the old material is abhorrent to me, but I will try to organize it differently."[9]

Jones, residing in enemy territory, had just one letter from Freud in 1915, though he had correspondence with "the ever-faithful Rank," Sachs, and Ferenczi. In December he reacted to news that Rank was to be editor of the army newspaper in Krakow: "About Rank I am very sad, it is the saddest personal news of the war to me, and I do hope that things will go lightly with him." Jones, 40 years later, wrote: "Rank's absence [1916–18] was a serious blow to Freud, with Abraham and Ferenczi at a distance, since he depended on him for essential help in his editorial and publishing activities." In his Freud biography, Jones credits Rank with "a special flair for interpreting dreams, myths and legends . . . truly vast erudition." He mentions Rank's contribution to *The Interpretation of Dreams,* adding: "Rank would have made an ideal private secretary and indeed he functioned in this way to Freud in many respects." And: "For years Rank had a close almost day-to-day contact with Freud, and yet the two men never really came near to each other. Rank lacked the charm, among other things, which seemed to mean much to Freud."[10]

Freud tells Ferenczi of Rank's army assignment with the *Krakauer Zeitung*, the only German daily in Galicia: "I will certainly miss him sorely, and there's no way of telling how he will be replaced for the journals."[11] On December 23 Rank visited Krakow. Freud did not pressure him to seek a billet closer to home. Oliver's wedding took place, and Rainer Maria Rilke joined the party—"charming company." Freud adds (to Ferenczi, Dec. 24) strong criticism of Jones, who had published an essay on war that refers the reader to Freud's recent paper, but "itself is an unconcealed rendering" of Freud's "Thoughts for the Times on War and Death," that is, plagiarism. Ferenczi responded, "Jones's tendency to plagiarize is familiar to me; he once appropriated my essay on suggestion in a similar way. His originality is (as I know from the analysis) inhibited; for that reason he has to satisfy his ambition in this way. Despite all that, he is a good boy, only one has to correct him in this respect." Ferenczi's conflict with Jones dated back to 1910.[12]

1916. On January 6 Freud told Ferenczi of Rank's leaving for Krakow, "quite insecure and sad, and I certainly let him go with regret. The Society evening yesterday was quite disgusting." Out of Freud's "grumpy mood" came an idea about the artist: "a remnant of the old technique of modifying oneself instead of the outside world (see Lamarck, etc.)." Ferenczi agonized about Gizella and Elma until Freud stopped him: "Analysis should enter in before or after an act and should not disturb one during it. . . . So, act now, as swiftly and decisively as possible, and refrain from analysis now, or treat it as an extra enjoyment without real influence."[13]

Krakow Zeitung ¶January 22, 1916 (official publication of the Royal
and Imperial Fortress Command, Military Postal Service 186)
Lieber Herr Professor!

As I informed you by postcard, the typewriter would be extremely valuable to me since there are assistants available to whom I could dictate my editorial contributions and my own materials. The rickety old one we have is too slow and loud for me, and is usually taken. I'd be very grateful to you, i.e. to your daughter and the Association, if I could have the typewriter, which only I would use. There's an opportunity for someone to go to Vienna today, thus sparing me the trouble of transport—I won't get a leave "for acquiring the typewriter" until February—so I ask you to kindly give the machine and accessories to the bearer of this letter, Vormeister Abriel, if that's acceptable to you. When I visit Vienna, I'd somehow compensate your daughter and the Association with one of our two office typewriters, which aren't fully utilized; I'd handle the Association correspondence from here, to the extent that our friend Sachs can't do it expeditiously. In any case, many thanks for your efforts and please forgive me for troubling you with such things. But how I should make amends to your daughter—I don't even dare come to Vienna.

If I do come, I hope I can tell you everything. Just this much today: I have a very interesting, by no means subordinate, but quite exhausting job here. Though in many ways it contrasts favorably with our beloved Vienna, I'm not yet reconciled with life here (although I can work and borrow books in the very fine library).

I'm sorry not to have any news yet from you about Vienna, things psychoanalytic and your sons. Yesterday two officers from the local general staff visited who know Imago *(one even a subscriber!). Apparently my news is delayed or hasn't even arrived (military mail).*

Please give my regards to your family; very cordial greetings to you.

Respectfully yours, Rank

Krakauer Zeitung ¶March 16, 1916

Lieber und verehrter Professor!

I thank you for your detailed letter of March 10 [missing] and am sorry to learn the story of the lectures. I noticed that you brought the lecture series to an early close—without "General Theory of Neurosis;" the semester usually lasts until Easter, of course. In any case you've certainly completed a significant piece of work, and I look forward to seeing the proofs. May I ask about the news in metapsychology, and if there is none, may I ask whether you are working on something new? Once again, I'd certainly like to participate in the internal progress of analysis to an extent, as in the good old days, though unfortunately only from afar. Having gotten the proofs for the two journals and through Sachs' truly selfless activity and reporting, I'm of course up to date concerning external events. Now things go acceptably with publishing, and otherwise I really couldn't do it better.

I've had a couple of bad days behind me—actually not yet behind me—when I felt very bad mentally. Please consider this new situation an excuse, and the exhausting job, if my letters leave something to be desired in number and maybe content, too. Under the circumstances, analytic work, sorely missed in scattered lucid moments, is out of the question. Recently Wilamowitz spoke in Berlin about the beggar Hauser[14]

(I'm familiar with the lecture's content), and reminded me of a world no more in existence. Constant reading of newspapers and magazines gives me ample opportunity to collect material. Have you gotten various clippings I sent (sister in Bern) and the recommendation for the Engelhorn novel Fine Threads *by Bahner? I also enclose an announcement for the "Movement."*

Next week my supervisor will finally return from leave and I'll try to get one myself, since it was promised me.

What do you hear from your sons? Is Ernst still where he was? And Martin? I've heard nothing from my brother for some time. At your convenience please give my greetings to the Society members.

With best regards to your family and cordial greetings to you.

Respectfully yours, Rank

Krakauer Zeitung ¶March 22, 1916

Lieber Herr Professor,

Many thanks for your extremely kind words [missing]; all the more since I don't need to take advantage of your kindness now. It's hard to say what's actually wrong, though as an analyst I should know. But then things would be different. So far, my analytical skills have failed me, or more precisely, they've expressed themselves only negatively, making things worse.

I'm glad to hear things are well with the Press again, and that you have good news from your family warriors. A few days ago I got a card from my brother, from Lemberg; he seems to be traveling more now.

I got all the pieces for Zeitschrift, *and saw the Bern group's announcement. The issue is really very elegant. Prochaska [printing office] just needs a push, and I'm sure things will go forward if you write him. I've seen this again with* Zeitschrift; *Heller's indolence, of course, always must be expected.*

Hitschmann wrote me recently that you should be "beaten" or "stabbed," and criticized me for my "military" intervention; due to various inhibitions I couldn't go into action until now. Now I see you've helped yourself.

With best regards to you and your family, and cordial greetings.

Yours thankfully, Rank

Krakauer Zeitung ¶May 8, 1916

Lieber Herr Professor

I hope you got my postcards from Warsaw, though I was told at the post office there was little hope. Anyway please accept my heartiest congratulations, belated though they may be [Freud was 60 on May 6].

I spent a few days in Warsaw, among the loveliest ever: various circumstances contributed. I traveled with a group of local physicians, some I met here, and some warmly recommended by Jekels and Nunberg; one turned out to be an old friend of Hitschmann. All showed great respect for psychoanalysis and its advocates, even some understanding of the field. The Congress proceedings themselves were neither more nor less interesting than all the other Congresses. At any rate, one saw and heard a great many experts. The presentation was fabulous and the reception very agreeable.

The city, with its unique life and activities, its luxurious apparel and dining, is interesting, extraordinarily. I saw a lot—of the inner workings of the German administration, too—and spoke with many well-informed people. Not to forget: I was in the Yiddish Theater, where I concluded that the splendid use of "Flatter" is but a pale imitation of the linguistic richness and originality of authentic Yiddish. At some point I hope to tell you things more interesting for us.

Today I received the latest edition of Imago; I still haven't got the Zeitschrift. Nor have I heard from Sachs for the longest time. I'm curious as to what will be with Heller. Things should go better now. Has he made any official announcements—concerning his discussion with R? Or is he again letting everything sleep?

What do you hear from your sons, and how is your son-in-law? From Fräulein Anna I know that you have undertaken a successful attack on the old Holzmann. If you need anything else from the library, just turn to him.

Many thanks for the last missive.

With best regards to your family and to you. Gratefully yours, Rank

Krakauer Zeitung ¶June 7, 1916

Lieber Herr Professor,

Today I'm finally getting around to answering your pleasant news of May 29. Meanwhile I was in Lemberg, where I met my brother and spent very pleasant days with some other acquaintances as well (among them, two Viennese physicians and Dr. Nelken). So far, things are going extremely well for my brother. He looks splendid and feels very well. Still nothing new with me.

For the success against Heller, we may congratulate you and ourselves. Anyway, the most difficult thing is always the battle over every positive point for the individuals, who our [...] chief of staff Sachs must lead—hopefully with as much success. Sachs also has to settle the matter of honoraria, and I'll ask him to do this soon.

Hopefully you have again received news from your sons. Perhaps you'll find the trail of the vanished Brecher too in Bad Gastein!

Has Tausk been called to Vienna, and is the Association still meeting?

With best regards to your family, and best greetings. Thankfully yours, Rank

P.S. Many thanks for the June missive. The military postal address delays and complicates everything. Simpler: Dr. Rank. Dunajewskigasse 5. Editor, Krakauer Zeitung.

On June 25 Rank expressed concern at hearing nothing from Freud or Sachs for a long while. He had an eye problem acting up that he considered to be "only" a nervous condition. Depressed and vegetating, he took part in various sports for which he had time. In Vienna just after Easter he had seen Freud, who told Ferenczi, "I was very pleased with him although he can't do anything for our cause now."[15] Then came a letter from Freud.

Hotel Bristol, Salzburg ¶July 26, 1916

Lieber Herr Doktor,

Today I received your postcard. As I already wrote, I returned from Gastein dissatisfied after a stay of 22 hours, and have taken up better lodgings here with wife, sister-in-law, and daughter. This means giving up the intimate connection with nature that I otherwise seek in the summer, but this summer is bad. The many problems with food, and meager choice of lodgings make one glad for what can be had here: stillness, beautiful paths, and urban comforts in lodgings and lifestyle. I've already completed the first lecture of the Neurosenlehre. *I'll work to finish the new edition of* Everyday Life *[1917], which Karger wants, and no more.*

With the journal came a malheur *[misfortune] for which again Heller is to blame. After many admonitions, our dear printer finally sent something—not the complete edition, but a first or second galley. Then he denied having received the draft mailed on May 31. Frau Z. thinks he could not have waited so long with the printing. He probably got the impression from Heller's behavior that he needn't worry about it much. Since Sachs had left, I had to redo all the corrections, but got them two days later, meticulously done, so I could bring them unchanged to Fischer before traveling. Since then*

I've heard nothing from Heller and gotten nothing; of course I didn't fail to inform him of my stay here.

The Dutch edition of Psychopathology of Everyday Life, *[edited] by Stärcke, which looks very good, is the only other news.*

By the way, during a night of insomnia (a rare occurrence with me), a whole theory of the legend occurred to me, based on your solution Helen = city [see n17]. Since then, nothing more has come to me. If you arrange a meeting on the long trip during your leave, I'll tell you about it. Just note that it is a case of symbol reversal—not the city for the woman, but the reverse. That can't be insignificant.

It seems that we can expect Ernst on leave. From Martin we receive news from time to time. He seems not too upset.

I'm glad reports of your subjective state now regularly sound pleasant.

Cordial greetings. Yours, Freud

P.S. After two years, Dr. Brecher was on leave for one day in Gastein, and we met him just on that day. He is unchanged, lost in dreams, out of this world—and, incidentally, stationed in Zell an See [Austria].

Freud agreed to reserve two hours daily for Ferenczi's analysis in Vienna while on leave during the summer; they would also work together and share at least one meal, but "technique will require that nothing personal will be discussed outside the sessions."[16]

Dr. Otto Rank Krakow ¶July 28, 1916

Lieber Herr Professor,

Many thanks for your detailed letter of July 2, which crossed with a second postcard I sent to Salzburg. At first I thought you were only traveling through, but then, who knows what's happening this crazy summer! Anyway, I'm glad you are as content as one can be now, and I wish you only good weather—or may one not do so?

I did predict the malheur *with Heller, if you recall. Precisely for that reason I wished to travel to Teschen [location of printer, Prochaska, in the Carpathians] which unfortunately wasn't possible then. I knew that one can't allow the statement to stand indefinitely. Hopefully the matter will follow its own course further, thanks to your kind intervention. Meanwhile, not knowing of this, I had the issue copied once by Heller himself and once by Frau Fischer.*

Would you kindly convey the various translations and new editions to Sachs, who will be in Vienna again on July 30? Maybe they'll fit in this issue; there is certainly room toward the back.

Your comment on the Helen legend interested me greatly. The reversal of symbols, stressed as well in "On Courting Cities" ["Um Städte Werben"],[17] always seemed an important element in understanding the issue, but I never reached the specific solution; so I'm all the more eager for it. Coincidentally, in the last few days (I just noticed it was precisely a month ago, on June 28), in a situation similar to yours—but more in a half dreaming state, and therefore not thought out—I had an insight concerning another unsolved Homeric theme: Penelope's weaving.

A recently married woman here, sewing curtains for her husband, who is stationed in the field, remarked in conversation: "I always have hope that he'll come back when they're finished." I believe she's been working on them for a very long time, and suspect she awaits his return with feelings of doubt. I was "thinking" about the following (not thoroughly): the sewing is a compulsive neurotic oracle—He shall not return (but he shall return—ambivalence): hence the undoing of the weaving. Here lies Penelope's ucs. unfaithfulness,[18] so manifold in her. As symbol of a city, she must sooner wish that he [Odysseus] not come. I've recently thought a lot, passionately, about Homer again, and ordered the new book by Wilamowitz, The Iliad and Homer.

Recently I came across a charming motif for an ex libris slip: in E. T. A. Hoffmann's novella The Choice of Bride which you must read, if only for the theme of choosing the caskets. You'll easily find the scene: it contains two fine psychological themes (renouncing the woman in favor of the book; wish-transforming a magic book into everything wished for). A well-known Viennese painter who is here now is tormenting his unconscious about how to represent these themes symbolically in a painting, but I've been able to help him.

Otherwise my mood continues to be good. My brother is here just now for two days, on his return trip from Vienna; there he was able to arrange things—I cannot say satisfactorily, but at least to an extent. I really enjoy my dog—a magnificent specimen of Lou's favorite breed.

The prospect of meeting you in the summer is so tempting that in my [...], which are taking on a more and more tangible form, I have almost become shaky. Where might you be in the last week of August or the first week of September?

I'm very glad to hear of the good news from your sons. Today I sent a feuilleton to Fräulein Bernays in Vienna that I think will interest her.

With best regards to your family and cordial greetings. Yours, Rank

On July 22 Freud told Abraham, "We saw Rank in Vienna recently; he was happier than formerly because of certain private improvements, otherwise, naturally, unchanged."

Salzburg Hotel Bristol ¶July 31, 1916

Lieber Herr Doktor,

Your idea that Penelope's behavior contains ambivalence, the leaning toward unfaithfulness, for which the later legend directly reproaches her, is so striking that it keeps me from working today, without, of course, my being able to add anything. One suspects more behind this. How the weaving and undoing come into this is not transparent. Given its origin, weaving must represent the genitals, the undoing their exposure. Anyway, your insight again shows that your work on Homer is destined to be important. During your leave you should not neglect to [...] in Asia. Maybe you can visit the real Troy; perhaps then you'll have another good idea.

What I wanted to tell you I can also write. Poetic mastery consists in sexualizing—let us say—a historical theme, putting a woman in place of the city. The story does that. There must be reasons for not wanting to recall historical events in full. A symbol differentiation comes up, and legend-form drives this on, lessening awareness of the symbolic (or actual?) relationship. Thus Helen is at first kept far from all human judgment. She is innocent, her conscious feelings don't develop with the situation. Oh, she's really not woman, but ever the city. In the end, this influence dissolves. In The Trojan Woman by Euripides she is wholly woman, sower of intrigue, defending herself against charges. Nothing now reminds one that she really was a symbol for the city. Also the non-aging of all these legendary heroines would make sense extended to city or country. One should look for similar examples.

Things go very well for us in Salzburg. The city is charming, to the forest [...] and all wishes fulfilled. I've finished two new lectures. We expect Ernst on Aug. 4, perhaps as lieutenant. I'll write Heller and Sachs today; just waiting for the midday mail. Ferenczi wrote today that he might spend 2 weeks vacation with me at the end of September. I look forward to good news from you.

Cordial greetings, Freud

Krakauer Zeitung ¶August 8, 1916

Lieber Herr Professor

Glad as I am that you like my idea, I'm sorry it disrupted your work. Thanks for your comment on the question about difference in symbols. I must think it over first, or better, let it rest, as everything with me is now resting, as I'm alone and with so awfully much to do. I'll really need my leave, which starts in 14 days. For now I'm sticking with my travel plans and will be happy if they come to pass. If so, I have a request: would you be so good as to send your friendly support a bit earlier this month, as an exception, to cover my expenses for food during the trip? Cordial thanks in advance!

If all goes as wished, I should have an opportunity to come through Budapest twice, though I could stop only on the return trip, Sept. 5, for the Danube Conference. Hopefully Ferenczi will be there. Where will you be? If I can't see you then, could we meet in the third week of Sept. in Munich, where a congress of psychiatrists (German Association of Psych. Medicine) is scheduled? Please write me about this, perhaps giving me an assignment so that I could travel there to report for the Zeitschrift!

Telegrams are arriving again by phone so I'll have to answer.

With best regards to your family and cordial greetings.

Yours, Rank

In September Rank would travel from Vienna to Constantinople for vacation via Budapest, where he attended a conference. On September 26 Freud informed Abraham, "Rank was here until yesterday evening on his return journey from Constantinople, where he had spent his leave, and was utterly enchanted by the Orient."

Chapter header

≈ Chapter 7 ≈

Krakow

1916–1918

I've become another person, one less interesting but more normal. . . . Analysis suddenly makes out of a man who has remained childish, therefore basically carefree, another who really becomes conscious of all responsibilities.
—Ferenczi to Freud, July 10, 1916

Ferenczi, 43, sought help for his choice of wife from Freud, who favored Gizella (Frau G.) over her daughter Elma while trying to seem impartial. Ferenczi's analysis, the only one by Freud of a member of the Committee, was done in three intense but brief series plus many letters that reveal the workings of Freudian therapy. Sándor and Otto, 11 years younger, edited the *Zeitschrift* with Freud and took a more liberal stance on the Committee than Abraham, Jones, or Sachs, who resisted innovation.

Ferenczi met Gizella Altschul Palos early in life: her family and his were close, and his younger brother married her younger daughter. Sándor's affair with Gizella began in 1900: he was a 27-year-old bachelor; she was a 35-year-old wife and mother. Around 1910 Ferenczi took her into analysis, which, in those days, might be a few weeks of sessions. In 1911 Ferenczi analyzed Gizella's older daughter, Elma, who did well at first. Then her suitor committed suicide. Ferenczi's concern and liking for her turned into passionate love; he begged Freud to take over the case; Freud did in 1912 and addressed the issue of transference versus real love on her part. Ferenczi hoped to marry Elma with the approval of her mother, still his occasional lover. The four principals exchanged comments in and outside of the consulting room and showed each other letters not meant for sharing.[1] Freud, a father figure, regarded Gizella as Ferenczi's Oedipal object and best choice (Ferenczi was 15 when his father died; as an adult he seldom saw his mother). Elma married another man, moved to the United States, later separated and returned to Hungary. In 1916 Ferenczi had two periods of analysis with Freud. Gizella continued the affair while selflessly supporting marriage between Elma and Sándor. His letters to Freud recount ailments, moodiness, sexual details, fantasies, self-analysis, deference, and gratitude.

Rank, 32, now separated from his professional partners, edited the army newspaper in Krakow. Freud's son, Oliver (Oli), 25, would be stationed there as an engineer. In August, Rank showed him "the beautiful parts of Krakow for two days: he was quite impressed, indeed enthralled."[2] Rank's next letter to Freud, in October, describes symptoms of manic-depressive (now bipolar) disorder.

Krakauer Zeitung ¶October 4, 1916

Lieber Herr Professor,

I'm still not really over the shock, and only today am I getting around to informing you that decisions have been made over my head: I'll have to remain here.

My mood is not good at all, partly because of this, and partly for other reasons, and now after every high [Rausch, "mania," "intoxication"] the letdown [Katzenjammer, "hangover"] comes in full force. I have less inclination than ever to do anything; I haven't so much as glanced at any of the fine books I brought along. Far from it!

I hope to be able to send you a better report on my mood next time.

With best regards and greetings. Yours, Rank

Krakauer Zeitung ¶October 18, 1916

Lieber Herr Professor!

Once again I had the pleasure of having Oli here for two days as my guest. I enjoyed his visit all the more, having been very depressed recently and withdrawn from everything. This freshened me up some, and I gladly noted that the brief visit did him a lot of good too, mentally and physically. The matter in which initial steps were taken had to be postponed to a later time.

Here nothing's new. At least I've begun reading, and next will try working, though Heller won't take the trouble to answer about the 2nd. Ed. [of The Artist]. Your dream has come to a sudden end, while other things go forward.

What's new in Vienna since the sessions? I've heard nothing from Sachs about them. Is Ferenczi still there?

Please specially thank Fräulein Bernays for the splendid book by [Claude] Farrère,
which in its sharp realism contrasts so agreeably with the lush sultriness of Pierre Loti.
With best regards and cordial greetings. Yours, Rank

Krakauer Zeitung ¶November 9, 1916

Lieber Herr Professor!

Forgive my not writing for so long, but till now I've had to deal with business cor-
respondence, specifically, about our new apartment in Vienna; unfortunately, despite
all efforts, it can't be held any longer.

So, again without a base. Besides that, I've been unwell a long time, and mentally,
too, I feel so tired I don't know where I'll find the energy to start all over again. You
are right, of course: one should be able to be happy even without sufficient reason. But
it often seems to me that I've reached the opposite pole, where one is depressed even
without sufficient reason.

Nevertheless I was glad to hear you've made good progress in literature and lec-
turing. Hopefully your practice is also [...]. Is the Nobel Prize in Medicine not to be
awarded this year?

Here, unfortunately, there's nothing new.

Cordial greetings. With thanks, yours, Rank

Freud confirms to Ferenczi, "Rank again seems very depressed in Krakow,
perhaps materially very stressed. It is really too bad about him." He scolds
Ferenczi for vacillating to the point where Gizella pulled back and 10 days
later, after multipage letters were exchanged, says "It seems to me you're now
using your analysis as a means of confusing your affairs, as you earlier used it
to delay."[3]

Internationale Zeitschrift für Ärtzliche Psychoanalyse [Krakow] ¶November 18, 1916
Lieber Herr Professor!

Thank you so much for your comforting lines. [Most Freud letters to Krakow
are missing.] You're right in many respects, as with the Krakauer Zeitung, *I realize*
more and more, but try in vain to change things. Maybe once again I can pull myself
together after all. Too bad, the trite saying that one is as young as one feels applies here
as always.

Allow me to be frank; please leave aside your kind intentions concerning the Heller
dream book. Carrying out your generous intentions, which I deeply appreciate, would
in this case mostly fortify my guilty conscience, which of course is not your intent.

And living a bit better or worse is really of no consequence now. [Freud probably offered a stipend; the book of essays on dreams never appeared.]

Since you write nothing about your two absent sons, I assume you get ongoing good reports. With your son-in-law in Hamburg things seem less favorable? Well, I'm glad you'll be seeing a larger family circle gathered around you. Please convey my best greetings on all sides.

Forgive me for depressing you with my private worries. I've kept them to myself a long time and wanted to go on that way, but such a mood can't be hidden forever. Anyway, I don't believe one can only strive forward. I'd have been destroyed by my success.

With cordial greetings. Thankfully yours, Rank

Krakauer Zeitung ¶December 3, 1916

Lieber Herr Professor!

Heartfelt thanks for the kindness and concern you conveyed to me through your son, who arrived safely here today. He's dealt with everything now, and I hope he'll soon feel comfortable here, although I can't offer as much as I'd wish since I'm still pretty much down.

Many thanks for the psa. news. Everything else I've of course heard in person—in detail and with great interest.

Best regards and greetings. Yours, Rank

Krakauer Zeitung ¶December 6, 1916

Lieber Herr Professor!

The military career of your son, who moved in yesterday, actually began today; he's getting his uniform, and has to sleep in the barracks for the first time—mandatory in the initial period—for now in the unit quarters, until a place is made in the first year quarters. For now he'll take his meals in the barracks, non-commissioned officers' mess, where I know the food is good. Meanwhile, I'll keep his things for him until his life is in order. He sensibly chose to accept this inevitable unpleasantness with humor, which I observe his doing in a way to be emulated. He feels very well and looks forward to upcoming events. Of course I'll keep in contact with him and keep you fully informed if he doesn't manage to. For now, for simplicity, please address his letters to "Krakauer Zeitung, First Year Freud."

With best greetings in his name and from me. Yours, Rank

P.S. I'm taking the liberty of sending, through Heller, a recently published novel by [Oskar] Schmitz The Refugee, which I recommend despite its somewhat daunting length; at least start it—I think you'll be as surprised as I was.

Freud read the book and praised it highly to Ferenczi: "I judge it more favorably than you and, above all, I consider it genuine."[4]

Krakauer Zeitung ¶December 12, 1916

Lieber Herr Professor!

Today I visited your son in the barracks, and can say I found him cheerful and well. He says he hasn't felt so well in a long time. Today he took part in military exercises for the first time; everything went well. For now he's not allowed to go out—but presumably can in a few days. He'll probably have to live in the barracks; he's already well beyond the uncomfortable stuff.

I've given him all the news. He has nothing special to report. After the initial training period of a few weeks he'll likely go to the school in Krems [Austria].

Sorry I have nothing to report except that my name has been submitted for promotion to sergeant; but I'm constantly feeling bad.

For some time Adler has been doing psychiatry in the garrison hospital—and haunts the cafés of Krakow.

With best regards and greetings. Yours, Rank

Krakauer Zeitung ¶December 19, 1916

Lieber Herr Professor!

Thanks for your kind letter, which corroborated my view of Schmitz. Such a thing can only be genuinely reproduced, but not substantiated. It's a synthesis of "Analysis of Phobia in a Six-Year-Old Boy." I still haven't gotten the promised dream literature, and ask only because I fear it's been lost. The post office, as usual, doesn't know.

The registered package for Oli arrived today; I'll deliver it tomorrow when I see him. He's fine, a paragon of freshness and enjoyment of life.

About the peace treaty and the prospects you attach to it, I agree with you completely.

Heller's in action again. I didn't understand what you wrote about an essay by Rubiner: is Zeitschrift für Individualpsychologie *still appearing, and what sort of Swiss publication is it? Who are the publishers?*

With best wishes to you and your family during the Christmas holidays. Respectfully yours, Rank

On December 22 Freud wrote Ferenczi that Wilson's peace initiative, "which should be taken more seriously, has had its share in bringing about a more life-affirming mood on my part."

Krakauer Zeitung ¶December 29, 1916

Lieber Herr Professor!

I'm glad I can report to you that today my promotion was approved, effective 1 January. There's a chance I'll be promoted to lieutenant very soon.

Otherwise everything here is unchanged and if it stays that way I might go to Karlstadt in early spring (February–March) to visit a health resort, to combat the physical ailments at least.

Your son is fit, cheerful, and content—a splendid soldier. The registered package for him arrived today. What news from the rest of your strapping warriors?

With best New Year wishes to you and yours.

Gratefully, your Rank

Krakauer Zeitung ¶January 21, 1917

Lieber Herr Professor!

Many thanks for your last letter and the current package. I just found time to write you since I'm still waiting for pleasant results of the event for which you so kindly congratulate me. I was supposed to travel to Romania at the beginning of the month— as a war correspondent—but had to postpone the trip for personal reasons. Maybe I'll go there in early February, and it's not impossible that I can be in Budapest with you at the same time.

The news from Heller didn't surprise me since I am becoming more and more convinced that in the long run it's impossible to work with him.

Just as before, your son is doing very well here. What are your other warriors doing?

My brother is now on leave in Vienna. He'll probably find more going on there and do more himself.

Best regards and greetings. Yours, Rank

On February 5, Rank said his crisis was not over: "Again, many thanks for your truly fatherly concern and your kind words, which are always a great comfort to me." Jones wrote Freud that he was newly married to the celebrated composer and singer Morfydd Owen: "She is Welsh, young (23), very pretty, intelligent, and musical."[5] On February 27, Ferenczi told Freud, "I've corresponded with Rank about a family matter (nephew ill in Krakow). His letter was friendly but showed decided depression." That same day, Rank, expecting to be in Vienna soon, wrote Freud that he was "looking forward to breathing some analytic air again." On March 2, Freud wrote Ferenczi that Rank was "in good shape again" and expected to see them both soon. Freud also addressed Ferenczi's concern that he would not have children with Gizella: "You wouldn't have had a child if you had been able to marry Mathilde"; Freud's eldest, a prospect for Sándor at one time, proved to be infertile. Long plagued with symptoms of hyperthyroidism, Ferenczi spent March through May in a Semmering sanatorium, 70 km from Vienna.

Krakauer Zeitung ¶March 23, 1917

Lieber Herr Professor!

Back from Warsaw, where one can live very well, I found your kind package awaiting me, for which many thanks. Quite a few proofs for the Lectures, *and the journals accumulated, too. I'll likely need at least a week to finish the backlog—lots of correspondence—so I can't think of starting anything until next month.*

For your sister-in-law I've gotten some of the requested yarn—under very amusing circumstances about which I'll write her myself when I have time. I'll ask about the rest here and then send everything together.

What do you hear from your sons? How are you and your family? The little one better again? His spring exuberance was probably premature; at least I stuck the whole time in deepest winter, and caught a cold, too. Have you heard from Ferenczi?

Cordial greetings. Yours, Rank

On March 24, Ferenczi asked Freud to tell Gizella that he wants to marry her, but needs to rebut her likely objection that Elma's return would turn him around and recapture his love. "I really believe that my intentions have finally matured . . . even the fact that I want to get Frau G. by way of your mediation seems to have a symbolic significance."

Krakow Fortress [postcard] ¶April 6, 1917

Lieber Herr Professor!

Many thanks for your card. I was so sure it had already been published—at least as an indirect discussion—but now subject to such tricks of memory, I don't wonder any more. In the 5 Apr. paper I found an announcement of lectures by Pfister in Berlin on 11 & 12 April. I drag around all day with unpleasant symptoms of neglected influenza, and will eagerly use the Easter holidays for being sick.

How are things with Ferenczi, from whom I hear absolutely nothing?

Cordial greetings. Yours, Rank

Krakauer Zeitung ¶April 9, 1917

Lieber Herr Professor!

Still not well, I'm using room-rest to flirt a bit with psychoanalysis. Most important, I've reread in context the third part [Lectures]: not only with great pleasure, at one sitting like an exciting novel, but with uplift and much profit. The value of this third part is, as you yourself said, greater for advanced than novice readers, whose feelings one can't imagine, since even we, presented with the imposing and instructive edifice of psychoanalysis, are awestruck when it suddenly comes in its entirety.

You can imagine my feelings when I approached The Artist, *that awaits its further fate. Whether because I simply wanted to paralyze this impression or whether there really is something in it, I found on reading it through that, apart from a few obscure spots, tasteless passages and errors, it's not as dated as it seemed in memory and through my personal development, and apart from a few excisions, modifications and amplifications, a new edition can and must remain as it was (assuming it needs a justification at all), given a preface or afterword to set myself outside the work and say what it really is: an attempt, within the framework of psychoanalysis, though at a later stage with other means and on a smaller scale, to work back from the analytically recognized structure of the psyche toward a corresponding external developmental pattern and to use the artist (understood here in a broad sense similar to the sexual concept) as a necessary mediator between the outer and inner worlds that coexist in mutual enmity. At the moment I see in this the only possible approach to the matter, but would gladly have your opinion. It would be remarkable were I to return now to my lit[erary] beginnings. Personally I've nearly overcome one of my most serious inner crises, if only fate will be a bit kind. If not badly mistaken, I sense the harbinger of an inner freeing, hopefully with practical outcome too, if I can overcome the last remaining problems that have defied my efforts.*

Heller has been remarkably friendly and forthcoming since I was last in Vienna, where he tried to interest me in his concert business. He answers every letter promptly, apologizes for a lost message, and asks where he can send me money: a strange illness whose study would be a task for Ps.A. I only wish the journals could gain from this since I cannot do anything from here. Sachs can pile as much on my back as he wants to—it hurts all the time anyway.

I'm sorry the typewriter [returned by Rank] arrived so late—I didn't know you needed it. Maybe you can use it for Metapsychology, *which still needs some work.*

Had a letter from Oli who says he's doing well—I assume the same about Martin, who's on leave. Please give him my hearty greetings. How is Ernst?—I hear things will be definite in 14 days.

My brother has an assignment in Lemberg [Lvov], and I hope to see him here soon. Thanks for the recent letters.

With best regards to all of your family and with cordial greetings.

Thankfully yours, Rank

Krakauer Zeitung [postcard] ¶April 11, 1917

Lieber Herr Professor!

First Lieutenant Engel, who is going to Vienna today, thoughtfully brought a box of cigars for you. I took the liberty of having the second box, Engel's own, brought to you as well, asking that you kindly have the cigars denicotinized at his expense since he can no longer smoke any others. I seem to recall that you have some experience with denicotinization, i.e. you know where it's done and maybe can have it done quickly. Please excuse this imposition and don't let your enjoyment of the weed be soured by the thought that these may be the last. I hope that won't be so.

With cordial greetings. Yours, Rank

Krakauer Zeitung ¶April 20, 1917

Lieber Herr Professor!

Many thanks for your kind lines. I hope you're feeling all well again. I was glad to hear the good news of your son Ernst and Ferenczi.

Unfortunately I can report nothing so good about myself. The favorable wind of fate, about which I rejoiced too soon, and which you hoped for too, burst out in hurricane force, stirring up everything, from which it's very hard to save myself. I hope to succeed, but it's doubtful without inner damage. With fate it is just as I said to you in Vienna: it shows its favor like Roller in The Robbers [Schiller, 1781] who wants to save the leader from the gallows. As for what you say about my simile of life, I've experienced it too often to ignore it; but I never knew how to appreciate and value luck because I presumptuously wanted to change noun into adjective. Or to put it better, I never knew how to use it. Luck forsakes a neurotic temperament.

Anyway, again I'm torn away from everything—thrown back from all that germinated since my last trip to Vienna, including work that I'd just begun to befriend. Please tell Sachs not to be annoyed at my latest broken promise: this time it's neither laziness nor mood, but really vis major *[greater force]. As soon as I can I'll send him something, but he shouldn't count on it for the next issue.*

I'm delighted to hear the typewriter was received with such open arms; but it deserves as much, for it's precious: unobtainable new, used ones cost 3–5 times the original price. And so there won't be any misunderstanding, I'll take the liberty of mentioning that 100 of the cigars are yours, but the other 100 belong to First Lieutenant Engel, in whose name I'm asking you to have them denicotinized since, if I'm not mistaken, you are in connection with the firm. But in spite of all this, it seems very uncertain when we'll be smoking the big Panamas.

Today I received the last of the Lectures.

With cordial greetings to your family and you. Yours thankfully, Rank

P.S. For some time I wanted to tell you that you can, of course, seal your letters to me.

Gizella balked at the Ferenczi-Freud proposal: she would yield the bridal honors to Elma and stay with her husband. She virtually promised Sándor's hand in marriage to Elma. He rallied to persuade Gizella to accept him, to take June and July in the country and work out an amicable separation from her husband.[6] A letter from Rank to Freud, May 3, mentions his slow recovery "from some really hard blows," anticipating their effects will be "integrated and dissolved somewhere in general experience."

Krakauer Zeitung ¶May 8, 1917

Lieber Herr Professor!

With great regret I heard you were not feeling well. I hope this subjective bad mood on your birthday—something I recently experienced myself—has now happily passed. As for the digestive difficulties, I can only imagine how you're reacting to the available food. Right now I'm planning, and will probably go to Karlsbad in summer after all. Isn't it possible you'll come too? If there's any such hope, please let me know the time period; I'd arrange to be there then, and would be fortunate to spend time with you again. As for the rest, I've now recovered. Fortunately, despite my hypersensitivity and nervousness, I have a thick skin and am as strong as a horse, as I saw again this time. I hope to find my way back to work soon, although your news of Heller, i.e. production of The Artist, *is not exactly encouraging.*

A few days before your letter I had a direct communication from Jones, quite short, and another invitation which tempts me more and more to give in as soon as possible.

Many thanks for the news of your warriors and your family.

I heard the news from Stockholm immediately after the announcement, and only wondered why the award is called the "Nobel" since the recipients certainly do not

*behave as the word would suggest. [No prize in medicine; Freud had hoped for it, if
only to annoy his opponents.]*

*Otherwise, I'm enjoying the spring bursting out now in full splendor in the glo-
rious environs here. From my new lodgings I have a wonderful view of the Wawel
Castle and the Vistula all the way to the Carpathian Mountains. Here I hope to find
peace again and the capacity to work too.*

Cordial greetings. Yours thankfully, Rank

Rank was offered a position with a publishing consortium (Präger) but
was not inclined to accept; the position would begin after war's end (May 31).
Freud reports to Ferenczi that he got a most interesting letter from a German physician: Georg Groddeck, who became a favorite of Ferenczi's (June
3). Despite Rank's lack of interest in Heller's concert arranging, the next letter reveals a budding impresario.

Krakauer Zeitung ¶June 17, 1917 [typed]

Lieber Herr Professor!

*Today I finally got time to write, even breathe—and it won't last long. This is the
greatest* Koppdraih *[Yiddish, "head-spinning"] in history. I literally haven't a single
free minute. Now I'm a concert manager extraordinaire: on assignment from the War
Press Command, with which I am in contact several times a day by telephone and
telegraph, I'm arranging a series of concerts and performances. First it was the Front
Theater, and then the Front Concert Ensemble. Yesterday at midnight at the station
I met the Court Opera Ensemble, which performs today and tomorrow. The Front
Cabaret is coming for the weekend. So far, no arrangements with the Front Circus.
I'm involved with military film showings and the opening of the Polish opera season.
Amid all this, the* Zeitung *has disappeared, and everything associated with it. I have
to arrange all these affairs from the ground up, with a thousand difficulties and petty
obstacles in an unmitigated state of chaos.*

My telegram address: Hellerersatz-Krakau [Heller-substitute-Krakow]!

*Nothing else new. Hopefully the butter and bread got there safely. Next week I go
to Warsaw.*

Cordial greetings to you and your family. Yours, Rank

*[P.S.] Yesterday I spoke with a woman I know who is going to Zakopane [Poland],
and who was at the Lake Csorba [Hungary] last year, where, however, she didn't find
the service ideal. Hopefully you'll have a better experience this year. Yours, Rank*

Krakauer Zeitung ¶July 7, 1917

Lieber Herr Professor!

Many thanks for the mail, which I found on return from Warsaw. It was very nice there, but so expensive I had to flee. As Bernstein and Sokolnicka informed me, a psychoanalytic association is just being set up there, but while I was there, some new problems arose. I have a lot to do here as my colleague is on leave. Whether and when and where I'll be going is still uncertain.

Hopefully you found everything as you wish and I'd gladly get your confirmation of that. In Warsaw I saw a photograph of Csorba; judging from it, I was very impressed.

What do you hear from your sons? Here everything is the same. I didn't get anything for your daughter in Warsaw, but have some remainders for Frl. Bernays.

Best regards and cordial greetings. Yours, Rank

Freud met Gizella at Csorba, "suffering and old-looking. Talking with her is a pleasure. I learned she has taken the decisive step with her husband; everything else seems unsure." Having read her letters from daughter Elma he tells Ferenczi, "because of your infidelity to Elma you have inflicted a deep wound on her and confused the possible future with demonic dexterity. But nothing else can be done. If Elma comes again you must forget that you can be something other than a father to her" (July 6). About that time Freud's nephew Hermann Graf, the only son of his sister Rosa, died in combat in Italy; "Grief was beyond description."[7]

Rank visited Csorba briefly in August, where Sachs and Ferenczi spent weeks with Freud, and Eitingon just a day.[8] On August 21, Freud wrote a congratulatory note to Gizella, since she would "finally make a beautiful life for yourself and for him. I am enormously happy about the easy outcome." Ferenczi, anticipating his engagement, mistakenly put his next letter to Freud in the envelope for Rank, and vice versa. Freud thought Ferenczi had gone crazy (*meschugge*): "I'm supposed to reserve a room in Budapest; you still owe me 300 crowns." Freud realized the mistake and returned the letter. Rank forwarded the Ferenczi letter to Freud unread: it spelled out details of Gizella's divorce. Freud shared another family concern with Ferenczi about his son Ernst, 25: "The little rascal got himself (in Graz or Agram) a little gonorrhea, which must now be clandestinely undone."[9]

In several short letters Rank reports on his travels during leave, including hiking with rucksacks and camping out and a September fortnight at a scenic spa in Germany, where he ate well, gained weight, and finished the *Artist* revision and a collection of papers on mythology. In Hungary on behalf of Präger, "I spent a little too much time with writers, who in Budapest belong to the dregs of humanity. Ferenczi was very kind, as usual, and is in good shape. He feels well and fit for work" (Oct. 10). Freud had not heard from Martin since an offensive in Italy on October 23.[10]

The following shows that Freud could deeply confide in Rank.

Krakauer Zeitung ¶November 6, 1917

Lieber Herr Professor!

Many thanks for your letter and enclosure. You spoke to me from the soul, but what can one do? Actually, perhaps something can still be done. I should get to Vienna at the end of the month, and then I'll talk with you about it.

After making a mess of the last chapter of the book on mythology I started work on Homer. I'm looking through what I've done thus far and am organizing the rest of my notes. The mechanics of work go well, but when I try to write anything it seems unclear and awkward. I lack concentration and [...], without which one simply cannot work well. But I hope at least to produce some preliminary material.

I was very glad to hear your good news. It's really no surprise that there are so many patients.

From Oli, who presumably isn't set up yet, I've had no word. Hopefully, though, you've heard from Martin. Please convey my best greetings to Ernst, as well as my best regards to your family.

Most cordial greetings. Yours with thanks, Rank

On November 18 Ferenczi pours out ambivalent feelings about Gizella to Freud. He hadn't shared his misgivings with her as in the past. He details dreams, fantasies, physical symptoms, analysis. Citing Groddeck, the psychosomatic specialist, he vows, "I won't let myself be made a fool of by these hypochondrias anymore. It is, after all, a pure attempt at *scaring myself away* from marriage." He thanks Freud for his tenacity in this and proclaims his enduring love of Gizella. Freud replies (Nov. 20): "It's not a matter of choosing a wife. She's already been that for 15 years, became that when she was young and beautiful, has aged with you, and that should not be a motive for casting out one's wife after so many long years. It's now only a matter of transforming an uncomfortable marriage into a contented living together. Incidentally—she is today, with all the deficiencies of her—merely physical—age, still worth incomparably more than most of the glossy women who get married. And finally—you know that yourself. What otherwise eludes you serves as a just punishment for you and, as such, will again satisfy an inner need." Freud is "worn out, and am beginning to find the world repulsively disgusting. The superstition that has limited my life to around February 1918 seems down-right friendly to me." He long held a premonition based on numerology that he would die at 61.

There were bread lines and riots in Vienna and Budapest, for which several military brigades were brought back from the front, but Freud's family was relatively comfortable, receiving gifts of groceries and cigars. Psycho-analytic journals could not be published for lack of paper. Freud had nine analytic patients: "I work all day, quite sovereign, with nine fools, can hardly control my appetite, but I can no longer find the good old sleep."[11]

Freud reported to Ferenczi on December 27: "Rank was here over the holidays for a short leave, not in the best shape, very much attached to the newspaper, where he is now the only mover. We took ourselves back to the old times for a few hours." He concludes, "Kind regards to Frau G. and you, and many wishes for 1919." With this slip Freud skips 1918, the year of his anticipated death.

≈ Chapter 8 ≈

Active Therapy and Armistice

1918

*Freud saw that everything appearing today as inner conflict—however senseless
it seems—was once, in the history of human evolution, an outward reaction
serving some good purpose. From this came attempts to reconstruct prehistoric
evolution from the ontogenetic psychology known through analysis. The real,
though unavowed, aim of this book is to show the psychological impetus progressing
from outside inward and constantly mounting, making the artist both possible and
necessary in cultural evolution.*
—Rank, Introduction to *The Artist*, 1918

I n this postwar edition of his first book Rank wrote, "The passing slice of
time has enriched the author in years and experience, but also led mankind
to the brink of monstrous cultural catastrophe." He stated that *The Artist* is
based on the "secure foundation of Freudian psychology . . . a complete and
finished science" and on "those direct philosophical forerunners of psychoanalysis, Schopenhauer and Nietzsche, for many ideas, if also the tendency to
speculate and overreach to grasp the whole, which may be explained by the
author's youthfulness." On January 21 he thanked Freud for his "comments
and corrections" on the text, which Freud had also mentioned to Abraham.[1]

Krakauer Zeitung ¶February 6, 1918
Lieber Herr Professor!
    *Many thanks for your missive today. Indeed, for the last few weeks I've felt better
than I have for a long time. On the double holiday I visited acquaintances in Central*

Galicia in the country (2 hrs from the railroad), greeted with the Polish hospitality that puts all Western European versions to shame. For two days I lived in glory and joy, i.e. eating, sleeping, and walking. I've been promised a package from there next week, which I've decided to send to Vienna—if it comes—and I'll be happy if it suits you.

As for my service, as before, I can't complain. Due to new train connections, Vienna papers don't arrive the same day, but the next, so we have no competition. Each day I routinely call Vienna at 9:00 A.M. If possible, I finish work around 11:00 A.M.—today, as usual—and then have the rest of the day. But I still fail to use it as I should.

Recently I recommended to Heller an engagement in Brest-Litovsk! The minutes of the proceedings there remind me of a pun by [Julius] Stettenheim: "Pax vobiscum [Peace with you] becomes "Pax schlägt sich, vobiscum verträgt sich" [The rabble riot; "with you" is quiet].

Isn't it strange, by the way, that now, with the future looking darker than ever, my mood has improved? Doesn't that show it's independent of external events, which, by the way, I always "knew"?

Re lieutenant—I have to wait for the February promotion. Ernst must by now have been granted his three-month leave to attend university, his entitlement with the new decree. Please give Martin and Oli my greetings, and my regards to everyone at home.

Yours, Rank

On February 17 Freud wrote separately to Abraham and Ferenczi about a new booklet, *War Neuroses and Psychic Trauma,* by Ernst Simmel, M.D., a German neurologist in a hospital for military casualties who used both psychoanalysis and hypnosis. Freud commented to Abraham that Simmel "has not gone the whole way with P/a, takes essentially the cathartic standpoint, works with hypnosis, which is bound to conceal resistance and sexual drives. . . . I think a year's training would make a good analyst of that man." To Ferenczi, Freud added, "it shows that German war medicine has taken the bait," and it is "no less significant than Groddeck." Later in the year, having read the book and met the author, Abraham cautioned that Simmel had not moved beyond the early, cathartic "Breuer-Freud point of view, has strong resistances against sexuality," and believes that sexuality had little or nothing to do with war neuroses.[2]

Krakauer Zeitung ¶March 4, 1918

Lieber Herr Professor!

Today at last the lieutenantcy came, which hopefully means the end of my military career in the World War.

Many thanks for the news! How is Oli, from whom I hear nothing—not even his address, and Ernst, who hopefully will still get the promised study leave? Has Martin become a first lieutenant?

The Artist *should appear soon, since Heller indicated this was a priority. He should get* Mythology *printed; I asked Sachs to bring him the ms. Perhaps you'll kindly remind Heller at your convenience. I wrote him that we shouldn't wait for war's end, as production costs are constantly rising—which apparently made an impression on him.*

Zeitschrift *(proof) is very elegant this time, and Jekels' "Macbeth" is fine both in content and presentation unlike most* Imago *articles, which leave something to be desired in one respect or the other.*

Won't you allow yourself some ease at Easter? I'll try to travel a bit, maybe to Warsaw, where there should be plenty to do. Sorry my packages to you were shipwrecked this time by the suspension of military leave. The man I sent to Poland and Vienna stayed longer and goes out to the field tomorrow. I hope at least some bonbons from Krakow got to you safely. It was intended as dessert after everything else, but perhaps will meet with favor in its own right.

Best regards and cordial greetings. Yours, Rank

Krakow, a former capital of Poland, was a city where education, industry, sciences, and arts flourished, a site of fine museums. Austrian forces took it from Russia in August 1915. It was a secure and stimulating post for Rank, though he suffered from depression. He attended concerts as a music critic for the paper and met a psychology student and music lover, Beata Mincer, whose aunt had studied with him in Vienna, and told her about *The Artist*. She was 11 years younger than Rank. Their relationship continued for much of his tenure in Krakow, unmentioned to any correspondents.[3]

Krakauer Zeitung ¶April 10, 1918

Lieber Herr Professor!

I got here from Vienna in the snow, and on the trip—in an unheated coupé—caught a powerful cold, on top of which the unhealthy Krakow climate and the obligatory spring illness laid me low in the last few weeks. Even now, despite the unusually beautiful weather—or maybe precisely because of it—I feel physically unwell. I long for some "country living" and peace, which could be doubly hard for me to obtain this year. Meanwhile, your pessimistic fears about places to stay have been partly fulfilled. For the first time, one begins to look ahead to the summer with dread—as formerly only with winter.

Otherwise, everything goes along as usual, which has the small advantage of excusing one from doing what little thinking is still possible.

What's new in Vienna and psychoanalysis? The volume of Zeitschrift *is ready, but* Imago *is in a logjam as usual. What's Heller doing? He's silent, despite various promises and though I've written him. Have you talked with him, or has he completely disappeared again?*

What do you hear from Martin? Won't things soon get moving there again? I wrote to Oli, but have no answer yet. And Ernst? My brother got a full month's leave (May) and is trying to arrange things so that he can remain in Vienna. Given the ongoing situation that's really the last resort.

[Max] Präger [publisher, R. Loewit Verlag; Rank's university classmate] will be here in a few days; I plan to travel to Warsaw with him, i.e. he'll be going with me since he can't go alone. Indeed, I'm very tired, but glad to use every chance to get away.

I've written to Lukatekowitz for your sister-in-law, but thus far have no answer. I hope to hear from you soon. Best regards to everyone in your home, and cordial greetings.

Yours thankfully, Rank

On April 8, Ferenczi told Freud that Elma was supportive of his plan to wed Gizella and would press her father for an amicable settlement, but Elma's sister and brother-in-law (Ferenczi's brother) strongly opposed it. By April 15 Ferenczi, calmer, said his pessimism had been excessive.

Krakauer Zeitung ¶April 20, 1918

Lieber Herr Professor!

I arrived from Warsaw today with Dr. Präger and take the opportunity to send off a few things. Life there is indescribable. I've physically recovered somewhat and feel more energetic. I came across a letter from Heller (about printing The Artist *and remuneration for same), which I could answer only with a few short lines. I'll comment*

on that and on psychoanalytic life in Warsaw next time. Today I'm up to my neck in
work.

Cordial greetings and best regards. Yours, Rank

The next letter reveals that Freud and Rank disclosed themselves emotionally to each other.

Krakauer Zeitung ¶May 4, 1918

Lieber Herr Professor!

Through my brother, who came through Krakow yesterday and has 5 weeks' leave,
I take the liberty of sending you a box of Trabuccos [cigars] and some fine butter—not
available for a long time here, either. Hopefully the package will arrive safely.

Otherwise, the last 2-3 days I began getting over the spring illness that plagued
me this year. My persistent inability to work, which gave me quite a guilty conscience,
doesn't exactly benefit from an innocent inability to work. Now it's been exactly 4
years (!) since, due to war, I stopped working on Homer; maybe I can still get back to it.

I enclose a few amusing clippings from the last few days; the typographical error is
certainly the nicest. Please keep these, as I collect all that material. For your informa-
tion I enclose Heller's note, which I answered appropriately. (Please return it when
convenient.) Since then he's been silent, and I'm happy not to hear from him.

The more frequent exchange of our emotional states, which you encouraged re-
cently, would doubtless affect me favorably if I didn't fear affecting you the opposite
way with my almost constant reports of bad mood. Interestingly, I occasionally think
my time in Krakow has not been the worst in my life, and maybe even better; some-
times I'm afraid I could end up looking back on it longingly. At the moment, though
it's just the opposite—and very much so.

I hope Fräulein Anna has fully recovered; I also hope to hear better things about
Fräulein Bernays' condition. Engel's leave in Abbazia goes marvelously. I heard an
anecdote from there (a true one) from a comrade who just returned, but it must be told
in person. Hopefully soon.

Cordially yours, Rank

The cigars and butter were probably a gift for Freud's long-dreaded birthday, following which he tells Ferenczi, "The nice superstition with 62 now
finally has to be given up. There is indeed no relying on the supernatural."
In this letter Freud praises Ferenczi's three recent draft papers as "show-

pieces . . . testimonials of total mastery. The one on equivalents to masturbation makes a good beginning with a theoretically as well as practically significant theme, that of active therapy." This innovation in practice and theory
was increasingly associated with Ferenczi and Rank. Along with end-setting
in treatment, they gave full credit to Freud—in humility and, no doubt, for
support against likely criticism from other analysts.[4]

The paper in question is "Technical Difficulties in the Analysis of a Case
of Hysteria (Including Observations on Larval Forms of Onanism and
'Onanistic Equivalents')."[5] Therein Ferenczi reports the case of a wife and
mother, intelligent, motivated, and with good insight, who, after a good start
in analysis, got stalled. All his efforts to no avail, Ferenczi set an ending date,
as Freud had with his Wolf Man case.[6] While professing her love for him,
which Ferenczi interpreted as transference, she remained stuck. He discharged her "uncured." After "many months" she returned, only to repeat:
initial improvement leading to impasse. She left, then returned for a third
try. This time she mentioned erotic genital sensations while relating her
love fantasies. Ferenczi noticed that she kept her legs crossed for the whole
hour while she lay on the couch. "This led us—not for the first time—to the
subject of onanism, an act performed by girls and women for preference by
pressing the thighs together." As before, she vehemently denied such practices, but Ferenczi decided to forbid the crossed legs because she "discharged
unnoticed the unconscious impulses and allowed only useless fragments to
reach the material of her ideas." He considered it to be subliminal or "larval"
masturbation. She complied and the effect was dramatic: she became tor-
mented, tense, and restless in the sessions. Astonished and pleased, Ferenczi
says her fantasies "resembled the deliria of fever, in which there cropped up
long forgotten memory fragments" that led to childhood traumas and the
source of her illness. But once again she stalled. Ferenczi surmised that her
autoerotic behavior continued in her daily life so he extended the prohibition to the whole day, including pleasurable touching of any parts of the body,
acts he called "masturbation equivalents." Eventually she agreed that she had
been "wasting her whole sexuality in those little 'naughtinesses.'" Her sexuality found "the way back" to the normal erotogenic zones; for the first time she
found satisfaction in marital intercourse. Many hysterical symptoms were
explained and cured.

This led Ferenczi to a technical innovation, "active therapy," prohibiting
larval onanism and its equivalents in analysis, because the "apparently harm-

less activities can easily become hiding-places for the libido" that make it more difficult for patients to bring disturbing material into consciousness. Ferenczi—who, unlike Freud, did not consider most masturbation to be harmful—banned it for therapeutic gain. (For an inhibited patient to masturbate with pleasure for the first time would be progress—if consciously erotic, not "larval," or unconscious.) "We owe the prototype of this 'active technique' to Freud himself," Ferenczi wrote, not citing a reference. Freud would direct a stalled anxious patient toward an anxiety-provoking situation to "free the wrongly anchored affects from their connections. We expect from this measure that the unsatisfied valencies of these free floating affects will above all attract to themselves their qualitatively adequate and historically correlated ideas." He concludes: "Besides observation and logical deduction (interpretation) psychoanalysis has also at command the method of experiment."

Eager to link their new psychology with natural science, Freudians borrowed terms from chemistry, physics, biology, and medicine, for example, *analysis, current, larval,* and *circulation:* Ferenczi argues metaphorically that, just as the peripheral blood pressure goes up when certain vessels are tied off, so, by shutting off certain paths of discharge of excitement in suitable analytic cases, the rise of pressure may "overcome the resistance of the censorship." Finally, the "new direction of the current" is not dictated as with hypnosis, "and we gladly let ourselves be surprised by the unexpected turns taken by the analysis."

Krakauer Zeitung ¶May 14, 1918

Lieber Herr Professor!

I gladly thank you for two letters, especially the first, with news of your summer vacation and Interpretation of Dreams, *and would be happier if you hadn't barred those topics from the second.*

Concerning ID, I agree completely, only suggest incorporating the metapsychological continuation of ID in an appropriate place. Regarding literature, our journals since the last edition should be especially reviewed for that purpose (including the discussion sections). I'll examine my collection here, and when convenient, in Vienna, I'll consult my notes there. Bibliographic matters like this are hardest of all to handle under the current situation, and from a distance.

From Heller I was prepared to hear such things and won't fret about him; that way one won't get upset, with the same outcome.

Re my leave, due to details of my assignment I have no information for now. Csorba would certainly be beautiful, and in many ways help me recuperate. I'll take this opportunity to ask for Ernst's address in Abbazia as soon as you know it; I'd like to ask him about some acquaintances.

I've waited months for the Homer proofs, and a cue on further work. I must immerse myself in the material by reading, but have no copy here. Recently I'm tempted to do the section on Homer the poet-personality; I can't work on the historical sections now due to lack of concentration and reading. Maybe it'll work out?

Otherwise, I always believe and hope it's the right conditions, now missing, that would make me fit for work, and I think I know what those are. And they aren't hard to arrange, and my comment on the Krakow Jews relates to the fact that I didn't bother to create the conditions, when I could have, given some good will, as the saying goes, and some adaptability. Whether being able to work only under certain conditions is a defect I won't presume to decide, but for me I think so. Anyway, I've seldom been so randomly free of external restrictions as now, but have never been so aware of my inability to make use of the situation mentally. Of course, in its regressive tendency, this is a highly neurotic trait, as perhaps is the need for a particular environment. I've suffered from periodic depressions as long as I remember, but could always compensate and overcome them with an appropriate lifestyle. The last two years, due to the extraordinary situations and experiences, these have been not occasional but constant; I kept silent about it because, despite my psychoanalytic insight, I couldn't bear to ask anyone for help—fate has so often sentenced me to this—because the few attempts to help imposed upon me with heroic sacrifice from various sides only made things worse.

Though you write that it's the younger generation that makes the difference, I, despite the numerical contradiction, admit belonging to us elders. To wit, in the last few months I've aged rapidly, as good observers around me have repeatedly said; and the bodily fatigue from which I can't escape has, beyond its undeniable mental origin, another root in this. Please take these lines for what they are—a frank confession of my current mood, which, like today's weather, can change overnight, and hopefully will.

> *Best regards and cordial greetings. Yours thankfully always, Rank*

Krakauer Zeitung ¶May 25, 1918

Lieber Herr Professor!

All typesetters in Krakow have been on strike for two days, and since we share printing presses we're forced to a standstill; we can't guess for how long, but it's increasingly distressing. The situation is not good, especially because a staff change is going on. I'd have been in Vienna this morning, but decided to remain at my post, as by coincidence both Engel and the printer have gone to their rooms and I have to deal with everyone here by myself.

At Pentecost I spent a few days in the mountains (Tatra), which did me a great deal of good; had the strike started a day earlier, I'd probably still be there.

Yesterday's sensation: two (!) letters came from Heller with the same date; they outdo each other in self-criticism, apologies, and promises for the future. As you can see: a dramatic success for my Heller-designed handling system. He goes with what I want. Today I'll ask as much of him as possible. Your judgment on the purely literary section of Homer was very useful since sometimes I get lost on my own. I'm working more, but things go very, very slowly.

It's a pity about Reik; he seems to have developed so much recently. I got the proofs for Tausk's work, but haven't read them yet. With this post I enclose a brochure which may interest you now, with the advantage that one can read it in ¼ hour. The nicest part, aside from the conclusion, is the Dostoevski quote (p. 76). Please add this little book to your dream library.

Instead of me will come "only" a prepared sausage; its arrival announced by telephone (or hopefully has been).

Best regards and cordial greetings. Yours, Rank

Krakauer Zeitung ¶June 5, 1918

Lieber Herr Professor!

Preparing the next section of Homer, about the triple time scheme, I've come across an apparent contradiction that I can't get past, though I feel it should be easy to solve. In individual fantasy activity, memories are falsified in the direction of ego-syntonic reality; in legends too this (of course) occurs, but inversely: to contrast the revered, great past with an empty or self-satisfied present. Indeed, this apparent contradiction exists in the tendency, basically the same—glorification of the past—and not in the mechanism, but nevertheless I can't escape an unclear feeling—there's something more here. In a word, may I ask in which direction I should focus my remarks?

Have your summer plans taken shape, and how long, i.e. when do you plan to be away from Vienna? A few days ago came news from Ernst; I'd asked for some. He complains about bad weather, and wants to go to the Tatra. From here (military command region), I can only recommend Zakopane to him, where one thrives at a fair price, but it's hard for civilians to get a residence permit.

Nothing from Heller since his booklet, and his wife wrote that he'll answer me after he returns from Germany. Meanwhile, typesetting for Zeitschrift goes slowly.

For ID I have a few little items in my collection here, mostly stupid—as if "dream interpretation" didn't exist.

Frau [Dr. Evgenia Kutner] Sokolnicka, who complained to me in Warsaw that as a neurologist she has to struggle with so many problems, wrote that she wants to go to Vienna this fall if there are possibilities for her there. She asks my opinion, reminding me of a remark you once made to Sachs, which raised her hopes that she could count on your support. I sketched the scene in Vienna, and promised I'd appeal to your kindness and get your advice. In Warsaw she's done a lot in a short time. She has interested and recruited many people for psychoanalysis (physicians, teachers, etc.) and organized lectures and courses; she claims some therapeutic successes too. I've seen that in Warsaw she fights against a wall of closed-mindedness and meanness; I spoke with various people there, including Bernstein, who is impossible, but who, as a respected neurologist, can discredit analysis just like the others—all the while believing himself to be a supporter. With people like that, one sees how likable the real opponents are.

Tomorrow my brother returns from leave on the way to his new post in Ukraine. It seems again there's not much cheer in Vienna. My mother is sick (pyelitis), and there are other unhappy details I need to learn about. Here things go as usual.

Most cordial thanks for the monthly allowance. Yours respectfully, Rank

Krakauer Zeitung ¶June 17, 1918

Lieber Herr Professor!

Many thanks for the hint, which hopefully will lead me further. Today I got the page proofs for Imago with the first chapter of Homer, and a letter from Heller in which he complains about the printer. One must be glad that so it goes.

My brother's visit has put me in a somber mood. He said he'd have to try to get to Vienna in the fall, otherwise everything will fall apart, and urged me to come back, too; perhaps together we can get something done. I'm still wondering if and how that will work, especially coming back, but also the rest, since I've finally given up ideas about working with Präger due to his (and Engel's) behavior. Life here is gradually becoming unbearable.

Given these somber auspices on all sides it is doubly difficult for me to appeal to your generosity, to make use of your repeated offer and ask for the loan of a few hundred crowns. You know what a struggle it is for me, despite everything, to broach such a request, and how heavily these things oppress me. I'm emboldened not only by the generous and detached attitude you always take in such matters, but also by the hope

that you'll consider this an advance on the amount for the next several months, which
in any case I use for the same expenses, though they've added up due to various things
happening at once.

Under the circumstances, I can't think of taking a holiday for the time being. Maybe
I can get sick leave with military lodgings somewhere. That would be best.

What do you hear from Martin, who is down there of course, and where has Oli
gone? Will you work until 15 July, or close up shop?

I hope you won't be offended by this frank request.

Cordial greetings. Yours thankfully, Rank

In the next letter Rank responds to two from Freud, the first provid-
ing the requested advance, the other with news of generous support for the
movement from Anton (Toni) von Freund, Ph.D., a wealthy Budapest brew-
ery owner. Ferenczi, his friend and therapist, referred Toni to Freud when he
developed an apparent psychotic reaction following removal of a cancerous
testicle. Unsure of his health, von Freund established a fund to support a psychoanalytic Verlag, headed by Freud, to be run by Otto Rank from Budapest.
That would end the onerous dependence on Heller.

Krakauer Zeitung ¶June 21, 1918

Lieber Herr Professor!

I really don't know how to thank you for your letter—its genuine warmth helps
more than anything to lift me up in this bad time; having that alone would justify my
request to you.

Meanwhile I got your first letter too: with your summer plans you inform me of
Dr. Freund's intentions. Amazing that once again, at a time of great desperation on
all sides, comes a ray of hope! I've had several truly uncanny moments in my life, and
thus believe all the more in the significance of such a coincidence. If something comes
of this—and I really feel it will—my practicum in Krakow will prove quite useful, as
I've become familiar with the printing business both technically and commercially. So
this seemingly lost time, which made me more practical and resourceful in relations
with people, has its value in that also.

I've overcome the hardest inner crises. For a while I've felt there'd be an upturn if
the external conditions, my environment, improved—now more likely than ever. I've
never been so close to believing that peace will come soon, and since, as you know, I've
not been too optimistic, perhaps this belief has something to it.

I'm glad your summer plans have solidified and that you'll be well provided for at the home of our kind neighbors. Amazing that your three warriors are all together in the South!

Profound thanks and cordial greetings. Yours, Rank

Rank and his brother, Paul Rosenfeld, brought their convalescing mother Karoline, 62, to Krakow in July: "My mother is feeling very well here, going to the well-stocked markets with mouth and eyes wide open—but also with purse the same" (July 25). Soon Karoline was thriving and he planned to visit Freud in Csorba (Aug. 10). On August 19 Rank, back in Krakow, expressed gratitude for the momentous day in Csorba, "with joy, pride, and thanks; a milestone not only in the history of the psychoanalytic movement, but also in my life, and inwardly I hope you'll excuse my negative comments, of which I'm now ashamed." He thanks "your dear ones and our friends" for the "beautiful day, which I shall never forget." This acknowledges the patronage of Anton von Freund, making Rank head of the Psychoanalytischer Verlag, with a good salary.

Writing from Abbazia, Italy, Rank says his hoped-for transfer there is not assured, but he is free to travel and will meet with von Freund in Budapest, which Freud said "will become the headquarters of our movement."[7] The International Psychoanalytical Association Congress was relocated from Breslau to Budapest, where the mayor and university and medical supporters would more than compensate for the loss of some German participants. Ferenczi, Rank, and von Freund formed an ad hoc committee, and Ferenczi told Freud "the goodwill and energy" of their patron and "Rank's ingenuity and skill complement each other very well."[8]

Budapest ¶September 11, 1918

Lieber Herr Professor!

You have heard by telegraph of the first Budapest sensation, the transfer of the Congress here, which hopefully won't displease you; the second is that my release from Krakow is being worked on with good prospects of success. In any case, the new direction is toward Budapest, and as much as I'd like to return to Vienna, I can't reject the idea that perhaps it's good to let myself be carried along by the Budapest tide. Meanwhile, I've arranged a compromise which makes possible my temporary presence in Vienna and prepares my permanent transfer. This proposal is too complicated and unready to be confirmed as yet. Anyhow, great things are happening here and we hope they'll lead to the general welfare and to our cause.

It was also a sensation and surprise—no less great—to be able to greet Fräulein Annerl ["Annie" Freud] upon my arrival in Budapest. She arrived fifteen minutes after me, at the same train station, so I was able to receive her in Budapest. Unfortunately we could spend only a few hours together at the home of Dr. Levy, and then returned to the station, where Fräulein Annerl, with heavy heart, had to take leave of beautiful Budapest, where it really felt good to be received with such kind hospitality by such people. Dr. Sachs is due here at the end of the week. I'll share my room with him and complete preparations for the Congress and for relocating the two journals.

Today I'll spend some time with Ferenczi, who I saw yesterday, and found fit and well. As for me, I'm not at the peak of health; I've recovered but little and miss my old work energy, which I could certainly use now. But I'm sure it will return, and that's great progress.

I wish you and Frau Freud the best relaxation, and especially weather as beautiful as we have here. Cordial greetings. Yours thankfully, Rank

Long separated from Loe Kann, Anna found another maternal companion in Toni's sister, Kata Levy, and was tutor-in-residence for Toni's young daughter. Kata was a social worker, analysand of Freud, and future analyst whose husband, Lajos Levy, friend and analysand of Ferenczi, was director of the Jewish Hospital in Budapest. As if these links between friendship and analysis were not enough, in October Freud began his analysis of Anna.[9]

On September 28–29 the Fifth IPA Congress took place in Budapest. Besides two participants from neutral Netherlands, all participants came from Austria/Hungary and Germany; there was optimism about the war ending. Freud spoke on lines of advance in psychoanalytic therapy. Ferenczi gave a paper on psychoanalysis and war neuroses; he had won a university professorship in Budapest and was elected president of the IPA. Rank presented "Myth and Folk Tales." Abraham and Simmel talked on war neuroses. A proposed new requirement that every analyst go through a training analysis was defeated. Freud thought it unnecessary; Otto Rank and Victor Tausk opposed the motion, which did not pass.[10] On September 30, Freud urged Ferenczi to "solidify the relationship with the man Providence has sent us at the right moment [Toni Freund, the new IPA Secretary], and with Rank, who can't be replaced by anyone else." On October 20 Freud mentioned that "Annerl's analysis is getting very fine, otherwise the cases are uninteresting."[11] This controversial father-daughter exercise was known to inner circles but was a well-kept secret outside.

Abraham reported disappointing news to Freud about a Berlin conference on war neuroses a month after Budapest. "The political situation made it impossible for Simmel and me to intervene successfully for our cause. Since an early peace was then anticipated, one could hardly expect a receptive mood toward new ideas . . . hostility from psychiatric circles has remained unchanged." More idealistic or less opportunistic than Freud, he explained his lack of disappointment: "I did not like the idea that psychoanalysis should suddenly become fashionable because of purely practical considerations. We would rapidly have acquired a number of colleagues who would merely have paid lip service and would afterwards have called themselves psychoanalysts." He commiserated with Freud about hardships, including famine, in Vienna, "about which we constantly read. Here, in East Prussia, we are tolerably well off in this respect. But the political future is dark."[12]

To Ferenczi, Freud lamented the death, on Armistice Day, of Victor Adler, founder of the Social Democratic Party, as one who would have been up to the challenge of rebuilding Austria. He was displeased about politics in Hungary, which soon quashed the Budapest plan. "No sooner does it begin to interest the world on account of the war neuroses than the war ends, and once we find a source that affords us monetary resources, it has to dry up immediately. But hard luck is one of the constants of life. Our kingdom is indeed not of this world."[13]

The Budapest Prize was a short-lived project launched by Freud, implemented after the Congress. He would pick the two best papers of the year (in this case the war years), one medical, one in the humanities, for an award of 1,000 crowns each. Ferenczi suggested Rank for *The Artist* or "Homer," but Freud declined: "*The Artist* is an old work, whereas I had my eye on the war years of 1914–1918. 'Homer' is only an introduction, which doesn't come into consideration for this review." The first scientific prize was divided between Karl Abraham, for a 1916 paper on libido, and Ernst Simmel, for his book on war neuroses. Theodor Reik's 1916 *Imago* paper, "Puberty Rites of Savages," got the humanities prize.[14] Freud's excitement about the Homer paper was offset by other considerations, and Rank was well provided for in the Verlag.

Rank and Beata "Tola" Mincer wed in Krakow on November 7. Rank, who had converted to Catholicism in order to legally change his name in 1909, converted back to Judaism so that a rabbi could preside. Ferenczi expressed surprise to Freud at the news (Nov. 24) and withheld judgment: "Let's wait and see!" Freud answered cautiously (Nov. 27) "Rank's marriage also didn't make a particularly favorable impression on me, but one certainly can't judge in these matters, not on behalf of another. . . . I can't do anything here without him." Freud was anxious about the fate of son Martin, part of a large contingent that surrendered to the Italians at war's end. Rank arrived in Budapest with his wife in early December, as the plans to relocate there were falling apart, along with hopes for political and university support for psychoanalysis. "He has, to *everyone's* surprise, brought home a little wife from Krakow, who up to now has not met with the approval of any of the friends." "Whether it will be a big mishap will appear only gradually." In this substantial letter to Abraham (Dec. 2) Freud explains how the largesse of von Freund was decimated by the revolution in Hungary from 2 million to 250,000 crowns, on which the interest of 10,000 would not go far, so the principal would be used up by the Verlag. "It's extraordinary how much money you have to have before you can do anything decent with it." He adds a piece of sad, shocking news from Jones, by way of Zurich, "that he has lost his young wife, apparently in the course of an operation."

Freud's dismay at Rank's marriage peaked on Christmas Day, when he wrote Abraham, "Rank seems to have done himself a great deal of harm with the marriage. A little Polish-Jewish woman whom nobody likes, and who does not seem to have any higher interests. It is quite sad and scarcely comprehensible." On New Year's Day he wrote Ferenczi that "Rank is plunging into work with his long-accustomed zeal, perhaps also to rehabilitate himself for his marriage. We will do the Verlag with Heller after all. . . . Even with all his weaknesses and shabbiness, the two of us do get along with him, and he can also show his better side. Toni has intimidated him too much."

Ferenczi reflected on 1918 as a year of upheaval leading to a test of strength. He wrote Freud in gratitude (Dec. 26), optimistic and grateful to be part of

an intellectual movement that is without a doubt a part of the future. Considered sub specie psychoanalysis, *the terrible events appear only as episodes of a still very primitive social organization. . . . To be sure, I find it shameful that the creator of the science that gives all values a new meaning has, after so many decades, not even found so much understanding in his own fatherland that the people,* in their own interest, *did not even look to him rather than to those who are ignorant. If ever a city undeservedly achieved recognition for having been the birthplace of a new idea it is Vienna....The Vienna school of P/a—with the exception of the incomparable Rank and Dr. Sachs—was also never actually on a high plane. I won't abandon the idea that you may yet move to Budapest.*

≈ Chapter 9 ≈

Eros Meets Thanatos

1919 and 1920

In psychoanalysis we act upon the transference itself, resolve what opposes it,
adjust the instrument with which we wish to make our impact. Thus it becomes
possible for us to derive an entirely fresh advantage from the power of suggestion;
we get it into our hands. The patient does not suggest to himself whatever he pleases:
we guide his suggestion so far as he is in any way accessible to its influence.
—Freud, "Analytic Therapy," *Introductory Lectures on Psychoanalysis*

Otto Rank and the Verlag did not move to Budapest due to political upheavals in Hungary, which also took away Ferenczi's professorship and much of Toni Freund's gift. Rank enjoyed the pun in "Lieber Freund" (friend) in a letter to Toni that already used *"du,"* the familiar "you."[1]

Lacking letters between Freud and Rank until 1921, our history relies on other primary sources. The Freud-Ferenczi letters of early 1919 bring news of James Jackson Putnam's death, the marriage of Sándor and Gizella in February, and diminishing hopes for the Verlag. Theodor Reik was hired to assist Rank. Martin Freud was still a prisoner in Italy: he was only able to send a reassuring Red Cross card in March, four months after Armistice. Ferenczi asked Freud to take a patient of his because (1) his work with her involved hypnosis, which barred shifting to analysis, and (2) she was having an affair with Toni Freund (both were married) and was suicidal. Freud had ten patients, including Toni, and demurred. "Toni is naturally much better than at home," Freud wrote, "but in neurotic defiance because I don't want to accept any more gifts from him. In some areas his primitive savagery has not yet been dismantled. . . . He has invited [lover] Frau Dr. D. to come to Vienna, but he gets frightened himself from time to time about the possibility that she could kill herself here."[2]

Freud wrote Ferenczi: "The discussions with Rank [*Leonardo* revision, etc.] are claiming much interest; he is working hard, but willingly. Such a Verlag gives much to do. His trip to Switzerland is now imminent, if he can get Jones there and learn more details, . . . New opportunities to invest money are opening up daily. We don't know anything about the big fund. Let's hope it hasn't gotten lost; Toni, who is at present angry at analysis, hasn't bothered about it, so it seems."[3]

Freud again praised Ferenczi's paper on active technique, now published: "pure gold, and can only be completely appreciated by the worker." And, "You will certainly learn about all our prospects and works through Rank, who is functioning flawlessly." The revised *Leonardo*, "the only pretty thing that I have written," was in press. In Zurich, March 24, Jones, Rank, and Sachs helped inaugurate the Swiss Society for Psychoanalysis, affiliated with the International Psychoanalytical Association. The society's board chair was Emil Oberholzer ("a *severe* neurotic," in Freud's opinion), Hermann Rorschach, vice chair, with Binswanger and Pfister among the members.[4]

Freud told Ferenczi "I miss Rank very much. . . . I finished a 26-page paper on the genesis of masochism, which bears the title 'A Child is Being Beaten.' A second one, with the mysterious heading 'Beyond the Pleasure Principle' is in process." Freud's masochism paper is based on six patients, including—disguised—daughter Anna. He speculated that his productivity was due to the spring, many colds, or the meatless postwar diet. "The Verlag is working valiantly, but under the stupidest impediments, which can't be removed as long as Rank is absent [Mar. 7–Apr. 11]. . . . That rascal Rank is having a good time in Switzerland . . . he certainly took into account in all his arrangements the uncertainty of our situation. Just as his work up to now has been altogether flawless."[5]

Ernest Jones wrote Freud from Switzerland, "Rank I find greatly improved, more independent, self-confident, and manly. I admire his quick brain and sure judgement. We got on splendidly together, and I think you may feel safe in leaving things in our hands, we agree about everything and shall have done a great deal of business before we separate." Decades later, Jones tells it differently: "I never knew anyone change so much." Rank had become "a wiry tough man with a masterful air." He says that Rank went through Swiss customs with a large handgun that he pulled from his pocket saying "Just in case." Jones diagnosed "a hypomanic reaction to the three severe attacks of melancholia he had suffered while in Krakow." Further, "I always regretted that the war interfered with the arrangements he had made to come to me in London for analysis; afterwards he could not be spared from Vienna."[6]

The day after Rank's return Freud informed Ferenczi: "Jones is totally with us, very warm, unfortunately aged, depressed to the point of illness" (Apr. 12). On May 28 Freud told Jones, "Rank is fighting like a lion" for the fund created by Toni Freund, though the Hungarian government was blocking its transfer. On July 28, Freud wrote Jones (in English) from vacation in Bad Gastein, encouraging him to come to Vienna: "As for business apply to Rank, who is bound to wait for his babe there. He is doing all the work, performing the possible and the impossible alike, I dare say, you know him for what he is, the truest, most reliable, most charming of helpers, the column, which is bearing the edifice. I have given him full power to decide as I recognize his superiority in managing these intricate practical matters." Jones replied on August 7, "I am fully in accord with your opinion of Rank, and have boundless admiration both for his capacity and his character. We are in regular communication over our mutual affairs, and are both confident about them in spite of the difficulties."

Jones planned to go to Basel for a week with Sachs, then to Vienna for a week with Rank; Freud was going to Hamburg to see Sophie but hoped Jones could stay long enough for a reunion after five years apart. They met in Vienna in September. There Jones met Katharina Jokl and married her a few days later. "Kitty," a schoolmate of Sophie Freud Halberstadt, was Jewish and an economics graduate.

Viktor Tausk: Shooting Star

A journalist, lawyer, and magistrate who became a physician, psychiatrist, and analyst, Viktor Tausk was born in Slovakia in 1879. The divorced father of two sons, he joined the Vienna Psychoanalytic Society in 1909, participating actively. Brilliant and multitalented—he wrote poetry and plays, acted, translated, played the violin—Tausk became intimate with Lou Andreas, 16 years older than he, known for her closeness to Nietzsche and Rilke. Freud, her analyst and teacher, may have been jealous of their relationship. In her *Journal* Lou comments about Tausk—Freud's "most outstanding" follower, and Rank, obedient, less colorful. Tausk was handsome, dashing, extroverted.

A military psychiatrist during the war, he sought personal analysis with Freud in 1919. Uncomfortable with Tausk, Freud refused, recommending instead neophyte analyst Helene Deutsch, a psychiatrist then in analysis with Freud. An attractive woman with a new baby, Helene and her husband, Felix, were friends of both Tausk and the Ranks; Helene and Otto were both 35, five years younger than Viktor.

Tausk was a fluent, spontaneous theorist while Freud had to pace himself, mistrusting Tausk's virtuosity. Priority for ideas and rivalry were ever present. Tausk might use the analysis to appropriate ideas still in the formative stage. Perhaps Tausk accepted Helene thinking that she would be more conduit than buffer. Indeed, much of her analysis with Freud was spent on Tausk. After three months, Freud told Deutsch to stop. Three months later, on July 3, Tausk shot himself. Newly engaged to a woman he knew he should not marry, barely solvent, depressed by the war, he could not go on despite his love for his sons and his sister. He left a farewell note to Freud that was respectful, gracious, absolving. So was the obituary Freud wrote—unlike some informal remarks to confidants.

On July 6 Freud wrote Abraham about vacation plans for a month beginning July 15: Martha, recovering from influenza, would go to a sanitarium while Freud took his holiday with Minna in (Bad) Gastein; Anna and Margarethe Rie—also in analysis with Freud—went elsewhere. Rank would stay in Vienna: "He is expecting to become a father soon." Freud continues, "Tausk shot himself a few days ago. You remember his behavior at the Congress. He was weighed down by his past and by the recent experiences of the war; he should have been married this week, but could not struggle on any longer. Despite his outstanding talents, he was of no use to us." Freud wrote similarly to Lou, and in reply she called Tausk a "frenzied soul with a tender heart" who called himself "an unhappy wretch." She agreed that he was a threat.[7]

Unlike Rank, Tausk was a son with lethal potential; to rid himself of the Oedipal threat Freud enlisted Helene Deutsch for Jocasta's role, but Tausk continued to threaten. Freud rarely refers to counter-transference, which he first wrote about in 1910: "the patient's influence on the [analyst's] unconscious feelings."[8] In the Tausk-Deutsch triangle with himself Freud presumed to make such influence conscious and neutralize its untoward effects. Yet in the lecture quoted in the epigraph to this chapter, Freud concluded, "The damaging results attributed to psychoanalysis are restricted essentially to passing manifestations of increased conflict if an analysis is clumsily carried out or if it is broken off in the middle."

As Toni Freund neared death, Freud's sadness was compounded with frustration at the collapse of major funding. Freud appointed psychiatrist Max Eitingon to the Committee, to replace Freund.

Thanatos, Eros, and Oedipus

Freud's *Beyond the Pleasure Principle* (*Jenzeits des Lust-Prinzips,* 1920) introduces death and aggression as drives contending with sex—a major change in his libido theory. Influenced by the war, it invokes biology as the underlying impulse toward death. Freud addresses recurrent nightmares, especially those of returning veterans, acknowledging that not all dreams are pleasure-seeking wish fulfillments. Following—but not acknowledging—Simmel and Ferenczi in *War Neuroses* (1919), Freud theorizes that anxiety dreams are efforts at mastery of trauma and loss through repetition. He finds an analogy in the *fort-da* game of his grandson, who seemed to handle mother's absence by acting out a lost-and-found ritual.[9] Biology supports psychology on the principle that things in nature do not happen by accident. Extrapolating to human psychology Freud claimed that mistakes are not random but result from unconscious wishes—forces to be understood and reckoned with. Since all living things die, he reasons, there must be a biological urge, a death drive—coexisting with the libido [Latin, "desire," "lust"], the life drive.

Combining art and biology, Freud created a new psychology of individual and social life that would have scientific credibility beyond the academic, narrow experiments in laboratories, classrooms, and hospitals. Having used the Oedipus myth to confirm unconscious motivation with regard to sex and aggression he now added biological drive to the latter.

Sophocles' *Oedipus* develops as a one-day judicial inquiry with witnesses. A plague rages in Thebes. Messengers return with the oracle's word: the plague would end only when the murderer of Laius is found and banished. An inquiry begins. The legend is summed up by Freud in *The Interpretation of Dreams* and here, with slight elaboration, by Rank in *The Incest Theme*:

Oedipus, son of Laius, King of Thebes and of his wife, Jocasta, was exposed immediately after birth because an oracle had revealed to his father, eager for offspring, that he was destined to be killed by his son. The infant, once exposed, is rescued by shepherds and grows up as a prince in another court, until, unsure of his origin, he consults the oracle and is advised to avoid his homeland lest he become his father's murderer and his mother's husband. Upon leaving his new home, he encounters King Laius, his unrecognized father, and kills him. Then he arrives in Thebes, solves the riddle of the Sphinx that is bringing doom to the city, and is rewarded by the Thebans as liberator: he is made king and receives the hand of his mother, Jocasta, in marriage. For a long time he reigns peacefully and with honor, and he has two sons and two daughters by his mother.[10]

Freud compares the "process of revealing" in the play to a psychoanalysis. He describes the traditional view of the "tragedy of destiny," where the effect "is said to lie in the contrast between the supreme will of the gods and the vain attempts of mankind to escape the evil that threatens them." The lesson for the observer is submission to "divine will and realization of his own impotence." Freud proposes that our interest in the play, and its power to move us, lies in an emotional connection: "It is the fate of all of us, perhaps, to direct our first sexual impulse towards our mother and our first hatred and murderous wish against our father. Our dreams convince us that that is so. King Oedipus . . . merely shows us the fulfillment of our own childhood wishes."

A footnote to the fourth (1914) edition of *The Interpretation of Dreams* says this "indication of the childhood impulses toward incest" has brought more criticism and denial than any other psychoanalytic proposition. In the fifth (1919) edition Freud adds that the Oedipus complex "throws a light of undreamt importance on the history of the human race and the evolution of religion and morality," with a reference to *Totem and Taboo*, part 4. In that work the overthrow of the patriarch by the sons led the latter to civilized restraint due to guilt for their deed. Notably, Freud addressed only the unconscious hostility of son toward father and its sexual source. He ignores the conscious, lethal hostility of fearful, cowardly Laius toward the son; he ignores the filial love for adoptive father Polybus by Oedipus. The actions of Laius, who sacrificed an innocent baby to save himself, and of Oedipus, who unselfishly leaves his beloved parents to avoid harming them, are not morally or psychologically equivalent. Many years later psychoanalyst Lili Peller urged us to change the adjectives and our thinking: instead of "real" and "adoptive" parents, we should consider them "birth" and "real" parents—an insight beyond that of Freud the biologist.[11]

Freud labored to extract the scientific truth from imaginative literature, folklore, and primitive customs. Oedipal patricide happened. It was not conscious, but was a fixture of man's unconscious. In myths, fate was divinely ordained and inexorable. For Freud—atheist and scientist—fate expresses a biological imperative. Integrating myth and biology, Freud formulates a universal family drama. The horror felt watching Oedipus comes from our unconscious wishes. Psychoanalysis makes us face up to them. Exoneration requires acknowledgment, acceptance, transcendence. What daughters go through is not so clear. We are unconsciously, biologically driven, our conscious will a negligible factor.

Otto Rank: Deputy and Family Man

Unlike Tausk, Rank was no threat, as Freud and Lou agreed in 1913. Smart, likable, diligent, and discreet, Rank was admired and sometimes envied for his scholarly output, managerial skill, and closeness to Freud. The Ranks' spacious apartment next to the Verlag office served as a place for social events that Tola hosted for Freud, including a visit from Lou. Upstairs lived Rank's divorced mother and his brother. Soon a favorite of Freud's, Tola was credited for an idea in his paper "The Uncanny." She studied psychoanalysis and became a child analyst like Anna, who was just a year older; they worked together in the Verlag. When daughter Helene was born on August 23, 1919, Tola was 23, Otto 35. Helene became Freud's surrogate granddaughter, since he then had only grandsons.

It was a hard year in Hungary. Fearing an invasion by surrounding armies (Romanian, Czech) supported by the victorious Triple Entente (UK, France, Russia), the Károlyi government resigned, giving over power to the Communists under Béla Kun. His Red Army regime lasted only 100 days, swept out by Miklós Horthy, the rightist admiral whose "white terror" brutally suppressed the "reds." With the Treaty of Versailles, Hungary lost almost two-thirds of its territory, leaving the population sympathetic to fascism. Ferenczi's professorship was revoked, even his membership in the medical society (along with that of 21 others) because of "Bolshevik" affiliation. Psychoanalysis faded into the background. There were food shortages, and no meat. Toni, being treated near Vienna, was failing and demanded eventual euthanasia. Freud wrote: "He scolds and complains a lot, cries for morphine, but is very often as tender and witty as ever. Euthanasia is easy if one doesn't want to kill the patient directly."[12]

The Freud-Abraham letters sum up the year. "Rank is really outstandingly competent and keen," Freud said about Verlag developments. "We are delighted to be able to work in our *jardín secret* while the storm lays waste to everything outside" (Feb. 5). Ferenczi yielded the IPA presidency to Jones. Abraham: "Rank sent me his book on myths. His achievements are truly amazing" (Nov. 23). Rank's collected prewar essays were the Verlag's fourth publication, the first being the book on psychiatric casualties of war.

On November 19 Rank traveled—with frustrating delays—to England via Holland for the Verlag and Jones's new Psychoanalytic Press, returning via Berlin and Leipzig on January 2, 1920. "Reik is being declared incompetent by both ladies [Anna and Tola]."[13] Freud wrote Jones that Toni Freund "is dying a slow and painful death" and that Martin Freud had married Ernestine "Esti" Drucker. Articles for *Zeitscrift* were "flowing in from all sides," and "I am nearly helpless and maimed when Rank is away." Freud thanked Jones's "young wife" Kitty (27; he was 40) for her letter of introduction.[14] Jones wrote impatiently about Rank's delay: "His having to wait in Holland is largely his own fault, but one cannot wonder that so much contact with the political atmosphere of Vienna has impaired his contact with the outer world." Loe had been "extraordinarily kind about Rank. She would even have gone to Holland (her homeland) to help him over the tedium of waiting, only that her husband is ill." Freud queried Jones: "In your remarks on Rank I noticed a harshness which reminded me of a similar mood regarding Abraham. You used kinder language even during the war. I hope nothing is wrong between you and ours."[15]

1920. Jones replied on January 16: "You may rest quite assured, as you must be already from talking with Rank, that I have no harsh feeling towards him or Abraham. Some momentary impatience on my part, of no importance, must have produced the impression on you." On January 20 Freud wrote, "Freund died this evening, a heavy loss for all of us, no better man among us. But we must not pity him!" On January 26 Freud wrote again, leaving the worst for last. Regarding Freund's funeral and Jones's dying father: "I wonder when my own turn will come. Yesterday I lived through an experience which makes me wish, it should not last a long time. My daughter Sophie—perhaps you remember her, or am I wrong to recall that your young wife knew her in school days?—died in Hamburg of a rapid *Grippe*-pneumonia, such as are now becoming frequent again in Middle Europe. She was not yet 27, leaves a despondent husband and two boys, the younger a babe of 13 months." Martha wanted to go immediately to Hamburg, but trains were unavailable. "I am deeply distressed and sure of the good feelings of my friends."

Jones commiserated on February 2 and the relationship warmed as Freud reacted to news of Jones's father's passing: "I was about your age when my father died (43) and it revolutionized my soul."[16]

An essay by Havelock Ellis provoked Freud to complain that it contained "the most refined and amiable form of resistance and repudiation calling me a great artist in order to injure the validity of our scientific claims (which is all wrong; I am sure in a few decades my name will be wiped away and our results will last)."[17] The warming of the Freud-Jones relationship appears in their letters in March: "Yours always affectionately" from Jones, "With sincere love to you and your wife," from Freud. Jones visited Vienna for the first week of April. On April 24 he sent thanks from London and asked Freud's help in convincing an "obdurate" Rank to accept a stipend from the English press because his salary, "which never was a big one, has so diminished in buying power as to make his existence very precarious. . . . He absolutely refused." Jones proposed to use part of a modest inheritance from his father to give Rank £50 annually ($140). On May 2 Freud wrote that he got Rank to accept, at least "for this year, 1920." Praising Jones, he adds, "I trust I would have been able to act the same way as you when I had grown wealthy but unfortunately fate has never put me to the trial." Soon afterwards Freud could announce happily that Eitingon made a gift of one million crowns ($5,000) to the fund "and so put an end to our most pungent fears." That enabled a raise for Rank of $60 annually, to almost $3,000.[18]

In the third volume of *Freud*, Jones recalled the ups and downs of the Verlag and his Psychoanalytic Press: "What is certain is that the *Verlag* could not have come into existence at all, or survived for a day, without the truly astounding capacity and energy, both editorial and managerial, with which Rank threw himself into the task. It was four years before he ever got away from Vienna on any sort of holiday, taking with him even then a mass of material to deal with. The five years in which Rank continued at this furious tempo must have been a factor in his subsequent mental breakdown."[19]

This foreshadows Jones's "psychiatric" explanation of Rank's departure from the movement. Freud shared a relevant observation with Ferenczi,

"The Verlag is laboring on 10,000 external difficulties, and Rank, who is as well behaved as ever, does seem to me to be depressed and not properly capable of accomplishment. He is very probably a periodic [manic-depressive]."[20]

A rare glimpse of Rank's private life comes in a letter from Ferenczi to Freud. Rank had written to Freud about Dr. Eugenia Sokolnicka (1884–1934), the Polish analyst who became a member of the VPS. She went to Ferenczi, who wrote about her to Freud. Anorgasmic in sexual relations, "she always indulged in self-gratification. Rank's wedding made her fall unhappily in love with him after the fact, although, where she might still have had an opportunity to do so, she was unable to love him totally." Apparently she and Rank were once romantically involved. Ferenczi tells Freud (June 4) that active therapy—prohibiting masturbation—did not work in this case.

Freud and Minna spent a month from July 30 at Bad Gastein, where he finished *Group Psychology and the Analysis of the Ego* (1921), while Martha went to Goisern with daughter Mathilde's family. Then Freud went via Hamburg (home of widowed son-in-law and two grandsons) to The Hague, for the Sixth IPA Congress, September 8–11. Ferenczi chaired the meeting, where Jones was elected president. There were 62 members, including newcomers Georg Groddeck and Melanie Klein, and 57 guests, including Anna Freud and Beata Rank, who traveled with the Professor and Rank. Frau Rank received Freud's ultimate compliment: "She is like a daughter, not just a student."[21]

Freud's planned trip to England with Anna was foiled by a visa problem, so they toured Holland instead and he returned home via Berlin on September 30.[22] Freud had mostly English-speaking patients and complained, "I now write no letters at all during the week. The six hours of English a day make me so tired that in the evening I am of no use for anything more." Ferenczi's mother was celebrating her eightieth birthday; all nine of her living children were present (three had died). Sándor, who had not seen her in six years, was glad for the reunion. Freud said, "My mother is between 85 and 86, which not infrequently causes me concern. It is incautious to get so old. . . . In March, Martin is expecting a son, the way it should be after wartime." He hoped Ferenczi would accept Rank's invitation to travel to Vienna around Christmas, but finances did not allow it.[23]

Rank began treating a few patients sometime in 1919. By the end of 1920 he had three or four regular hours, which helped his income. Eric Hiller had come from England to help coordinate Verlag and *Journal* publication. The Committee decided to send circular letters (*Rundbriefe*) twice monthly or more. Each site—Vienna (Freud, Rank), Berlin (Abraham, Eitingon, Sachs), London (Jones), and Budapest (Ferenczi)—would send identical letters to the other three.

Jones, a new father, wrote in his first Rundbrief, "Following the fashion of other analysts (Rank, Hitschmann, Flügel, etc), we began with a daughter. The doctor . . . observed that the child's first reaction to this world, before the cord was severed, was to suck her thumb! I wonder if this happens in the womb itself as a preparation for the arousing of oral excitability for the nipple." Rank's Rundbrief closing: "*Last not least* [in English] we express to Jones our hearty congratulations, along the same lines. His allusion to the other analysts who began with daughters is probably to be understood as consoling; all the more remarkable that Jones names only those who also ended with these daughters, and not the other, possibly even more important analysts (of course Freud himself above all) who didn't rest satisfied with the first daughter."[24]

Rank asked Freud (Oct. 16), "I hope the little analytic joke I allowed myself with Jones at the end won't displease you too much."

≈ Chapter 10 ≈

Rising Tension

1921

The Committee hoped to set up a spring meeting around Freud's sixty-fifth birthday, but he was not eager, and the group finally met in September for a ten-day outing in Germany. At Rank's suggestion they adopted the familiar *du* with each other (except Freud): "I already *duze* with Ferenczi, Jones and Sachs, who does so with me and Jones, and as I gather from letters, Ferenczi does with Abraham."[1]

Ferenczi's letter to Freud on January 6 asks support from him and Rank for his patient, Dr. Solkolnicka, who was moving to Paris. Her personality has improved, though "she still feels insulted by Rank's behavior at the Congress." Would they endorse her by letter to the French publisher, Payot, and to Freud's translator there? That would enhance the outcome of her analysis "and take much of the danger out of her lethal [suicidal] intentions." Ten days later Freud gave sour assent: "*We both* don't like her, whereas you evidently have a weakness for the disagreeable person." Freud explained that he declined a spring meeting because it would seem to treat his sixty-fifth birthday as his last! And he was too busy: "I will have foreigners [analysands] who lie in wait for every day, who can't extend themselves, and whom I have to exploit as irreplaceable as long as they are here."

Though in Austrian currency he was a millionaire, Freud actually was poor—with a mere quarter of his prewar worth. He was helping Martin, Oli, and son-in-law Max; he worried about Martha, who, unlike the wife of a civil servant, would have no pension when he died.

Terrible inflation followed the war. The supply of crowns (Kroner) increased from 12 to 147 billion between 1920 and the end of 1921. In 1919, 100 crowns dropped in value from 11 Swiss francs to less than three.[2]

Freud explained to Eitingon—a financial supporter—on January 23: "I'd need to increase Rank's salary by 10,000 K/mo. . . . He's really sacrificing himself, since he can only support himself adequately by offering 3 to 4 hours of analysis daily. I won't presume to take these from him for a salary increase, as he rightly says he gets great stimulation through contact with the mother earth of psychoanalysis." The next day Freud reproached Jones: "I do not agree when you get moody and harass Rank about trifles like misprints, etc. which can nowhere be avoided." He relates excitedly that evidence supports his theory that *Hamlet* was written in conjunction with the death of Shakespeare's father in 1601.[3]

In reply (Feb. 3) concerning Rank, Jones admits that some issues arise, but "I give myself more self-criticism than I do anything on his side." His good feeling for Rank is such that he "cannot imagine any difficulties ever arising important enough to be referred to you." Ferenczi advised Freud (Feb. 7) to have Rank tone down admonitions to Karl Abraham in the Rundbriefe. Abraham wanted to dismiss Hans Liebermann as manager of the Berlin Psychoanalytic society, but Eitingon and Sachs outvoted him; Abraham said he'd resign if the issue came up again. Evidently Rank sided with the majority. These are the first notable strains in the Committee.

To Jones, Freud wrote (Mar. 18) "Rank is as excellent as analyst as in mythology, he could take such patients whom I must decline, even English ones." Rank was treating two English-speaking patients (from Australia and Africa) daily, "and succeeds quite well." Rank needed these, "to keep up his touch with the source of our knowledge." Freud goes on, "I said to Rank your authors should not indulge in mysterious hinting that the solutions, the meaning, is evident, but should condescend to write down what these interpretations are. It is a kind of discretion of which we have no use in analysis." Jones replied, "not so much one of social discretion as the fear most young writers have to write what they think is elementary. . . . It is only assured authorities that dare to be elementary" (Apr. 1).

On April 3 Martin and Esti became parents of Anton Walter Freud, named for Toni Freund.[4]

To Eitingon (May 23) Freud reports giving Rank 1,000 Swiss francs

(100,000 Kr., or $900). Rank's annual salary of 180,000 crowns (about $1,000) was still too little. "It is not easy to work with Jones, and Rank has times when he is not as active as otherwise. He now gives four [analytic] hours daily although I have urged him not to exceed two." They brought 4,000 crowns per day, which equaled 100 marks, or $24 (about $6 per session: probably $4,800 per year for 20 sessions x 40 weeks). Freud also gave Frau Rank 1,000 marks ($240) for her work. In July, Jones reports that the Verlag paid Heller 65,000 marks ($15,470) for the rights to all the psychoanalytic works.[5]

Eitingon managed to visit Freud on his birthday. Before summer vacation, Freud finished *Group Psychology and the Analysis of the Ego*, his major work of the year. The gift of the manuscript to Rank indicates his significant role in its development. According to the Jones biography and several letters, Freud was increasingly focused on the prospect of aging and death. He left Vienna for Bad Gastein with Minna on July 15 while Martha and daughter Anna went to Aussee. They all met at Seefeld on August 14 and spent another month; Freud had several visitors, including Ferenczi, and, for the first time since before the war, A. A. Brill, from New York.

In the next letter, Rank refers to Freud's oldest daughter, Mathilde, then 34, and her husband, Robert Hollitscher. Childless after a miscarriage, she took charge of Heinele after Sophie's death.

Wien I, Grünangergasse 3–5 ¶July 25, 1921

Lieber Herr Professor,

Many thanks for your friendly card, promising all good for your recovery. Hopefully things will continue to go as they've begun. Here, vacation mood comes only gradually. We have a psychoanalytic visitor at least weekly—the latest an enjoyable stopover with Sachs, with whom we plan a return visit in Semmering on Wednesday (which serves well as a Sunday). We hope this will be a chance to see the Hollitschers as well.

Thus far only the two Rundbriefe enclosed have come, about which I have no particular comment; Jones's hasn't arrived. If it does in the next few days, I'll send it so we can deal with it on August 1.

I've received and read the Abraham paper that he mentioned; since it's the Congress piece known to you, I won't send it. Besides, I find it beneath the classical heights one expects from A. It gives the impression of being patched together (a defect of many Congress presentations!). Then I read Jones's awkward artifice, presented like a schoolboy, the doubtless correct point of view not sharply elaborated (I didn't hear the presentation!). But anyway, worthy enough. This unclear elaboration seems to be a defect of most psychoanalytic papers now that address mono-symptomatic neuroses, e.g. Feldmann's paper on blushing (disregarding the dismal German) shows obscurity that can be penetrated only by a reader who already knows more than the author. (In this respect Jones's paper is much superior pedagogically, because it's more primitive!) I enclose two shorter manuscripts that came: one worthless, Kolner's interesting but crazy.

I'm constantly busy with two issues of the Zeitschrift; they progress slowly. By contrast, the Italian edition of Three Essays will be ready soon. You'll get corrections directly from the Verlag (as will Ferenczi and Bernfeld); if you have a comment, please send it with the specific page to the Verlag or to me. The 4th and 5th volumes [Freud, Neurosenlehre (Collected Papers)] are being printed by Prochaska. In the new 4th volume won't we need to say that the major analysis is absent and appears in the 5th? And should this be a publisher's note, or would you write a few words as preface?

Otherwise, there's not much to report about the Press, except that it gives me more and more to worry about. Things with Harz won't last forever, of course, and then we'll be without locus and staff there. Most important, it's so clear that the Verlag suffers from too much improvisation. Although no business operation can begin without space and personnel, we actually started from the tip of the pyramid and now hang in mid-air. Something has to happen this fall, the more so since we may have to do some things elsewhere. What will happen, I don't know. In any case, we must talk about this. I do think the Verlag can develop and succeed financially; but now one has to invest a lot. I got Hiller interested in the still due Pound-expenses.

My practice proceeds according to plan; an hour of English a day doesn't make a summer. Sure, I understand more and more, but I sense my speaking abilities are getting proportionately worse and worse. By the way, Mrs. Brierley recently said she wrote you about the Brunswick Psychoanalytic Clinic. On July 15, Miss [Caroline] Newton appeared punctually at my office, and we agreed to begin on October 1, at $5.00 per hour. Incidentally, she immediately asked for one of my books—apparently to find out whether I analyze the way [Leonard] Blumgart does. Anyway, many thanks for the case, which is going to help a lot.

I still haven't found time to work on the 2nd ed. of Myth of the Birth of the Hero [1922]. A few days ago I sent Deuticke the first half, corrected in the winter, to get myself to gulp the second, trickier half! Then I'll look through the material for the book on children, which, beside the regular affairs, will fill the fleeting weeks of summer.

Have you already written to Stärcke? He starts vacation on 29th. Róheim got his prize a few days ago.[6]

With cordial greetings, also to your sister-in-law, and my wife includes herself, and best regards to the Deutsch family. I am, Yours, Rank

Wien I, Grünangergasse 3–5 ¶July 28, 1921

Lieber Herr Professor!

Jones's letter [Rundbrief] was sent to you from Semmering [70 km s. of Vienna] with Sachs' comments added; I'd like to have them as well. Today I found Abraham's letter here. I'd like to answer it on the 1st, if possible. Translation and publishing matters I'll deal with as soon as I know your basic opinion; I believe nothing stands in the way of these translations. From Ossipow, whose address I had to get, no answer yet. The Spaniard paid 130 pesetas (13 10-peseta bills) for Group Psychology and the Analysis of the Ego *and* Beyond the Pleasure Principle. *If I receive no instructions to the contrary, I'll send half to Lissa and Kann.*

Miss Turner, head of the Brunswick nest, recommended to me a new [female] patient for the fall; she asked that I accept her at half fee due to special circumstances. I'll refuse and say that my schedule for fall is already full; perhaps I'll recommend someone else. Levi Bianchini wrote that he hopes to print the Introductory Lectures, *I & II soon (in Naples). From Hermann I received another short paper on the role of similarity in Hume's psychology.*

Yesterday was very beautiful in Semmering, but the excursion made us aware of how much we miss such lovely summer weather here in Mödling. We found your daughter looking very nice, although we're sorry to hear she wasn't feeling well.

With cordial greetings. Yours, Rank

Imago [Mödling (14 km s. of Vienna)] ¶July 30, 1921

Lieber Herr Professor!

Yesterday I got your letter of the 26th (and another with enclosures). I hasten to answer your card of yesterday that came today [all missing]. Let me assure you that your speculations are unfounded. It's just that for me the most important man in the universe, the dispatcher, was on vacation, and coincidentally Harz (who's not here) also had lots to do, so things went slowly. And we had to deal with visitors from Leipzig and then Zurich, since Steckmar and Blumot must have our new books. Storfer is very fine and reliable, and does what he can under the circumstances. And summer slows everything due to vacations. Finally, it was never my intention, nor is it now, to hide anything from Heller. What I wrote about the Verlag was all I can say now, and if that sounds cryptic, the problem is, I don't know how these problems can be solved. On Wednesday I also spoke with Sachs about the Verlag: he spontaneously expressed the same concerns before I could broach these issues. In a word: we can be reassured about things at the moment (all dealt with in the meantime; Storfer was here yesterday), but the near future remains troubling due to space and personnel issues, of course closely tied to finances.

Unfortunately I must share another not so happy matter. A letter from Ferenczi came a few days ago with news of his mother's death, and a hint that his ailment may be more serious. He gave up Tegernsee [Bavarian spa], and hopes to undergo a thorough examination by Dr. [Felix] Deutsch in Vienna (blood, urine, x-ray). He intends to go to Garmisch (unless Dr. Deutsch suggests something else). Ferenczi came to Vienna yesterday; I won't see him until tomorrow, but my wife, who put our Vienna apartment at his disposal, found him not very well. I just heard (by telephone) from Frau Deutsch that his condition is neither trivial nor dangerous: a kidney problem was found, but the tests are incomplete. When I hear more, I'll tell you, of course. The Ferenczis plan to stay in Vienna until Tuesday.

And now to your letter, which I'd like to use in the Rundbrief. I await the foreign Rundbriefe sent to you, along with your comments. I don't think it matters if it's sent out 1–2 days later, since we will have communicated with Ferenczi and Sachs.

In her letter to me, Miss Turner, the head of the Brunswick Clinic, said she hoped she could get in touch with you. She wants to write you soon, and come to Vienna herself! I did not agree to this (letter and answer enclosed).

Several weeks ago I renewed our old exchange agreement with Dr. Schultz, editor of Mitra. *I think that will suffice—or do you also wish to subscribe?*

Something unfortunate may have happened with Dr. [Monroe] Meyer, too. Before we left I wrote Jones, asking Hiller to forward the answer to Dr. A. Then Jones wrote that Meyer should translate the article by Westermann-Holstijn in the festschrift under way, and Hiller told Meyer. Hiller told me yesterday (he was here since I'm not going into Vienna) that Meyer, annoyed, said he'd only translate your works. Jones and Hiller may find this strange, but they don't take Meyer's neurosis seriously enough. I wrote Meyer an apology, mainly because Hiller hadn't asked him to work at the Verlag as I promised: this doubtless caused the irritation. I further promised that I'd write to Jones again, and asked him meanwhile to translate the French articles (vol. 1), since he claims to do this perfectly and since Jones supports publishing these articles in English, too.

Sachs noted—and understood—your hint. I'm glad you're feeling so well; hopefully this will continue. I feel much better since I gave up the illusion of that pleasant summer weather reaching me here.

With cordial greetings from all of us. Yours, Rank

Writing from Vienna to Freud on August 1, Rank reported that Ferenczi's health problem would require lifestyle changes and might result in an atrophied kidney and that Dr. Deutsch had not confided this to the patient. Regarding the Verlag, Rank continued to worry about space and personnel as well as money. Ferenczi wrote to Freud, "I can't describe to you in how touchingly caring a fashion the Rank and Deutsch families have exerted themselves on my behalf" (Aug. 7).

Mödling, August 6, 1921

Lieber Herr Professor!

Thank you for your letter of 3. August [missing] especially for the kind dedication, which pleased me more than some personal success. In any case, I recognize happily that the larger world, not considerate about your vacation, still encircles you, and I gratefully participate in the attention. In France there seems to be a move afoot that could be significant. The Indian has already been sent a journal prospectus, his book discussed by Jones. Ossipow is prepared to take over the translation of Introductory Lectures; *from the Verlag so far I've heard nothing.*

As for the mutilated passage, there is unfortunately nothing I can do since all editions of Introductory Lectures *are of course printed from plates; I don't understand the passage myself. Perhaps you can reconstruct it after all.*

So, now that business is taken care of I go eagerly to my Goethe interpretation, which in a way makes sense of the mystery of this much-talented writer. That is, it makes comprehensible not only his writing of literature (feminine orientation), but also his other talents, in terms of identification—just as we understood the varied aspects of neurosis in terms of identification. Furthermore, the entire interpretation is available for all to see (if one knows), in the following passage [Xenien 6]:

From Father I have my stature,	*(collector, pedant, etc.;*
And the serious view of life;	*identification with father)*
From Mama a happy nature,	*(= writer; identification with*
And joy in telling tales.[7]	*Mother)*

You ask, incontrovertible? It almost seems so, if one takes into account the poet's feminine, even popular, nature (long hair, flashy clothes). I'm pleased to find things as I suggested in the Incest *book: the incest complex not only constitutes great material for the writer, but also a main source of his productive energy ("giving birth to works," i.e. book-children of the father, of course).*

I do think the gist of my last comments on totemism offers much to explore; I haven't put it clearly. Maybe we can discuss this. I made some notes (Deuticke has already printed half of the 2nd edition of Myth*).*

Two more fruits of reading may interest you: the enclosed interpretation of a legend, which you'll want to read for its geographic relevance. And in the same issue of L.E. I found a quotation from Thomas Mann's drama Fiorenza *[1919]. "Is then the one who is strong a hero?!—No, he who is weak, yet has such passionate spirit that he wins the crown anyhow: he is a hero." Nicely suggests that the hero essentially is a poet (liar).*

Finally, two news items. 1) Reik writes from Semmering that he's staying there on doctor's advice (lung catarrh). Do you know about this? 2) A gentleman from Barmen [Germany] asks for an analyst in Copenhagen! I don't know of anyone. The one who once sent us an article, whose name I forgot, is certainly not a real analyst.

I hope you have long since overcome the passing illness that is now raging in our house and has also had me in its grip for a week.

With cordial greetings to you and your sister-in-law from both of us. Yours, Rank

Rank's *Incest* book has many references to Goethe, including a chapter, "Goethe's Love for His Sister," but he probably found the "Xenien" lines later. They are from a set of epigrams by Goethe and Schiller, some sharply satirical; this one comes from the milder group (*Zahm,* "tame").

Prof. Dr. Freud Bad Gastein ¶August 10, 1921 [first Freud letter since 1916]
Lieber Doktor

Our beautiful summer stay here will soon end; Sunday the 14th we depart and on the 15th begin our stay in Seefeld Spa (Tirol). My unwellness is in fact long gone, as I hope is true for your family. The world has left us alone in recent days; I have nothing to enclose. Mrs. Riviere wants to come for analysis in January. [Édouard] Claparède sent a tender card in answer to my thanks—that's all. I hope I've fixed the spoiled text, though I was bewildered and have a growing dislike of stereotypography. The paper on occultism is done; I'd have no time to do it now. Van Emden and his wife are here, and my niece, Lucie Wiender, with her two boys, eight at table, gregarious life.

It's still too hot to walk. Yesterday I accidentally fell right into Heller's arms, who, accompanied by his wife, crept up on me, now gray, fat, and aged. He was all tenderness, bestowing on me promises & pathological symptoms as confirmations of P/A—found me looking 10 yr younger—he was blissful. I was mean enough not to say a word about what could divide us. I knew nothing about Reik. If he is worried, the fund will gladly assist with a big contribution.

I have no objections to your interesting discussions comparing myth and primeval history. It all depends on the fact that in the totem, as in the social contract, the primal facts are retained in negative form; that the parents can be replaced by animals remains a problem, but perhaps that is a foundational given, i.e. needs an explanation from somewhere else entirely.

I enclose the germ of an invasion into your own private territory—an attempt to unveil from a diagram the mystery that is Goethe. This is a reaction to reading the long G-biography by E. Ludwig [1920], which adduces so much human material, but still reveals no clue leading to the poet. The objection made concerning our PA psychographies applies much more seriously to this and all other non-analytic ones. Of course I would be interested in hearing of comments about the notes. You'll easily find the trail leading here from the analysis of the Sandman [in Freud's essay "The Uncanny," 1919]. I'm hoping to arrive at the Seefeld spa on the 19th. Re German visas, I'd want to know when you'll be traveling and when we can send you the passports, as well as relevant details. Also, the dates of our Congress need to be set soon.

The name of my youngest [grandchild] in Berlin is Gabriel. They say he looks a lot like his father [Ernst]. Cordial greetings to you and your wife. Yours, Freud

Wien, August 13, 1921

Lieber Herr Professor!

I thank you for your letter of the 10th and acknowledge receipt of both manuscripts, which I can't read yet since I'm really busy: I take revenge by sending a manuscript that came to the editor, which I got yesterday. I sent it separately; it contained the enclosed letter. I also got another article by Franz Pollak, Prague (in Zeitschrift [Vol. 4] in press he has a paper: "The Cure of a Schizophrenic through Analysis." It contains only the bare facts, but for a psychiatrist this is "solid enough." I think it is acceptable, with some editorial cuts.

Pargot wrote the enclosed outburst; before answering, I'd like your response, though I have no doubt about what to write, namely, this doesn't concern me at all, he has no monopoly, and last, he should have acted faster. Please return the letter. Apropos of

Heller: the Spaniard wrote that he has acquired the rights for volume IV. Do you know this?

Monroe Meyer wrote that he is satisfied, and will translate the French papers, but hopes to get the German later. The Verlag is very grateful for your correction of the spoiled text; otherwise the whole thing would have been long delayed. I don't think the blame lies with the plates: we had the plates corrected before our edition, but apparently overlooked this passage. And now to the new edition of volume 4, without the long case history; in our opinion, the omission should be mentioned in the book, perhaps after the table of contents, etc., unless you wish to write a preface. Concerning the article "On the Prehistory of Analytic Technique," Storfer pointed out to you that it's written in the 3rd person; you made no response; was that intentional?

Jones writes that he wants to discuss the English editions with me (sequence, volumes, etc.). Hiller left yesterday for vacation in the Salzkammergut, and it immediately began to rain! Poor guy!

As for me, on a free Wednesday recently I did the major revision of Hero Myth. I was amazed at how nicely our previous knowledge (prehistory) can simply be appended to it. Of course a few new problems came up that can be dealt with later. But I'd like to discuss one with you now. In the hero myth, why is the truly totemistic (protective) role associated only with the mother (infant), whereas totemism is mainly a father problem? The tendency of the myth—letting the old, primal father live again and setting up the mother to protect it [child] from him—plays a major role; but it can't be the whole story. Behind this the question seems to arise: how can humans replace the parents (the father) with an animal (or plant!) in the first place? Maybe this comes just from the mother (maternal animal) and the pact with father would be: "If you were like mother, you would spare me, and I would respect you." It is perhaps a feminine role associated with father, as shown, e.g., by the myths of Zeus, who carries (protects) Dionysis in his thigh and Athena in his head, and the myth of Kronos, who carries his children in his belly (like the mother). Of course, the other side should not be overlooked. That the primal father who swallows his offspring compares with a predatory animal. And it's likely no coincidence that, in the pact with the father, swallowing up (the sacrifice) has its place (behind all of which again is the primitive/infantile sexual theory of eating). I hope I've expressed myself clearly, and would like to know at least whether you see a problem there too, so that one can get the meaning of the myth. This time I have, as it were, allowed myself to follow the myth itself, rather than adducing knowledge gained from elsewhere, for I have seen how faithfully the myth has preserved the old circumstances.

Next, another brief scholarly contribution. Abraham sent me his essay on father *rescue and asked for comments; since I'd like to hear your opinion, as would Abraham, I enclose a copy I made for myself. I must admit being irritated for a moment that an analyst like Abraham could fail to recognize analytical problems in such a way; I only hope this irritation doesn't show in my letter. Of course I know very well this doesn't solve the problem; I just wanted to suggest the problem itself (of course, fear of retribution also plays a role in the dynamic understanding of the rescue fantasy; indeed perhaps it represents the point of transition from the son into the father role— the point where the meaning of patricide can be transformed into rescuing father, etc.).*

Finally, the practical question of the German visas. In connection with his departure, I asked [Walter] Schmideberg to enquire in the German consulate; based on that information, I'd suggest the following as simplest and safest. You should send your passport (or passports) with enclosed, completed form, and a photograph, to the German Passport Office, Rotenturmstrasse 19, Vienna I, certified, with accompanying letter in which very briefly, without detailed reasons, you request certification of your passport and certified return to your current address. For trips of up to 4 weeks, no entry permit is required; one gets the visa automatically. This is not only simplest, but also the correct way postulated by the Passport Office. Getting involved would create difficulties for me, as it did last year, since they only give the visa to the passport holder. That's reliable, and if you start two weeks before departure, there will be time. Of course I'd be happy to undertake any steps you might desire, and you know it's not for personal convenience that I make this suggestion. This is prescribed by the Passport Office, and I think it's best.

About our meeting, I've urged Abraham, as well as Sachs, who was here yesterday while traveling through, and who will be in Berlin on Monday.

The Rundbrief for the first was written by you and me only; nothing from Jones and Abraham! I had news from Ferenczi that he's better. I've heard nothing more from Reik; I'm writing him today.

Now, last not least [English], our hearty congratulations on the new grandchild— to you and your dear wife, who just sent our little one such a nice gift. Hopefully it will be possible to see little Gabriel in Berlin [born to Ernst and Lucy, July 31].

I hope to hear of your arrival in Seefeld. Please convey to your family our cordial greetings and best wishes (especially for weather).

I'll permit myself to enclose a few lines for your daughter. Cordially yours, Rank

Rank seems confident as theorist and manager. He presents a major theoretical question; Freud's answer, if sent, is missing. Rank just finished revising *Myth of the Birth of the Hero* (2d ed., 1922). The first edition, 1909, preceded

Freud's *Totem and Taboo,* now integrated. Rank develops the material with a greater role for mother in nurturance, and constructive rebellion by the son in lieu of patricide. At 37, father of a 2-year-old, Rank shows more independence from Freud.

In *Totem and Taboo* Freud described the path from primeval horde—a strong old male, several females—to small group cohesion and solidarity: social organization. The sons, expelled by the patriarch at their sexual maturity, banded together to kill him. The young assassins then regulated their society because of guilt and the need for cooperation. This avoided mutual destruction in pursuit of the females, who become sexually untouchable within the extended family or tribe. The unifying totem symbol protects, and is protected by, group members and descendents. The second unifying principle of totemism is sexual exogamy: marriage outside the family or tribe.

In the final chapter of his revised *Hero,* Rank describes father-son and fraternal hostility as "competition for the tender devotion and love of the mother." The erotic relation of Oedipus and Jocasta is downplayed in most hero birth myths, which focus on infanticide and patricide. In these myths a "step-motherly" figure, often an animal, cares for and sometimes nurses the child. The hero, whose birth and survival occur against great odds, comes to see father as inimical and feels he owes nothing to his sire. Mother protects the child, as when she takes Zeus to a cave and the goat nurses him. "Thus the mother returns in the hero myth as a protective, nourishing totem animal, while the old, pre-totemistic, primeval father, with all his primitive characteristics, lives on in the sire." The exposure myth, for example, the story of Oedipus, symbolizes birth but also contains the cruel act of the primal father and his wish—expressed "through the oracle"—that the child had never been born. Citing a 1918 article by F-J. Nejmark, Rank concludes: "Thus revolution against every form of tyranny ultimately felt to be oppressive is in the end a revolt against paternal power."

A letter from Rank to Freud on August 18 suggests that Eitingon is the logical choice to succeed "poor Reik" as partner in the Verlag. On August 25 in a Rundbrief, Rank mentions a visit from Smith Ely Jelliffe, American psychiatrist and co-editor of the *Journal of Nervous and Mental Disease:* "He acted very sincere, tried to get chummy, but on the next day he was seen by the Professor in Stekel's company. The Professor considers him to be a dangerous, unscrupulous American." Freud mistrusted Jelliffe and his co-editor W. A. White because of their links to Carl Jung.[8]

Imago Mödling, August 25, 1921

Lieber Herr Professor!

Thank you for the three letters of the 16th, 18th, and 21st [missing], the last arriving today with the Rundbrief enclosures (I got all three late as they were addressed to Vienna). I immediately wrote our Rundbrief, enclosed.

News from Brill is very surprising; his coming is perhaps just as crazy as his earlier silence. Anyway, I'm very curious. Maybe he'll go to Berlin too and I can see him. Your account of Jelliffe is very amusing; the Havanas are indeed the best thing about America! I've used your other news freely for the Rundbrief, as you'll see, just adding a bit.

I had already pressed the staff before your complaint; I found the printing-houses are suffering from all the vacations. Typesetting of Ferenczi's book has been delayed, You'll of course get everything that comes. On the other hand, you probably already got the first section of the English Beyond (for possible corrections).

Yesterday I got from Deuticke the first corrections of Myth, *the ending of which I still don't have ready. If you'll permit, I'd like to send you the corrections to look over; for the first half (introductory material) I'll just send page proofs. When the Interpretation [final chapter] is being typeset we'll probably be back in Vienna.*

We're very glad to hear that you're feeling so well in Seefeld, and hope that things go well for your wife and daughter.

> *With cordial greetings—to family as well—from both of us. Yours, Rank*

Wien August 29, 1921

Lieber Herr Professor!

Many thanks for your kind lines, which held such good news about your stay and your state of health. Unfortunately, I can respond only with negative comments in this regard. For 2–3 weeks I've felt physically unwell and suffer extreme fatigue, which is certainly not normal. And I have heavy worries about the Verlag, so relevant just now since the situation with Harz has intensified and he wants the premises vacated in September. I wrote him that I must travel in September; I tried to delay it until October, but don't know how things will end up, even less how the problems might resolve. If he remains adamant, I don't know whether I'll be able to stick to my current travel plans (Sept. 13 departure).

Fortunately the one analysis, all-English, ends tomorrow, so I'll reschedule the other (ends mid-Sept.) to an hour in the evening and can spend the day in Vienna and try to bring some order into the Verlag situation.

Please send the first section of the English Beyond *back to Hiller (Weissgärber-länder 44–46); he's waiting for your corrections. Hiller will take care of the Sanskrit corrections for the English edition. Unfortunately, I've already returned my galley proofs—there were too many trouble spots: often the typesetter didn't put insertions and additions in the right place. So, after all, I'd just like to show you the 2nd corrections after I've checked them and find nothing wrong so you're spared from corrections for a while. Searching for typographical errors can never compete with searching for mushrooms [Freud's passion]!*

Cordial greetings to you and your dear family. Yours, Rank

A letter of September 8 from Rank thanks Freud for "comforting lines that I'll certainly take to heart" and dwells on the problem of finding office space. He refers to Freud's letter of August 31 and card of September 5 (missing). Rank says he'll travel directly to the Committee meeting (Hildesheim), as he is unable to make anticipated stops in Berlin and Leipzig. Ferenczi (from Groddeck's sanatorium in Germany, to Freud, September 9) was annoyed that Rank's plan changed: Tola was not coming. Therefore Gizella went back to Vienna and Jones's wife to London. "If we had known that, we would have organized ourselves that way in the first place."

Ferenczi was asserting himself more. When Freud reported excitedly about the first contact from Georg Groddeck in 1917, Ferenczi was skeptical. Publication of Groddeck's somewhat ribald *Soul Seeker* (1920) brought a protest from the Swiss Society about the Verlag's editorial judgment; Rank and Freud wrote a 10-page letter defending the book. However, as Freud's enthusiasm waned toward the psychosomatic specialist, Ferenczi's grew. Groddeck dubbed himself "wild analyst" at the Hague Congress, and the name stuck. Before the Committee outing, Ferenczi visited Groddeck for somatic as well as intellectual benefits. The two were close in age; Ferenczi established a more egalitarian relationship with Groddeck than he had with Freud, who "was too big for me, too much of a father." Ferenczi resented Freud's dismissal of Groddeck but failed to change it.[9]

The Committee—minus Rank, who came later—met Freud in Berlin on September 20, then went to the Harz Mountains for a 10-day tour led by Abraham. Jones later recalled that at one mountain vista Freud tested the members for fear of heights by having us "lean forward against the rail with our hands behind our backs and our feet well back, and then suddenly to imagine that it was not there." Each passed the test; "I naturally asked Freud if he had ever suffered from that particular fear. He said he had as a young man, but had conquered it by will power. I remarked it was not a very analytic way of dealing with it, but it was of course long before the days of psychoanalysis."[10] Freud's overall theory hardly ever mentions will, which, with thinking and feeling, constituted the nineteenth-century "faculty" theory of mind.

Jones's disparagement of will is telling. He had just rejected a paper on Bergson and Freud because the author wrote about similarity, not difference. He wrote Freud, "I fear that your Life Instinct in *Jenseits* will lead to your being claimed an adherent of self-creative evolution and vitalism; it will be said that you have found out the error of materialistic determinism. But you are proof by now against misunderstandings, and can also rely on us to correct them for you."[11]

In October Freud's caseload was dominated by American and English analysands. The former, six M.D.s, were Albert Polon, Clarence Obendorf, Abram Kardiner, Leonard Blumgart, Monroe Meyer, and Horace Frink (Freud's ill-fated favorite); the Brits, translators referred by Jones, were Joan Riviere and the Stracheys, James and Alix. Freud routinely had six sessions per week with a maximum of nine daily clients—none on Sunday. Having forgotten a tenth commitment, he asked the Americans if one would accept analysis by Otto Rank at half price. None would. The six spent an anxious night: would Freud draw lots? Send someone away? The next day Freud happily declared a solution from Anna, "a mathematical genius," who reasoned that 6 x 5 = 5 x 6: if each one gave up an hour, all six could have Freud. They agreed, and the standard five-session week was born. Besides analysis, the visitors attended lectures by the Viennese training establishment; Freud told Jones that Rank's lectures (presumably in English) had "impressed all of them immensely." The training roster grew in the coming months with guest speakers, including Abraham, Ferenczi, Roheim, and Sachs.[12]

The year had begun with Freud resisting the celebration of 65 years. Eitingon, visiting him on May 6, presented the gift of a bust by David Königsberger. Freud called it "a ghostly threatening bronze doppelganger," which he thought Eitingon had ordered for himself, "otherwise I wouldn't have sat for it last year." In March Freud had felt "a step toward really getting old. Since then the thought of death never leaves me at all, and sometimes I have the feeling that seven organs are vying with one another to make an end of my life."[13] At year's end he wrote Ernst and Lucie: "I never realized that the older one grows the more there is to do. The idea of peaceful old age seems as much a legend as that of happy youth. Much of my time is taken up with refusals and information to all corners of the world; everyone wants to be analyzed by me, yet not one patient is leaving before the end of February." To Jones: "The Americans are now doing much better, they may be good for something."[14]

Chapter 11

Favorite Son

January to July 1922

The hero claims to have acted alone in accomplishing the deed [patricide]
which certainly the horde as a whole would have ventured upon.
But, as Rank has observed, fairy tales have preserved clear traces of the facts
that were disavowed. . . .
The poet [myth maker] who had taken this step and had in this way
set himself free from the group in his imagination, is nevertheless able
(as Rank has further observed) to find his way back to it in reality.
For he goes and relates to the group his hero's deeds, which he has invented.
At bottom this hero is no one but himself. Thus he lowers himself to the
level of reality, and raises his hearers to the level of imagination.
—Freud, *Group Psychology,* Postscript B

The lines above endorse Rank's concept of the creative type: poet as hero. Freud presented the manuscript of *Group Psychology* to Rank, in gratitude.[1] In 1922 the two seemed closer than ever in thought and feeling as Rank and Ferenczi sought to improve the outcomes of psychoanalytic therapy.

Continuing its academic program of 1921, the Vienna Psychoanalytic Society met on alternate Wednesday evenings, often with foreign analysands and guests; Rank served as vice chairman. Committee members debated issues with increasing acrimony in the Rundbriefe, especially on administrative matters—publications, personnel, and finances. There were conflicts about nonmedical analysts, a novel by Georg Groddeck, telepathy, and homosexuals. Should homosexuals qualify as psychoanalysts based on relevant merits?

Only Rank sided with Freud in favor. Jones was adamantly negative, afraid the movement would be discredited. Even Ferenczi said, "These people are too abnormal."[2]

The seventh edition of Freud's *Interpretation of Dreams* appeared, for which Rank sent congratulations (May 20) "and cordial thanks for informing me of my undeserved and ever increasing involvement in that volume."

In the Freud-Jones relationship, strains involving Rank grew between the Verlag and Psychoanalytic Press. Mrs. Joan Riviere, a translator, therapist, and difficult patient of Jones, had come to Freud for analysis; there were acrimonious letters between the two men. On February 27, Jones announced the birth of son Mervyn that day: "typical *Judenbub* [Jewish lad], but with blond hair and blue eyes."

Freud wrote Jones about Mrs. Riviere on March 23: "In my experience you have not to scratch too deeply the skin of a so called masculine woman to bring her femininity to the light. I am very glad you had no sexual relations with her as your hints made me suspect. To be sure it was a technical error to befriend her before her analysis was brought to a close." Freud also complained that the Press issued its first two volumes late, and in "gorgeous leather-binding. The contents do not correspond to the cover." Reminding Jones that subsistence depended on sale of the English books and journals—the Verlag made no money—he concluded with a wish that "these offsprings of the Anglo-Viennese alliance shall thrive as do the other two you raise in your house." (Jones and his Viennese-Jewish wife now had two children.)

Jones assured Freud that he had no such sexual temptation in twelve years and, should it occur, "I have no doubt at all of my capacity to deal with it." Regarding lateness, Jones praised Rank as "wonderful, better than anyone I know," but Rank's pushing harder "would accelerate matters more than anything else" (Apr. 1). On April 6, having consulted Rank, Freud faults Jones for his "personal interference in every little step of the process" (supervising five editor-translators). Freud wondered why "you should want to do it all alone and suffer yourself to be crushed by the common drudgery of the routine work.... Obviously misprints and arrangement of lines should not be objects of your interest, it means anal gratification as you have pointed out yourself." With Riviere, Strachey, and Rickman now working in England, things should speed up: "You will be served like a master and feel like such.... Pardon my meddling with your affairs but they are ours and mine too, and Rank is too meek to oppose you in these quarters. My broad shoulders as you say are better to lift this weight." Years later Jones recalled, "The innocent allusion to Rank, which evoked what novelists term a mirthless laugh, showed me that Freud never saw the overbearing letters I was constantly receiving from him."[3]

Freud replied on May 11 apologizing for his initial criticism of Jones. "I do not wish to sow discord between you and him, I am willing to drop the matter and to give up my attempts to interfere with the activity of the Press." On June 4 Freud scolded Jones for mistakes made in Mrs. Riviere's analysis; he praised her as translator and editor, and her "uncommon combination of male intelligence and female love for detailed work." She complained that Jones sent edits of her work to the printer without her seeing them first. Regarding referrals from Jones, he will accept Mr. Kyrle, but not his wife, "whom you should send to Rank who is as good an analyst as any man I know." On June 10, Jones defended himself as an administrator and attacked Mrs. R., "whose tone was so full of rude and overbearing superciliousness." Freud pushed back (June 15): "Accuracy and plainness is not in the character of your dealings with people. Slight distortions and evasions, lapses of memory, twisted denials" showed up when Mrs. Riviere "was right and could not be refuted."

July 6, 1922

Lieber Herr Professor,

I write to you a day before my departure, exhausted by a thousand tasks—many completed and a few incomplete—and by the dog-day heat of the last week. You'll find all the Verlag news in the enclosed letter. Please don't misunderstand: I don't expect you to write one article after another. It was only said hypothetically.

On the other hand, I permit myself to disturb you with an article of mine, written during the last week of June, thinking specifically of a Congress presentation, which I've been urged to do from many sides (again today in the circular from Berlin). Disregarding the objective difficulties my topic entails, it's doubtful whether it would ever (possibly abridged!) be appropriate as a Congress presentation. I'd like your advice about this. Of course I'd very much appreciate any objective comments. Perhaps one point, vengeance on the same-sex competitor, will especially interest you: in the last few days, after the article was done, and indeed due to this insight, I was able to effectively eliminate the huge guilt feeling left in the final portion of the analysis of Dr. Blum's [female] friend. Thus, after all, I was able to conclude the analysis well (of course, in reality no decision was made). Please return the article to me in Seefeld as I'd like to discuss it with Ferenczi in August in any case.

Also enclosed are the two Rundbriefe that arrived today: Abraham seems in a good mood (although he didn't yet have my enclosed letter—or because he didn't: perhaps it came out less eloquently than I wished). Jones' charming/ironic comment about me to Abraham is apparently a reflex of his current orientation to you. But you are apparently so far removed now from all these petty details that I must again ask you to pardon me for bothering you with my article.

With best regards to your sister-in-law and cordial greetings to you. Yours, Rank

Prof. Dr. Freud Bad Gastein Wien, IX Berggasse 19 ¶July 8, 1922
Lieber Herr Doktor!

I'm sorry that so soon after you've begun vacation I must tug on the cord—not very long in any case—that ties you to your profession. I'm obliged to you for everything you've sent—the official letter as well as the private one. I feel I should apologize for Abraham's and Jones's little unkindnesses, for they were actually reactions applying to me, deflected to you. In themselves, I find them very unfair. Indeed, I remember everything you have written, and after working with you for about 15 years I can attest that you are not among those who need to vent their moods on their friends. I certainly hope you'll laugh about this, and that they, fully understanding the motivational context, will overlook any bad habits in their friends.

I'm doing exactly what you think impossible, writing one article after another since it's impossible to write several simultaneously. The first two, on the interpretation of dreams and on neurotic mechanisms, are outlined, the first half-written. Only one worry: the vacation may not last long enough to get everything done. Time passes so fast; one week gone, it's a pity about each day spent, they are so preciously peaceful, free and happy, and with heavenly air, the water, Dutch cigars, and good food—everything as idyllic as can be in the hell that is Central Europe.

When I finish this letter I'll go to the square to get a large envelope in which to put some items for you, including the short afterword for Little Hans, which you need. I'll then take a break from productive work to write the addendum to [Fanny] Lowtzky's essay and read your ms. I hope the second task will lift an old burden from me.

I'm never entirely sure if I did the right thing at the time, holding you back from the study of medicine. I believe on the whole I was right; thinking of my boredom during medical studies, I'm more certain, but when I see you by right firmly in the saddle of the analyst, my own responsibility falls away.

By the way, don't you think I'll achieve something special during vacation? The angler throws out his net, sometimes catching a fat carp, often only a few little whitefish.

Give my cordial greetings to the entire colony, but especially to your wife and daughter. Enjoy the vacation and the freedom to work, though they are not without conditions....F

Rank's manuscript referred to in the next letter was "Psychological Potency," published as a chapter in *Sexualität und Schuldgefühl* (*Sexuality and Guilt*) along with "Perversion and Neurosis" (1926). Rank was also working on his "dream book," *Eine Neurosenanalyse in Träumen* (*An Analysis of Neuroses in Dreams*) (1924), and collaborating with Ferenczi on *The Development of Psychoanalysis* (1923), which would rock the Committee.

Prof. Dr. Freud Bad Gastein Wien, IX Berggasse 19 ¶July 10, 1922

Lieber Herr Doktor,

Yesterday I read your whole manuscript. As you know, I don't like to judge the productions of my closest friends and colleagues because I don't want, through my criticism, to restrict their freedom, and because I only assimilate and master new information slowly. With your essay I'll make an exception, since you directly ask and since it is your first purely analytic work.

I don't think it's appropriate for presentation at the Congress. What a Congress lecture needs is little new, and that very clear. Your manuscript is very rich, not so transparent and lacks certain didactic considerations. It doesn't assume an impartial, naïve reader with limited receptive capacity. It would be impressive, but confusing. Apart from this I'd criticize it for mixing in and mentioning in passing, as if well known, important material that deserves detailed special treatment. This includes the discussion of the mechanism of healing through identification—nearly lost in the material; the establishment of a too-far-reaching identification, which is quite correct, but fails to remain within the bounds of desirable identification; the excellent recognition of affect gratification through the wrong object (highly characteristic for unconscious work, cf. the anecdote about the tailor who is to be hanged for the crime of the smith); the discussion of multiple identification in formal action, which is not very clear; the discussion of masculine protest, etc. Although the material is very valuable, the piece lacks inner structure that would allow the reader to grasp the whole.

So I think the work should be rewritten much more broadly, comfortably, and didactically, and that it would be better for you to toss the Congress a lighter morsel. I do not need to say that had the work been written by another person I would simply have declared it very good and valuable. Well, what shall I do with the manuscript?

I must regretfully accept the fact that we've now completed one third of our stay at Gastein. At least the essay on meaning will be finished today.

Cordial greetings. Yours, Freud

Prof. Dr. Freud Wien, IX Berggasse 19 ¶July 11, 1922

Lieber Herr Doktor,

You have the right to complain that I never leave you in peace. Today's reason is the following: I'll read Lowtzky's essay and write an editorial comment in an afterword. This isn't an easy decision. It'd be nice to delay it until I've read Flournoy's Spirits and Mediums, *which I brought along. While reading it, I'd probably arrive at a certain orientation. Can this be done now?*

Would this totally disrupt your plans for No. 3? [International Journal of Psychoanalysis] *Could you use something else for No. 3, e.g. my now completed comments on the theory and practice of dream interpretation? A 1–2 week delay would not suffice. I'd like time for thought, and Flournoy's book is thick. Maybe we could put L.'s essay in No. 3 and promise in a note an editorial for the next issue?*

I await your kind decision. Things still go well here. Prices are rising. The meal that cost 4500 on July 1 is now 6000!

Cordially yours, Freud

Rank had agreed in June to collaborate with Lou Andreas-Salomé and Anna Freud on a *Kinderbuch*, about sexual knowledge of young children. On July 13 Lou wrote him to say the project was not feasible. Instead of a compendium of Freud's relevant findings for those familiar with the subject, the book was to be for a general audience, so a different approach was needed. The amount of work would be too great, and she worried about publishing examples obtained from patients and parents. "Dear Dr. Rank, don't be angry with me!" She thanked him for his kind words on her acceptance into the VPS.

Seefeld Internationale Psychoanalytische Verlag ¶July 14, 1922

Lieber Herr Professor!

I must thank you for three letters and apologize for not answering the last one, with its pressing question; I spent all yesterday in Garmisch visiting my mother-in-law at the spa.

So I'll be quick to catch up with undone tasks. Of course Lowtzky's essay can wait until issue no. 4—all the more if we substitute an article of yours. I'd like not to separate the essay from the comments by several months. As for your work on dreams—though I don't know what's in it—I'm glad you've decided to publish it despite my book [the Press could not easily do both at once]. Otherwise, I'd interpret your reservations as a compulsion to work, whereas I've really never before in my life felt so lazy. To save time—necessary, with the lack of publications—would you send your work directly to the Verlag (certified). I'll give instructions on what to do with it. I'll send comments on Little Hans to the press today.

I especially thank you for your detailed comments on my paper and apologize doubly, since I well know your distaste for this kind of thing, understand it, and—you will grant—largely respect it. Of course I was relieved to see that you yourself respected the reasons that brought me to go beyond my self-imposed limits this time. What you've said about my work, I too have felt, but less clearly, and for that reason I appealed to your judgment. I wrote the paper in about 8 days so as not always to appear at the Congress merely as a functionary, but I soon realized it would not be appropriate as a presentation. Unfortunately, I know all too well that its greatest fault is the most difficult to correct; actually, it cannot even be corrected. Namely, I have a completely undidactic, even antididactic writing style, which in almost 20 years of writing I've not given up, and which I think it is pointless to resist. I'd regret most if you took such an analytic intermezzo as a reason for doubts about my career choice. The main thing, of course, is that I myself feel content and happy in my current position; I envy no one, and would wish to trade with no one. You least of all have reason to criticize yourself, dear Professor—you who have given me so much more than I can say, and daily, even hourly, still do.

Many thanks for enclosures in your first letter. The letter from the Gymnasium student is a precious document; pity it cannot be shared with the public (quite a tidbit for the Neues Wiener Journal). I got from Jones the paper by Brun and sent it on for translation; I enclose his letter again; also a card from Jones, which I answered today saying that the term "recurrent dream" doesn't seem appropriate for either type of dream; without explanation, the term means nothing specific to me. If you differ on this, kindly send a card to Jones.

Tomorrow at noon Sachs, with his English nightmare, will be traveling through; I'll speak with him. You still have the Rundbriefe. Kindly send them to me, with any comments for the Committee, before you leave Gastein. I won't write the next Rundbrief until August 1. Let's not think about that yet.

With cordial greetings, from my wife as well, to your sister-in-law and to yourself.

Yours thankfully, Rank

Prof. Dr. Freud Bad Gastein, Wien, IX Berggasse 19 ¶July 17, 1922

Lieber Herr Doktor,

Since I have your letter with me, I can answer you now that a new week has begun.

Business matters first: I got the beautiful copy of Dream *from the Verlag. The Verlag is marvelous, the Press still always behind. The new edition of* Beyond *is ready for proofing. Enclosed you will find: 1) two reports by Prinzhorn, with a letter. 2) my letters with my comments on the reports. 3) my article on dreams, which contains only comments on* Interp. Dreams, *but which should have the effect of speeding you along in the completion of your dream book [*Eine Neurosenanalyse in Träumen, 1924*].*

From [Honorio] Delgado I got a copy of the Revista *(IV:2) and a small book,* Algunos aspectos de la psicología del niño *(Child Psychology) [1922].*

[American psychiatrist Thaddeus] Ames is a sensible person. He says he's ready to work with you if I have no time. Thus, he and Frau Kyrle will be your solid foundations [analysands]. My other article, "Neurotic Mechanisms in Jealousy, Paranoia, and Homosexuality" I'm sending directly to the Verlag for printing. It may need some corrections since I didn't have on hand the comments on paranoia in the Schreber analysis. You haven't told me what I should do with your manuscript on potency. I'm glad you took my critique so well, but certainly want you to make a presentation, something purely analytical, so people will get used to this side of your activity.

Cordially; greetings to all, Freud

P.S. My manuscript is being mailed as printed matter.

Dr. Otto Rank Seefeld ¶July 18, 1922

Lieber Herr Professor,

I acknowledge receipt of both your registered items: letter and the manuscript.

I must clarify the latter, I must get clarification since I don't know if I understood correctly that you want "Comments on Paranoia" printed first, and then the "Comments on Dreams." Originally I had this reversed, and asked you to send the "Comments on Dreams" directly to the Verlag as well. What raised my doubts is your saying "Paranoia" will need corrections that you can't do without a copy of Schreber. If "Paranoia" is printed now, it will appear in early September, likely before you get the Schreber. Since two articles for the next Zeitschrift *have been printed—you should have gotten them—your decision is crucial. Perhaps you should send things directly to the Verlag, especially if "Paranoia" is not to be printed now. If it is, then "Comments on Dreams" will go in later. Given all this, shall I keep the manuscript or return it to you?*

Re Prinzhorn, I'd like to print both articles in the next issue under "The Move-

ment," but not without an editorial comment on the glaring bias in linking things (shaking out the sweet bits and boasting that he baked the whole cake himself). (The false logic of this comment illustrates the false logic of his bias.)

Please return my manuscript when convenient (and not registered); I have a carbon copy. My intention was indeed to make people familiar with my analytical activities. I doubt that I'll find anything else in the course of the summer; at the moment I'm empty as a squeezed out sponge and lazy as a full one. (This state is difficult to imagine, but real.) To my inquiry, Deuticke just wrote that he has only 99 copies of the Incest *book, but can't send a precise accounting. Our contract states that after production costs are recovered I'm to receive an honorarium of 500 (peacetime) crowns. Instead, he's offering me 500 German marks—which I find shameless. Especially since just in the last few days he's announced in the stock market paper the foreign prices for his press's publications; the price for the incest book in England is 12 shillings, about 70,000 crowns, or about 1000 marks—which he'll get by selling just one copy in England. Perhaps you'd be interested in the foreign prices for your books.*

[UK] Shillings	*Sw. Franks*	*$ [US]*
Jokes	8/6 8.50	1.70
Interp Dreams	12/- 12.-	2.40
Neurosis III	9/7 9.60	1.92

Since you left, the following manuscripts have come in:

1) An article by Flournoy on androgynous symbolism in India, a study based on his trip; it's a correct, schoolboyish report, nothing more. I'll have it translated; in this case he wants the original text to appear in Claparède (Archives de Psychologie), *otherwise certainly in French in* Imago! *Which would you support?*

2) Melanie Klein, continuation of her study on children, especially anxiety, would like you to read this theoretically fresh work; I assuaged her with autumn.

3) Frau Dr. Müller-Braunschweig on [...] (it's in Vienna).

Levi-Bianchini writes that he wants to translate your Leonardo *himself. Dr. Benedicty is willing to publish* Gradiva *without the novella, just with his introduction.*

News from here: I spoke with Sachs for 1 minute while he was traveling through; he'll come again in August to meet Abraham, coming from Arlberg, who sent me, before leaving Berlin, a nice card agreeing with my last Rundbrief and announcing a visit to Seefeld in mid-August. Since Ferenczi will be there too, we can celebrate "reconciliation" in Seekirche.

Hitschmann, who came yesterday, I waved to from afar; hopefully that's fine with him, as it is for me. I've heard that Helsen [...] is here. We're staying so gloriously far from town that we really know nothing of Seefeld; but we see Lampl's brother, the poor fellow, every day.

Hopefully you again have weather as beautiful as ours since today.

With cordial greetings from both of us; soon our daughter will be old enough to send her greetings too. Yours, Rank

Prof. Dr. Freud B Gastein Wien, IX Berggasse 19 ¶July 20, 1922

Lieber Herr Doktor

I wanted to write to you today about the enclosed letter, but didn't give myself license as the week was not over. Your letter, just received, relieves me of this conscientious consideration.

About Mrs. Riviere's letter, I notice the devilishly clever woman is probably correct in all her observations. Jones's reaction we of course understand, and Abraham's irritation probably stems from his envy of Eitingon, who has irrevocably attained the status of family member to which he aspired. But Abraham is nobler than Jones, and his irritation is less significant. Overall, these displaced affects are not desirable, and that they fall on you is really unfair and I think when Ferenczi is here you can discuss it with him. His receptive kindness fits him for the role of conciliator. Also, from the analysis [by Ferenczi], he has most influence on Jones.

Concerning the new arrangement of the collected [Freud] works, I await your opinion after there's something from J. himself about that. I won't resist much: the affair is starting to lose interest, but I don't think he'll actually finish anything.

I sent you the dream remarks since you might be especially interested in them, and since I hadn't thought to publish them immediately. I sent the other manuscript on neurotic mechanisms in jealousy, paranoia, and homosexuality to the Verlag on July 17 enclosing a note saying that it should be typeset for Zeitschrift 3 instead of the dream article you had announced. Thus any possible misunderstanding will be avoided. I'll arrange to do the needed corrections by asking the Verlag to send a copy here of the collection containing the Schreber analysis (I think it's volume three). It's of little concern.

You've said nothing about the dream remarks, hopefully because you haven't yet read them, and there's no hurry. Otherwise, you've no need to treat me with special consideration, as I've admitted doing towards you.

I quite agree with your position on Prinzhorn if you're not too harsh. In his letter he emphasized his inner compulsion for independence, and I answered that I saw no merit in that. You certainly won't feel embarrassed with Deuticke. I'll send back your manuscript from Gastein after all. If you have nothing else, then peel off something from the all-too-abundant contents for your presentation. I prefer Flournoy's presentation in translation rather than in French. I'll be glad to read any mss. you send.

I wish the best outcome from your meeting in August. Perhaps it's wholly good that I can be present only in spirit. I'm sure you've already discovered the wonderful forests of Seefeld. I know that little Helene's real birthday is during the vacation; Minna's amazing memory declares that it is August 22.

Cordial best wishes to you and your wife. Yours, Freud

P.S. I've already read here the idiotic article from Vienna on Interpretation of Dreams. Stekel is also touching on the topic.

Dr. Otto Rank Seefeld ¶July 24, 1922

Lieber Herr Professor!

Some items are accumulating, and I'd like to organize them before the pile grows with its customary incredible speed.

1) The letter from Kazan with indication—to be interpreted ambivalently—of the further spread of psychoanalysis in Russia. In the next Rundbrief I'll convey the most important things, so please return the letter to me, if possible, before you leave Gastein. I answered Mr. [Aleksandr] Luria politely and sent the books he requested.

2) The letter from Frau Lou Andreas, which again destroys my timid hopes of surmounting the problems with the book on children, though objectively I am of the same opinion.

3) A copy came today of Jones's letter to Eitingon—which you probably got also—along with a list of Congress participants responding thus far. If you have any comments, please send them so they can be included in the Rundbrief. By the way, the idea came to me today—not simply due to laziness—to write the Rundbrief; when Ferenczi gets here, perhaps with him, thus a few days after it's due (August 1), which won't be a problem in the summer.

4) The letter from Mrs. Riviere, which I enclose again after noting its contents. Of course I'd be glad to express myself concerning Jones's suggestions about the Collected Shorter Writings, but I must confess as openly as you that the matter is beginning to lose interest for me too. It's become impossible for someone in our position to express an opinion on all the various ideas; as soon as one does so, another suggestion comes in, and the result is just greater delay.

Incidentally, I happened to write Hiller today, who seems to have dreamed up new delays. If I had my way, I would really knock some heads together at the Press in Ber-

lin! The content of Journal no. 2, which arrived today, doesn't seem to be worth the sacrifices.

As for your manuscripts, everything is in good order. After the fact, I thank you especially for sending your work on dreams, which meanwhile I was able to read in a free hour. As usual, of course, you've brought together the essential things in a few concise sentences, from which anyone, based on individual experience, can infer the rest. However, I believe I can express more precisely the justification for my planned work in that very few people have sufficient individual experience, and your 10 Commandments of dream interpretation can surely bear further comment. I used the last few days, all under the star of subjective and objective cooling off, to begin writing the introduction.

We're all very well here, and I hope we will soon get accustomed to the fickle Seefeld weather. Wife and child are thriving; the latter will be three years old on August 23 (remembered almost exactly). While writing this, though, I wonder whether that's actually correct; I just can't imagine that in a few years the little one will be more perfect than now. She's already talking about so many things, and knows so much, and is interested in so many things, that there certainly can't be much left for later.

With most cordial greetings from both of us—to your dear sister-in-law as well.

Yours, Rank

"Ten Commandments" refers to "Remarks on the Theory and Practice of Dream Interpretation," in which Freud says, "The question of the value to be assigned to dreams is intimately related to the other question of their susceptibility to influence from 'suggestion' by the physician. Analysts may at first be alarmed at the mention of this possibility. But on further reflection this alarm will give place to the realization that the influencing of the patient's dreams is no more a blunder on the part of the analyst or disgrace to him than the guiding of the patient's conscious thoughts." Rank and Ferenczi surely found support in this for their active therapy.[4]

Prof. Dr. Freud B Gastein Wien, IX Berggasse 19 ¶July 27, 1922
Lieber Herr Doktor,

I enclose your two letters! Many thanks for the alpine postcard addressed to all the participants!

I received the copy of the letter to Eitingon. Concerning the list of presentations I'd say just that I'd not be happy to see my name on it, nor to note the absence of yours. Your manuscript will be sent today. The Verlag has shown me a pile of Hun-

garian crowns. Apparently 25 francs from somewhere (it's hard to keep track of all the income) have not yet arrived in Holland. I very much approve of your plan to let the Rundbrief wait for Ferenczi.

To remain polite with the Press is really not easy. I thanked Hiller for his efforts and asked that he make this delay the last. You've probably gotten Jones's suggestion. The only guarantee is for Mrs. Riviere to be involved in the affair, assuming longevity.

I didn't expect that my comments would overlap closely with your little book. Let's plan to publish simultaneously.

Starting in August my address will be: Hochgebirge Kurhaus Obersalzberg, Berchtesgaden; that is, unless political events make the trip impossible. Perhaps you'll soon be in Bavaria without even moving an inch. Perhaps it will be impossible to go from Bavaria to Berlin. Once again the devil is brewing something big.

I assure you little Helene will continue to develop even after August 23 [age 3]. The classic age is just coming.

Cordial greetings to Ferenczi. I wish you and your dear wife the best of weather: so far the summer wasn't even worth mentioning. Best wishes otherwise! Yours, Freud

In a letter to Rank from Göttingen, July 31, Anna Freud expressed regret that the *Kinderbuch* project with Lou had to be dropped but that everyone agreed, "including Papa." She reports that his *Group Psychology* was sent to the printer. In the 1923 revision Freud notes that it "was written under the influence of an exchange of ideas with Otto Rank" and his "Don Juan Gestalt."

In "Don Juan," Rank addresses the role of woman as nurturer, not just sex object. This would reflect his parenting experience with Tola. A major thesis expressed at the end applies to creators in general, not just poets, thus including Freud and himself. It foreshadows Rank's dialectical thinking about creativity in *Art and Artist* (1932).

Therefore we see that the poet embodies the double function of the ego ideal. Seen from the outside, the poet creates a new personal ideal for the masses, a creation to which he was driven by his inner conflicts arising from the formation of his own ideal. Dissatisfied with the ideal of the group, he forms his own individual ideal in order to proffer it to the group, without whose recognition his creation remains very unsatisfactory. . . . The pressure that the poet feels to solicit recognition of his new ideal from the group reveals that he created it not only to satisfy his own narcissism, but also to replace the old common ideal with a new one. . . . The tragedy of every great poetic personality is that when this aim succeeds, it must finally lead to disappointment instead of satisfaction, just as the primal deed does. The reason is that as his personal ideal is generally recognized and appreciated, it becomes established as another group ideal, the very thing that he wishes to shun. . . . Whenever we find distinct periods in the work of a poet, such a process of devaluation of the poet's previous ego ideal formation is at work.[5]

From the warm, indeed loving, embrace between Freud and Rank in 1922 the struggles of heresy and orthodoxy would bring the Committee toward fratricide.

≈ Chapter 12 ≈

Fratricide

August to December 1922

The Seventh International Congress of the International Psychoanalytical Association took place in Berlin, September 25–27. It was the
last attended by Freud, and the last time the Committee would meet
together. The famous photograph of the seven members was taken there.

Dr. Otto Rank Seefeld ¶August 2, 1922

Lieber Herr Professor,

*I hope you're safely settled in Berchtesgaden, as this year the political storms seem
to dissipate more easily than the real ones. Although you've not expressly said so, I can
assume the stay in Gastein suited you well; I'd be happy if you'd verify that. For the
rest of your stay I wish the best, especially for weather, weather, and again weather,
which, it seems, is as important for a summer holiday as money is for waging war.
We've set up our nest in the glorious forests here; we no longer notice the rain, and
are glad it brings beautiful mushrooms as a result, whose way of shooting out of the
ground seems like a legend from prehistoric times.*

*Yesterday the Ferenczis arrived, exhausted, to increase the colony. I made use of the
poor weather, right at hand, to write the enclosed Rundbrief, from which you'll learn
some new details. Here I need to make two points. 1) My Congress presentation, which
I put down on paper last week: the rain had started up again, as if in response to a
magic wish. It lacks only a middle portion, which will determine whether the whole
will be good or bad. The beginning is good: it starts with terminologically sloppy
expressions, e.g. designations for unconscious homosexuality etc. so as not to reveal
the hidden gap in our knowledge—a gap lying just behind. The conclusion suggests*

the cardinal point of the problem, the guilt feeling, but then strays a bit in a theory of perversions, ending with the analysis of the snake fantasy—which doesn't seem fully ripe yet. The middle portion crystallizes around an instructive case that shows, at times very clearly, the connections between perversion and neurosis, while sometimes leading to problems I can't solve. As a whole, the piece is more unified (and shorter) and direct than the first, confusing theme, and I have no doubt it will meet with your approval if appropriately revised.

After this extensive discussion, please allow me to comment on your Congress presentation too, since you must, after all, present something. My suggestion—I intend it as nothing more—derives from the wish to burden you as little as possible with a Congress topic, and makes sense only if you still haven't chosen one. In that case, I think your paper on neurotic mechanisms in jealousy etc. would be very appropriate; the apparent disadvantage—that it will appear in the next issue of the Zeitschrift— could be used to advantage if you spoke on the first or second day, since the journal appears on the third day when listeners would greet it gladly in order to read your comments. If this suggestion does not meet with your approval, please don't take it the wrong way; it's inspired only by good will and the desire to lighten your workload as much as possible.

I can't accept your suggestion that your "Comments on Dreams" wait for my book—not only because the date is uncertain, but also because there would be no objective basis for such an arrangement. I'm sorry if I expressed myself so unclearly that you reacted with this impression. From your comments I've gained some firm guidelines for the viewpoint and overall concept that I'd want to add. I especially take to heart the idea that in conceptualizing dreams one must never forget their wish nature, and that accordingly—even in analysis—one shouldn't overvalue them, a danger one can easily succumb to in the detailed monographic presentation of a topic. If it meets with your approval, I'd propose, as a compromise, that your article appear in the first issue of the next Zeitschrift, for which we'll need an article from you anyway. The second point, to repeat, is that Psyche und Eros has ceased publication, which is really a triumph for our good cause (hopefully you agree with my comment about that in the Rundbrief). I'm only afraid that now, beside neo-analysis, Old Stickler [Stekel] will make himself independent with pseudo-analysis.

After the adventures with the Press, my handling of which you'll find in the Rundbrief, Reik, in an attack of irritable jealousy, seems to perpetuate the summer of our discontent. You've surely received his Rundbrief/articles; I find this laudable, and will tell him so. However, he found it necessary to send me a separate dose of affect, in effect screaming at me as if I were at fault for everything, or had rejected all his suggestions, in which case he threatens to resign. He blames me for trying to get him to resign, but I don't need to say that I'm only doing so because he's not getting anything done (his last report to the Association, which I showed you, proved this again—one can't rely on him for anything without supervision and coaching). So I plan to write him, ignoring his private commentary, to say I agree with his Rundbrief on most points—just minor differences—and all the more since it suggests putting responsibility for the annual report in the hands of the Congress and officially placing responsibility for managing presentations in his hands, so I wouldn't need to do anything on either count. The more this ideal could be done, the happier I'd be, and I'd do anything to support him in this. I just await your answer before telling him. It's my personal conviction that even then he won't accomplish anything, but I'd give him a chance to prove otherwise. He's useful only for writing books—nothing else. Even when he deals with the Verlag as an author, he becomes insufferable—this is not my impression alone—and I'll spare you the depiction of how much patience is needed to deal with his neurotic moods. He walked out after telling me for the umpteenth time that he was already sick of his book, and that the longer the printing takes, the more we are forcing him to make large insertions and changes in the proofs. Then, through the Verlag, I returned the greater part of his manuscript—that is not in use at the printer—asking him to mark corrections. Meanwhile, as it is now, for technical and material reasons, the Verlag can't take on extensive, previously agreed proofs that the author can still indicate in the manuscript without losing time. Please forgive me for troubling you with these details, but I consider it my duty to tell you how I handled such a valuable analyst as Reik, and my motives for so doing.

Enclosed also is a suggestion from [Wilhelm] Reich, certainly one of our most diligent and valuable young workers. Perhaps managing the Congress presentations, which can no longer be handled by one person, could be improved by bringing him in this circle.

My woman patient is staying until the 19th, then I'll still have a whole month free. Many thanks for the news about Ames, which I've made note of. Miss Cole is coming to see Ferenczi for fourteen days—for "discussions," as she puts it.

I think I've bothered you enough for today.

With cordial greetings from both of us to you and your dear family. Yours, Rank

Prof. Dr. Freud Pension Moritz Salzberg, Berchtesg ¶August 4, 1922
Lieber Herr Doktor

I write to you from a charming studio with a view of an apple tree, a green meadow, and dark firs. It's wonderfully quiet. Eitingon, who was here last year, enjoined the innkeepers to make things comfortable for us, and this seems to be a success. Since you especially ask about my state of health, I first thank you for describing it to the others in the Rundbrief as satisfactory, and then admit to you that it's not so. The appearance of stomach troubles (recurring every year) in Gastein forced me to combine the bathing cure with Karlsbad's drinking, and given this combined effect of the curative powers, a peculiar physical exhaustion has taken hold. The stomach troubles, attributed by the wise to Gastein's radioactive drinking water, seemed almost gone upon leaving there, but recurred yesterday and leaves me unhappy.

All conjectures, pessimist as well as optimist, remain in play. In practice, we'll hold with the latter. That I've felt unsure about my health for a long time cannot have escaped you. I tell no one else about it, or I'd hear the usual insincerities. You are the youngest and liveliest among us, while one knows that an age so close to 70 is a very serious thing.

I don't want to fill your imagination with admissions suggestive of hypochondria, so I'll add that I'm mentally clear and eager for work. I'm now working on something called The Ego and the Id, *which has Groddeck as godfather. It may be just an essay or perhaps a brochure like* Beyond, *of which it is actually a continuation. The draft is going well, but awaits the right mood and inspiration, without which it cannot be completed.*

In order to have peace, and time to work, I've declined several lucrative opportunities that impressed me and should impress you, too. In Gastein I turned away the wife of a copper king; the fee would surely have covered the cost of our stay there. Here on the Salzberg [mountain], another American woman is begging for treatment; she'd have paid $50 a day since she was used to paying Brill $20 for half an hour in New York. (Incidentally, another demonstration of how Brill succumbs to the American dollar-drug.) But she won't prevail: I won't sell my time here. I'm thinking of unloading her on [Horace] Frink, who visited with his fiancée, an estimable woman, for six days in Gastein, and is coming to Berchtesgaden—not without ulterior analytical motives, for he is by no means well. I won't allow him to come up the mountain either.

From Gastein I sent you the ms. of your proposed presentation, registered. I'm so glad you decided on a different, more narrowly defined one. Perhaps you haven't fully appreciated the motivation for my regret, recently expressed, that I didn't permit you to study medicine. In that case I believe there'd be no doubt about the person to whom I'd bequeath the leading role in the psychoanalytic movement. As things stand, I'd wish that Abraham's clarity and correctness could be melded with Ferenczi's talent, and that Jones's inexhaustible pen could be added as well.

I take note of your kind proposal concerning my presentation for the Congress, and if necessary will refer back to it. I thought it would be most comfortable to make no plans and to take advantage of the notation "topic to be announced" so I can come up with something at the last minute. I can't direct my interests now: they are centered on the "I" and the "It." I noted the demise of Eros und Psyche. It came to an end with a renewed stench. The author was so kind as to send the last issue, with analyses—careless and idiotic in equal measure—of my analyses, but of course we have comfort in the fact that even this inferior publication will have an afterlife in another realm. We'll never be rid of parasites, but fortunately one can't catch typhoid fever from all of them.

I accept your characterization of Reik as correct; I've known for some time that he is not the one. I'm also sending you a secret memo that he enclosed when he sent the official one. He intended it partly as a continuation of his description and partly as an excuse. Anyway, promise him all possible assistance, but shouldn't we consider releasing him from his office if that is his wish? So his note will be a topic for our Committee; please bring it to the meeting.

There is another enclosure from Andace in Milan. Can it be combined with the article by Edoardo Weiss? I'll await your decision. (The enclosures will actually go in a separate envelope.) My wife, Anna, and Oliver should arrive tomorrow. The weather here, as in Gastein, is far from consistently pleasant, but not as bad as described in the reports from Seefeld, the Harz, and Berlin. We do still have a right to summer weather.

Minna sends you cordial thanks, and will certainly write to you herself. Cordial greetings to your little family, to the Ferenczis, and to all staying there previously.

Yours, Freud

P.S. Small request for proofreading "Neurotic Mechanisms," should you receive it soon. "Project into the blue" should of course read "project outward."

Prof. Dr. Freud Salzberg ¶August 10, 1922

Lieber Herr Doktor,

Since your answer hasn't arrived and I have no further alarming details to report concerning my health—organs are in better shape, but I am still plagued by fatigue—my letter will be no more than an accompaniment to the five enclosures, all of which you will find in the same folder.

1) Most important: the letter from California. It's good that I delayed comments on Lowtzky's article. The task will now be easier. The case described in the letter has conquered my resistance. On one hand it completely confirms the outlook expressed in "Dream and Telepathy;" on the other it contains a fact for which there seems to be no explanation other than conveyance of information from outside. I'd be fully convinced if the same thing happened to me, but I'm still in the regrettable position of the count in the Tannhäuser parody ["Such a thing shall not happen to me"]. The nice thing is that the scholarly and erudite writer of the letter has no reservations. The bride apparently identified herself with the insane man, and thought: "If he leaves me, I don't know what I'll do." This threat made its way to him, and he answered: "Just do it! Then I'll finally be rid of you," whereupon his awakened conscience—the only thing he understood—overwhelmed him with reproach. Please let me know your opinion.

2) [Nikolaj] Ossipow's article. You need to decide whether it should or should not be printed in the Zeitschrift as precursor to the book.

3) Your letter to Reik. No objections! This must be carefully considered at the meeting before the Congress. Shouldn't a way be found for Reik to resign from his position, for which he really seems unsuited?

4) The argument among the Italians. I share your opinion that in this matter the publisher has not overstepped his rights. If his preface isn't good, the translator's version is certainly no worse. Of course one must proceed diplomatically with excitable Latins.

5) Reich's suggestion is very praiseworthy. Couldn't the seminar take over the technical evenings and convene in the weeks left free by the society? This is also a topic for discussion by the Committee. Abraham intends to extend the Congress to four days. I'm inclined to decide as little as possible myself. In any case, if there's no other way, experience will show whether this can work. Jones again sent a new classification of the essays for the collection. I must insist that "Character and Anal Eroticism" belongs in the clinical section, and preferably also the continuation, "Transferences of Drives." On the other hand "The Dream as Evidence" will go very nicely in the applied section. Meanwhile, at least, nothing is advancing.

> *Cordial greetings to you, and your wife and child—*
> *and to all the meteorologists of Seefeld. Yours, Freud*

Seefeld ¶August 12, 1922

Lieber Herr Professor!

In your card you remind me that I still owe a response to your extensive letter. But it can only be answered in a certain mood—which the constant visits of friends in Seefeld doesn't allow. There's always coming and going of acquaintances—actually more coming than going. A few days ago Schütz treated us to some fun—we were on the glorious Eppzir railroad line with him and the Ferenczis. Then Sachs came yesterday, loaded down with two Englishwomen. On Monday we're expecting Abraham and his fellow-travelers; Federn threatens to come here from Zell am See; Nunberg has written a prescription for himself to come here for his health; and a visit from Bernfeld is just visible like summer lightning on the distant horizon! If things continue like this—politically, that is—maybe this pre-Congress will have to substitute for the real one. For me the whole thing has lost interest.

Anyway, I'm doubly glad you've been able to pass recent days so pleasantly, which here, alas, have been only figuratively humid; I wish you a speedy recovery, aided by the double curative effect. As for rejected temptations, it occurs to me that two days before my departure Dr. Steiner (from the bank) telephoned me with an urgent inquiry (on his own!), asking for your address, since American business friends of his, who had just arrived in Holland, wanted to consult with you and undergo an analysis in the summer. I gave him your address, saying I knew all efforts and temptations would be for nought (I think these Americans want to invite you to Switzerland).

I'll keep Reik's memo until Abraham is here, since he wanted me to show it to Abraham. I acknowledge Reik's self-criticism, but miss any criticism of his role as a conference presenter, where he behaved no better than Sachs, whom he condemns.

As for the Italian offer, I agree that your idea—to recommend Ed. Weiss—is the best. Given the still poor situation with the Italian books, we must not create any competition for ourselves there.

From the Verlag I got news that production goes very well. Of your books, Totem *(new—pocket edition) and* Introductory Lectures, III *will appear this month.* Diary, *and perhaps the book on the Id will come out before the Congress. The small Polish edition of* Interpretation of Dreams *will be released soon.*

Meanwhile, I hope you got the corrections for your Zeitschrift *essay. I too oppose extending the time of the Congress, and will inform Abraham.*

With most cordial greetings to you and your dear family. Yours, Rank
P.S. [from Hanns Sachs] Dear Professor,

Yesterday, after a rather adventurous trip, I arrived in A., and now, as the greatest vacation pleasure, I'm enjoying the company of R[ank] and F[erenczi]. With best wishes for a speedy recovery, respectfully yours, HS

As in the work with Ferenczi on therapeutic aspects of psychoanalysis, Rank is both fearless and respectful toward Freud, whom he challenges about telepathy and who remains gracious and firm in disagreement.

Seefeld *Imago* ¶August 15, 1922

Lieber Herr Professor,

I'm hurrying to answer your missive concerning telepathy. I'll save other matters until after I've spoken with Abraham, expected here today; then, perhaps, we'll send off a little Rundbrief together. (Sachs went back to Berlin yesterday.)

As you know, dear Professor, I am among those who are quite skeptical—since nothing of the kind ever happened to me—and the farther away the source of the report, the less I'll be convinced. Furthermore, the case itself seems to me, given its conditions, anything but clean: 1. an abnormal person, 2. apparently in a neurotic conflict, 3. certainly influenced by reading your article in Imago—["Dreams and Telepathy"] *which in this case seems not to have occurred simultaneously, 4. (a counterargument added by Ferenczi): his occupation at a first-aid station, which continuously receives such calls—a fact his fiancée or lover must have known. (Also, one more analytical conjecture of my own: for the young woman, the identification was made easier by the fact that in case of injury she could hope to be taken to "his" station, where she would be treated and saved by him. This situation would actually presume constant suicidal fantasies on her part, just as for him we certainly must also assume constant fantasies of eliminating her; it would of course be interesting to discover whether her other suicidal fantasies also involved falling down from heights.) Furthermore, this type of idea of eliminating someone cannot be established purely telepathically. It's just that the precise time remains as something inviolable, provided that everything is reproduced without (subsequent excessive) distortion. Even Ferenczi felt that this case proves nothing more or less about telepathy than hundreds of other reported cases, and it should not have shaken your resistance. As for me, I wouldn't even use the case. As I've said, I mistrust such "submitted" reports, and I don't think this is influenced only by the proximity of the "mine dog."* [Grubenhund: Hoax report to provoke interest.]

Cordial greetings from Ferenczi and me to you and your family. Yours, Rank

Seefeld ¶August 22, 1922

Lieber Herr Professor,

Having no word from you I'd almost be worried, if not for the fact that you've spoiled me to such an extent. So I assume that nothing happened worth mentioning, and you're enjoying the beautiful pre-autumn days, which we have here.

Ferenczi, with whom I've talked a lot on personal terms and scientifically, and with whom I get along best in both, leaves the day after tomorrow, unfortunately. I shared personal Committee issues, and he promised to try to influence Jones. We're both aware that we two are the only ones—even within the Committee—at work seriously with your psychoanalysis, especially in therapy, also generally; on both of these counts, things in Berlin and London leave something to be desired.

We decided first to start a scientific campaign against overestimation of the castration complex—manifested more and more—and we hope to bring Abraham and Jones over to our side as the first to join us; we think they are on the other side now. The campaign will of course stand in the sign of the Oedipus complex, in its deep, libido-theoretical meaning. Since we consider this correction very important, and believe it will deepen understanding of analysis in the world, we're of course eager to learn of your opinion. We prefer not to discuss this at the Committee as it's a question of scientific principles, not resolvable in friendly discussion, but through scientific argument. If you agree, then the Committee, while taking on a more "worldly" character (business, publicity, criticism, personal details, Verlag, etc.), would develop a scientific core, a very desirable element.

Conversations with various analysts here push me to get the dream book written; moving slowly—so important in demonstrating all that otherwise cannot be shown.

[One page is illegible.]

…because of the prices, but also due to shortages, and the expulsion of foreigners may occur any day. Since we're so near the German border, and while things, for now, cost only half what they do here, we plan to spend September in Bavaria until the Congress, going from there to Berlin. Meanwhile, Storfer is managing the Verlag as well as can be (enclosed is his last report)—and otherwise I have nothing to do in Vienna. Don't you find this the best solution under the circumstances?

With heartiest greetings to your dear family and to you as well, from both of us.

Yours, Rank

P.S. Should I deal with the enclosed letter myself or just send it on to Frau Stein?

On August 22 Jones sent a long Rundbrief about the Congress, reacting to Rank's of August 16 (coauthored with Ferenczi and Abraham).[1] "Rank's hammer has once more fallen, this time on London and, as it seems to me, very unfairly." Rank had claimed that Flugel's temporary absence left work undone: Jones said he himself had filled in. Rank claimed that Eitingon had not received the list of presentations; Jones claimed they were sent.

Prof. Dr. Freud Wien, IX Berggasse 19 ¶August 24, 1922

Lieber Herr Doktor

I won't leave you without an answer any longer since you're thinking about the interruption in transportation. My condition has gradually changed, the tiredness replaced by an unpleasant depressed mood, for which I find explanation enough in the news from Vienna (Moische and the sinking ship) and in concerns for autumn. On the evening of the 16th a telegram came reporting that Caecilie ["Maus" Graf, 23, daughter of Freud's sister Rosa], was in hospital with acute [suicidal] veronal poisoning. The next days, with all their vicissitudes, responsibilities, and arrangements, were pure hell. On the evening of the 18th she died without regaining consciousness. Dr. Deutsch had been summoned. My brother [Alexander], who arrived here a few days earlier, has gone back to Vienna for the funeral. I don't know whether my sister's condition will oblige me to do the same. Since then I've given up trying to make my stay in this beautiful place an idyll, and I place no importance on my condition.

Recently I've answered no letters, distracting myself by writing. I finished two essays "Psychoanalysis" and "Theory of the Libido" for Marcuse's Encyclopedia. Ego and Id is almost done.

Maus was a sweet girl, beloved by all, but hard to approach. Relations between her and her mother, with whom it is hard to get along, were poor. She had a serious suitor whom she was planning to marry soon, and against whom many objections could be raised. But we don't know what finally pushed her to the fatal step, for which she had been preparing since March. Nor do we know whether the tragedy is over with her death. In her despair, as we found in both of the previous circumstances, my sister is simply insufferable.[2]

I have of course also had concerns similar to those you express about the survival of the Verlag and our ability to remain in Vienna. I believe we can only wait and be glad we are away from Vienna for now. By the end of September much will be clear. If we leave Vienna, you should certainly join us. Our friends will certainly follow quickly; I cannot manage them alone. We ought to let Eitingon know the rest about the state of the Verlag. He is our immediate hope. Beyond that I know of no one.

I'm very glad to hear of your agreement with Ferenczi. For the moment I can't take sides in your campaign against the castration complex since I don't know your arguments. In any case, many things formerly close to me have strangely receded into the distance, which should not bother you younger and [...] friends of the present. I was surprised by the extremely sharp criticism expressed by both of you concerning the last telepathic dream. Everything you reveal is merely favorable circumstance rather *than objection; the only thing available is the argument that one has not experienced this oneself, but must take someone else's word for it. I've thought about adopting this dream for presentation at the Congress as no other topic occurs to me.*

Given the current situation, I find your plan to spend September in Bavaria entirely appropriate. If one returned to Vienna it would be hard to leave at the end of September. Concern about getting foreign currency is least justified. Please deal as you see fit with the enclosed letter from the American woman, and also with the inquiry from Lehmann.

Many thanks for the cards sent during mountain excursions, and for Ferenczi's letter; please excuse me for not responding.

Awaiting your swift reply, Cordially yours, Freud

[turn page] Over! For Frau Rank!

Salzberg ¶August 24, 1922

Dear Little Frau Rank,

I'd be very sorry if you were to renounce your [Polish] translation because of harsh criticism. Of course I can make no judgment about it, but since you yourself have certain revisions in mind, and are so diligently consulting other authorities on your language, I would think your translation could successfully defend itself against a violent process like that suggested by Dr. J [Jones]. Don't lose courage: that would not be like you.

Cordial greetings to you and to little three-year-old Helene. Yours, Freud

On the same day Freud wrote Ferenczi, "I have been very happy about the intensification of your intimacy with Rank; it promises good things for the future." Ferenczi responded on August 31, "The stay in Seefeld was, in fact, significant for me, since the unity between Rank and me, which was also never disrupted earlier, was sealed there. I hope we can find a little bit of time in Berlin to present our plan to you personally." On August 28 Freud sent a note to the Ranks with thanks for their condolence regarding Maus, adding that the tone of Jones's last Rundbrief was "no better."

[Seefeld] ¶September 3, 1922
From September 6: Tutzing am Starnbergersee,
Hotel König Ludwig—probably till Sept. 20, then Berlin.

Dear Professor,

I must thank you for your detailed letter of August 24 and for a brief note (re Jones's Rundbrief). From both I had the impression that in the irritating and ultimately sad mood of this summer, you have found tranquility in your work.

Since this is probably the last letter from Seefeld—on Wednesday we go to Bavaria—while I look back with a sense of melancholy on the larch-covered embankment, the Black Forest behind it, and in the distance the Wetterstein mountain face, in my mind's eye I must look back at everything that happened in the psychoanalytic movement around me in the last two months. Were it not for the fact that it would be criminal to compare current world politics with anything respectable, I'd compare the world situation to our small movement.

As you well know, the situation in the allied Committee was somewhat critical last winter, and improved only partly this summer. My personal relationship with Abraham, who was here with his family as our guest, is closer again, but on the other hand, we (Ferenczi and I) have become more critical of A. as analyst, who—to do a rating this once—we'd put on a level between Jones and Ferenczi. Judging from the patients who come from him to me, Jones doesn't seem to be on top of things technically, only partly due to his isolation (Ferenczi wants to speak with him and advise him to continue with his own analysis).

As I hinted to you, here in Seefeld a strong bond developed between Ferenczi and me, and your support strengthens my hope that it will prove fruitful. First we plan a collaboration [book] on the progress of psychoanalytic method; Ferenczi will write the critical part, and I the affirmative; I intend it to be situational-critical, with some positive aspects. I take the liberty of sending for your perusal a carbon copy of the first draft fantasized into the typewriter. It can only give a vague impression of what we want to do. We won't spell out details on technique, etc., but on the other hand our next works will be produced in this spirit; step by step, they'll fill out the program. The dream analysis book especially belongs in this; it goes slowly but surely, along with smaller works in preparation (the improved "psych. St." [...], my Congress presentation, etc.). We hope to confer in Berlin about the plan, of course only if we're sure you agree and support it. We're assuming Abraham and Jones will readily follow our lead, though they may not come through the process entirely unscathed.

So much for the report on the meeting of the Committee; we don't want to risk its safe and harmonious continuation through our initiatives, but rather to strengthen it.

While this took place during high season, Federn came about a week ago with Nunberg (and Dr. Neug[arten].). His visit, too, had political import, and since he reported Jekels had visited him recently in Zell and they discussed and decided various things with Nunberg, I called him the representative of the "little entente," to which he snorted an understanding laugh. It was about a Congress lecture (on the status of libido), canceled by Eitingon since it had been announced too late; Federn wants to publish it as an accompanying booklet. It also concerned my teaching at the Vienna Polyclinic, which I limited to giving a course on analytic technique of dream interpretation.

The main political issue was Federn's sense of having been insulted by Hitsch-mann and his (justified) criticism of Reik's meeting minutes (and also, as I'd long suspected, his irritation that Hitschmann is editor of Zeitschrift—*Federn is always offering to "Germanify* [verdatschen]" *the articles written by non-German authors!). He expected that he and Hitschmann would alternate as vice-president—as they do in governing the Clinic, so they shouldn't simply re-elect the committee by acclamation. He proposed to do the meeting reports (minutes) by writing synopses of the medical presentations himself; Reik would do the applied ones. Federn would ask support from Reich, who is willing to work. I said it might be more expedient if Federn replaced me as first secretary, writing meeting reports for the* Korrespondenzblatt; *Reik could serve as corresponding secretary—as is done in other groups. Another place on the board might be found for me. Aid from Reich, who has made himself noticeable elsewhere as well (the seminar!), would not be discouraged. (Reich wanted to visit me here, but didn't happen to find me in.) Then there's the crisis about Reik in the scheme of presentations; perhaps the Federn-Reich bloc could help here too (seminar).*

So, I think that after dealing in Berlin with international problems and Committee problems we'll still have to deal with the Austrian problem—unless by then it has disappeared, along with Austria itself.

*From the Verlag I have positive news again. The books sold out for so long are again available (*Diary, Introductory Lectures *in all editions, etc.), and in Vienna alone we are taking in 1 to 1½ million daily, which, despite adjusting the value, does add up to something, especially since Leipzig is doing even better. Storfer works fabulously, reliably, and prudently—you can't wish for more—so I'd make him head of the whole technical side and give him the corresponding position officially. He'll represent the Verlag at the Congress. The entire [English] Press must come under this same tech-*

nical directorship; I'll present two alternatives: it becomes independent financially or, if tied financially to the Verlag, as it is now (i.e. we pay for everything), it must be subject to our technical direction. Then we'll decide the production rate for English publications. I also wrote Heller a few days ago to show him, given the endless delays with new books, how ominous this tactic is materially: if the books had appeared earlier (on time), the Verlag wouldn't have fallen into financial crisis, since we'd have been able to apply profits from the English books. Recently he tried to put himself in a good light by saying that he had "privately" lent the Verlag 20 pounds. That won't do.

Zeitschrift and Imago VIII:3 are nearly ready, and—if the printers' strike that broke out Friday in Vienna ends—they'll be at the Congress; in every respect the Verlag will make a fine showing at the Congress.

I'm writing Jones privately to say he should ask Abraham, Ferenczi and Sachs, all of whom dared get close to me this year, whether I'm really the barking dog he likes to call me.

Dear Professor, please take this long epistle only as an informative report on my analytic activities in Seefeld, accepting it favorably if the mood you have described continues. Nothing will be decided or changed before Berlin or without your approval.

Most cordial greetings to the members of your family in Berchtesgaden and to yourself, and best wishes for the remainder of your stay.

Respectfully yours, Rank

P.S. The enclosed literary critique of Strachey's brother may interest you—or him. In L'esprit Nouveau *there is "a comprehensive description of Freud by Jan Epstein" (notice in* Literarisches Echo).

Prof. Dr. Freud Salzberg ¶September 8, 1922

Lieber Herr Doktor,

Situation report: The 6th day of miserable weather, the 4th of a persistent, dripping fog. I have finally acquiesced and had the rooms heated. Eitingon was here on days 3 and 4 and never saw the mountain. I hope the mountains are still there "latently." In the hotel a palace revolution is underway. Most of the staff deserted after the intervention of a gendarme. Today my wife went to [...] to see her sister. We—Oliver, Anna, little Edith Rischawy, and I—want to see if we can hold out until the 14th. For the night of the 15th/16th we have tickets for a sleeping car, Munich to Hamburg. Frink is coming up here every day from Berchtesgaden for analysis, usually with his very charming fiancée.

Eitingon abducted Ego and Id *and took it to Berlin; I wouldn't look at it for a few* months in any case. He thinks it should be published as a short volume like Beyond. But it's only 96 pages (2 bound sheets). While it was here a letter arrived from Erma-kow as well as the first part of the lectures translated by Wulff. I enclose the letter. In my answer I suggest that all correspondence be sent via Eitingon in Berlin, where the mails should be functioning regularly. Incidentally, there are no more concerns about the Russian editions. Farà da se; they'll take care of everything in Moscow themselves.

I've had several sincere discussions with Eitingon, and inducted him into the Jones issue, about which he knew almost nothing. We did not discuss the material condition of the Verlag, but I have the impression that he's not concerned about that, which is very good. If we have to leave Vienna because it becomes impossible to live there and because friends in need of analysis no longer want to go there, he offers us initial shelter in Berlin. If I were ten years younger I would pin all sorts of plans on resettlement. In September my health definitely improved, but I have no real certainty.

I'll also arrive in Berlin with Anna on the 20th or 21st. Eitingon thinks Committee meetings could very well be held in his home. We'll probably be busiest with the English problems. I'm much opposed to granting the Press any sort of independence, be it technical or financial. Considering its achievements during the last two years, it has destroyed any claim to independence! Jones will presumably remain in the directorship, but will be supported by Rickman, as he himself proposes; Hiller's position will probably go through serious [...], and Flügel will probably be replaced as secretary. Jones has shown himself to be very incompetent. In light of this external problem, the tempests in our local teapot certainly recede into the background.

I'm glad you can praise Storfer so highly. Finding the right apprentice is one of the duties and merits of the master craftsman.

As you know, your coauthorship with Ferenczi has my full support. The energetic, daring initiative of your joint draft is really gratifying. I've always feared I'm holding back those closest to me from expressing their own opinions, and am glad to see evidence to the contrary. There is much I do not yet understand, and other aspects seem too severe or too extreme or too sure. Of course, you still have not done any revisions. Since its [...] with Oedipus we can no longer do away with the "complex." Subordination to the therapeutic-technical point of view pits argumentation much too strictly against description, which is still indispensable. The castration complex, for example, has not yet been adequately dealt with descriptively, and accordingly should not yet be condemned. It should be of interest to you that the unconscious sensation of guilt also plays a major role in Ego and Id. But don't take the above comments as a critique yet.

Now I need only wish you and your wife and child a satisfying late summer in Bavaria, though I do not expect you will have better weather than we have here.

Cordially yours, Freud

P.S. The [postal] strike in Vienna is of course grist for the mill for our [English] Press, which now has an excuse if it remains unrepresented at the Congress. The issues of our Zeitschrift *now seem threatened as well. We've gotten no newspaper since Monday.*

Three brief letters to Rank from Freud follow, dealing with details of the Berlin Congress. The last invites the Ranks to lunch, courtesy of Mrs. Bijur and Dr. Frink, who drove Freud from Berchtesgaden. Years later Beata (Tola) Rank recalled that lunch. Frink's wife-to-be was wealthy, and had purchased a brooch for $2,000. Freud asked Tola, "If a woman has so much money, spends too much for a piece of jewelry, what do you think she would give to the Verlag?" Startled at the time, Tola laughed in retrospect: "Although I wasn't so wise, I thought to myself, one has nothing to do with the other." Freud's hope for "millions" from Mrs. Frink came to naught.[3]

The Congress drew 256 participants; about half were members of the IPA. Presentations were diverse and high-level. Rank presented "Perversions and Neurosis," publishing a longer paper with that title in 1923 in German and English. Rank addressed sadism, masochism, homosexuality, exhibitionism, and masturbation, which Freud regarded as deviant and unhealthy. Rank challenges this position, writing: "In masturbation itself there lies besides regression to an infantile autoeroticism an important psycho-biologic advance in the direction of permitting or affirming sensuality, which in consideration of the special tendency of neurotics to repress the sensual bodily components we may designate as healthy."[4]

As in his letters, Freud supported Ferenczi and Rank when they differed with him. Although they downplayed the castration complex, he proposed a prize to encourage more papers on the mutual influence of theory and therapy, the topic of their forthcoming book.

Rumblings of conflict in the Committee erupted in the Rundbriefe after the Congress. On November 1, Abraham wrote that the Committee was the opposite of a neurotic family: "Those people fight as soon as they are together and are full of love as soon as they are separated." Freud countered a charge by Abraham that Rank's last two Rundbriefe had not been seen by him.

"They contain nothing for which I am not also responsible," Freud wrote. He took seriously the conflict between Jones and Rank, convinced that Rank was a proxy target for anger at the Professor. Freud described himself as in the "uncomfortable but unavoidable position of criticizing my friend Jones, expressing my dissatisfaction with his actions toward various persons, finding fault with his actions as director of the Press."

Freud said he would not attend the next Committee meeting, so the members could "enter into direct relations with one another as equals." Further, "Jones should allow the brief analysis that he had with Ferenczi back then to be competed." The letter goes on at length about the possibility of moving the Verlag to Berlin, emphasizing that Rank is its sole director. "I find no reason to cast reproach on Rank, who as always is doing his best. I don't think it would occur to any of you to do so, were unrelated affects not clouding our friendly relations." Freud, symbolic primal father, somewhat ailing but very much alive, did not want to be "put in the role of old Attinghausen" (Nov. 26), who, on his deathbed, admonishes those present to remain united in their struggle for freedom (Schiller's *William Tell*).

Jones wrote a long Rundbrief response on December 4:

> Professor's conclusion is that Abraham and I display a neurotic response to a normal stimulus applied by Rank, so that the remedy would lie in our recognizing our neuroses on the one side and the impeccable correctness of Rank on the other. For me, on the contrary, the reaction seems much more a normal, though delayed, response to a long series of instances where Rank has shown grave discourtesy and lack of consideration. . . . Like Abraham, I could not believe that Professor actually read the Vienna Rundbriefe [co-authored and typed by Rank] and was surprised to learn from his letter that he did so. . . . If in these circumstances I, who after all have had some, need analysis, then how much truer must this be for Rank, who has had none.[5]

On December 15 Freud sent a four-page letter in his own hand to quash any suspicion that he let Rank speak for him. Rebutting Jones, he said, "In 15 years of consistently intimate working relationship with Rank the idea scarcely occurred to me that he needed an analysis. And with that let me shut up."

On December 20, Rank addressed the Committee in his own long Rundbrief, "for which I had to sacrifice an entire afternoon." Thanking Professor

for his support, he challenges "dear Karl" and "dear Ernest" on administration, finances, and the connection between the Verlag and the Press, which
he insists must be severed, letting the Press stand on its own. He writes with
authority, energy, and indignation, asking his colleagues

> to concentrate on the difficulty and responsibility of my position as intensely as
> I do every day and every hour. This is the surest way to keep you from finding
> fault with me in petty details or making difficulties for me, given that for years
> I've been doing almost nothing except fighting a series of immense difficulties
> in the interest of psychoanalysis. I believe I can say that so far I've been suc-
> cessful, not without despairing sometimes, feeling crippling exhaustion and
> tiredness, given the enormity of the task and my own small powers. In such
> times and situations I wanted our friendship to assist me, but each of my com-
> ments has been placed under the magnifying glass of critical judgment so I've
> been blamed when things did not go entirely smoothly. I think we should be
> glad that much is going well in the first place; where there are problems or mis-
> takes, we should help one another. I probably need not assure you that you'll
> find in me the old friend and helper of former days, but I ask that you not make
> me responsible for anything and everything that occurs in the psychoanalytic
> movement. . . .
>
> In a business, one hand and one will must direct everything. Then things
> either go well or poorly, otherwise nothing will happen at all! Perhaps you'll
> see in this another example of my autocratic tendencies, but there is nothing I
> can do about it. That's the way it is when one has to deal with various people,
> and the more people one has to deal with, all the more energetically must the
> one director know how to effect his will (obviously not in opposition to reason,
> but in opposition to the numerous opinions of the others). Can you imagine
> how it would be with a newspaper if one employee said he didn't like the font
> and that another should be used, if another employee criticized the paper, a
> third the contents, and a fourth the editing? Yet that is how things have been
> with the Press until now, and that is why it has accomplished nothing.

After several more long paragraphs, Rank joins with Freud to welcome the
Moscow psychoanalytic group, as they had the Americans. "I cannot imagine that the Muscovites are worse, analytically or personally, than the New
York group was upon its acceptance, and indeed it is precisely due to that
acceptance that we could influence that group over time." He reports that

Eitingon visited Paris and is favorably impressed with Dr. LaForgue, "whom our member Sokolnicka will try to assess." Rank concludes, "Heartiest greetings and best wishes for Christmas and the New Year, in the spirit of our old friendship."

As the Verlag separates itself from the English Press, Freud sides openly with Rank about who needs analysis. Battle lines are clear between the southern and northern contingents of the Committee: Vienna and Budapest versus Berlin and London.

Chapter 13

Birth of the Mother

January to June 1923

*Psychoanalysis has developed, as is well known, in the course of almost thirty years,
from a simple medical method of treatment of certain neurotic disturbances
to an extensive scientific theoretic system that is slowly but steadily growing
and seems to lead to a new interpretation of life.*
—Ferenczi and Rank, *Development of Psychoanalysis*

Schism increased in the Committee for months before it would meet—without Freud. In January the swords came out. Jones wrote to Abraham, "I have renounced the hope of leading the Professor to any sort of objectivity where Rank is concerned. One must recognize with regret that even Freud has his human frailties and that age is bringing with it one-sidedness of vision and diminution of critical power." Freud wrote Ferenczi that he and Rank had managed the divorce of Press and Verlag, "while Jones would rather see the old gloomy condition perpetuated. . . . The separation has not been easy for us either. . . . Jones is in many respects a personality unsuited to be a leader." For his part Ferenczi distrusted the English and the Americans, and he saw Abraham as one who "grouses about every formal triviality" and Sachs as too ready to "bury the hatchet."[1]

Freud had surgery on April 20 to remove a growth from his mouth. Attributing it to his beloved cigars, he minimized this, though suspecting it was more than leukoplakia. Without telling his family, he went to an outpatient clinic for oral surgery. There were complications. Martha and Anna were called. They found him sitting on a chair, covered with blood. He was assigned the only available bed, with a deaf-mute dwarf as roommate. Hours later, the bleeding started again. Freud's roommate rushed for help, probably saving his life. "My father, the dwarf and I spent the night together," Anna recalled. "He was weak from loss of blood, half-drugged with medicines and in great pain."[2]

Rank informed the Committee inaccurately on May 1, along with regular business: "The Professor himself unfortunately had to undergo a small operation last week; it was a leukoplakia of the oral mucosa (inside left cheek), caused by heavy smoking, that had to be removed because it annoyed him. The Professor had to interrupt his work a few days, having difficulty eating and speaking, but he finds himself well again and working for a few days." The lesion was on the right palate and jaw, not the left cheek. Felix Deutsch had seen it and thought it was cancer, but did not share that with Freud, though he probably told Rank.

A few days later Freud got a gift for his sixty-seventh birthday: the draft manuscript of Rank's *The Trauma of Birth and Its Meaning for Psychoanalysis*. Its dedication:

SIGM. FREUD
Explorer of the Unconscious
Creator of Psychoanalysis
Dedicated on 6 May 1923

Early analysts ignored both sides of the mother-child relationship, mother being passive and primarily the object of male sexual desire and competition. Rank brought a new perspective on mother as emotionally nurturing for the child and powerful in her own right. When the Berliners later attacked Rank, Ferenczi quoted Freud's first reaction to the book: "I don't know if 33 or 66 percent of it is true; in any case, this is the most significant advance since the discovery of psychoanalysis. Someone else would have made himself independent with this."[3]

But Rank was favoring therapy over research. For Freud, psychoanalysis was primarily a method of scientific research into the unconscious and the basis for a general theory of mind. "This need to help is lacking in me because I did not lose anyone whom I loved in my early years." Therapy was secondary and he disparaged it, although it provided his income: "Regrettably, only a few patients are worth the trouble we spend on them, so that we are not allowed to have a therapeutic attitude, but we must be glad to have learned something in every case."[4] Freud warned against a *furor sanandi*—a passionate desire to cure. Such aims were often diagnosed as reaction-formation. For instance, the urge to alleviate suffering might mask sadism; exaggerated militarism might cover up tenderness. Though he often broke the rules himself, Freud urged strict objectivity for practitioners, a blank screen suitable for scientific research.

> I cannot advise my colleagues too strongly to model themselves during the psychoanalytic treatment on the surgeon, who puts aside all feelings, even his human sympathy, and concentrates his mental forces on the single aim of performing the operation as skillfully as possible. . . . The justification for requiring this emotional coldness in the analyst is that it creates . . . for the doctor a desirable protection for his own emotional life and for the patient the largest amount of help we can give him today. . . . The doctor should be opaque to his patients and, like a mirror, should show them nothing but what is shown to him.[5]

Freud was as adamant about the Oedipus complex in a footnote to *Three Essays on the Theory of Sexuality* (4th ed., 1920). He regularly updated this important text, first published in 1905.

> It has justly been said that the Oedipus complex is the nuclear complex of the neuroses, and constitutes the essential part of their content. It represents the peak of infantile sexuality, which, through its after-effects, exercises a decisive influence on the sexuality of adults. Every new arrival on this planet is faced by the task of mastering the Oedipus complex; anyone who fails to do so falls a victim to neurosis. With the progress of psychoanalytic studies the importance of the Oedipus complex has become more and more clearly evident; its recognition has become a shibboleth that distinguishes the adherents of psychoanalysis from its opponents.

The Developmental Aims of Psychoanalysis

For Ferenczi and Rank, therapy took precedence over scientific research as the aim of psychoanalytic practice. The title of their 70-page *Developmental Aims of Psychoanalysis* was shortened to *The Development of Psychoanalysis* when Caroline Newton translated it into English in 1925. An American social worker who spent two years in Vienna, she was analyzed by both Freud and Rank and became a member of the Vienna Psychoanalytic Society. In her preface she notes that Ferenczi and Rank worked on the book in 1922 and revised it after the Berlin Congress. "Dr. Rank and Dr. Ferenczi are admittedly Professor Freud's most brilliant and original followers, but the *Entwicklungsziele der Psychoanalyse* attracted a quite special attention. Both men, in addition to their other great contributions to psychoanalysis, are particularly skillful therapists and this book offers an opportunity for practicing analysts to see the development of analytic technique and the special angles of two of its most successful practitioners."

The epigraph alludes to almost 30 years of psychoanalysis. Freud first used the term in an 1896 article. Recent years, however, brought "increasing confusion," due to major growth in theory, while "the technical and therapeutic factor which was originally the heart of the matter and the actual stimulus to every important advance in the theory has been strikingly neglected in the literature as well as in practice" (2). Ferenczi and Rank credit Freud often, even as they offer a paradigm shift. They did not take him for granted, and he read their drafts—with some misgivings.

Ferenczi's *active therapy* meant assigning or prohibiting behavior in order to bring out repressed feelings and memory. The *transference* to the analyst provides material for understanding *repressed* elements—memory and feelings. Transference develops in the analytic situation, opening pathways to interpretation and insight, but it includes *resistance*, the involuntary obstruction that contains essential clues to the neurosis and is a major focus of analysis. The term *acting out* refers to behavior to be stopped because it discharges feelings that must be dealt with in therapy. Common examples are drinking, tardiness, forgetting, pursuing an inappropriate relationship, and as Ferenczi discovered, unconscious sexual release. Acting out interferes with *remembering* and may involve a *compulsion to repeat*. Freud had written about *abreaction* (strong emotional reaction to an event or memory) in his work with Breuer. He wrote on repetition and remembering in 1914, and focused on it in *Beyond the Pleasure Principle* (1920). Ferenczi's active therapy, supported by Rank, made emotional experience—repeated in the session—central in treatment. Emotion, here and now, was more important for healing than interpretation.

In his chapter "The Analytic Situation," Rank introduces the element of time. He offers "a very general definition of psychoanalysis . . . *as an individually determined process of definite duration in the libido development of the patient*. The task of the analyst consists of watching the process of the automatic unwinding of the libido—which, like the organic process of healing, takes place within a definite time and contains crises" (6).

Rank calls the active therapist a "catalyzer." Citing Freud, he describes libido attachment to the therapist—transference—as a reproduction of the infantile attachment to mother, the resolution of which is "weaning of the libido" (12). To achieve this, the analyst sets a time for ending (13). The patient protests, claiming that the treatment will fail, when in fact it will only fail if separation is not accomplished. Some patients will try to prolong the ordeal, others to shorten it. Rank welcomes the regression and uses the resistance, which is reproduction rather than remembering. The following illustrates Rank's writing style, often hard to summarize. We see the beginnings of ego, emotion, cognition, will, early childhood issues, and relationship therapy.

The first phase of every analysis represents an education of the ego. . . . In a later phase, after the transference has developed, the libido, the development of which was arrested in childhood, fully unfolds; in the weaning or deprivation phase, the ego energy or forces proceeding from the new ego ideal again see to it that the newly awakened desires adjust themselves to reality. . . . Without the help of these ego forces, and without some natural egoism, the final task of psychoanalysis, the weaning from the cure, would be impossible. For in this phase the problem is to get the patient, with the help of the love for the analyst, to give up this love. . . . The libido, as it frees itself from the cure, seeks out new interests in life. We see the process of sublimation that in ordinary life requires years of education, take place before our eyes at the end of the cure in the shortest time, without any particular guidance being needed. (20)

Noting the ambivalence of patients toward separation at the end of treatment, Ferenczi and Rank concluded that these strong emotions derived from an earlier developmental period, before the Oedipal phase, that had not been adequately analyzed. "As a result, in some cases, the actual analytic task was neglected." This left a gap: "deeper layers of mental life" were unexamined.[6] The aim of therapy, they wrote, "does not consist either in the verification of the 'Oedipus complex,' or in the simple repetition of the Oedipus situation in the relation to the analyst, but rather in setting free and detachment of the infantile libido from fixation on its first objects." Interpreting all the patient's emotional suffering as fear of paternal castration is a mask, "a protection against further analysis."[7] The castration complex comes under attack.

Active therapy changed the emphasis from "wishing to understand every-thing at once, everything that the patient says or does and to explain it to him." It was a mistake—all too common—to interpret every dream as though the point were to prove the correctness of the theory. It was the "difference between seeking memories for the purpose of reaching the affects, and pro-voking the affects for the sake of uncovering the unconscious." Ferenczi and Rank transmit their challenge firmly but gently: "We can see why psycho-analysis as a science had first to go through a phase of understanding before it could come to a full appreciation of the factor of experience." Their chapter ends: "A correctly executed psychoanalysis is from this point of view a social process, a 'mass structure of two,' according to Freud . . . the analyst must take the place of the most important persons in the patient's environment."[8]

Ferenczi and Rank add, "We believe, moreover, in general that affects in order to work convincingly must be revived, i.e., made actually present. . . . The analyst must always take into account that almost every expression of his patient springs from several periods, but he must give his chief attention to the present reaction." They minimize the past, including "historical, cultural and phylogenetic analogies," putting the future in the hands of the patient who is "sufficiently enlightened about his past and present mental strivings." Analysts ought not be "filling the gaps in the memory of the patient with knowledge . . . a fatal mistake." Another common mistake: to equate negative transference with resistance, which must be analyzed; so must strong positive transference. They mention that ego analysis has been neglected in therapy, "for which Freud has recently given valuable hints." While noting the limita-tions of hypnosis, they value the constructive use of suggestion, ubiquitous in medicine.[9]

Ferenczi and Rank end their book with an encomium to Hippocrates via Freud and Darwin and to the benign kinship between art and science.

> The most important advance in psychoanalysis consists finally in a great in-crease of consciousness . . . such an important step in the development of man-kind that it may actually be regarded as a biologic advance that for the first time takes place under a kind of self-control.
>
> Under the influence of this increase in consciousness the physician, who has developed from the medicine man, sorcerer, charlatan, and magic healer,

and who at his best often remains somewhat an artist, will develop increasing knowledge of mental mechanisms, and in this sense prove the saying that medicine is the oldest art and the youngest science. (68–69)

Ernest Jones was vigilant about ideological fidelity. He tells of meeting Otto and Beata in Switzerland in March 1919, when she was four months pregnant. He wrote decades later that Rank "astonished me by remarking in a dismal tone that men were of no importance in life; the essence of life was the relationship between mother and child." He adds that Rank gave a paper at the VPS two years later about marriage, saying that relations between husband and wife "always repeated in essence those between mother and child (on both sides alternately)."[10]

'The Trauma of Birth'

When Helene was born in August 1919, Rank was 35, Tola 23. Jones became a father at 41 in 1920 to Gwenith. Sigmund and Martha Freud were 31 and 26, respectively, at the birth of Mathilde, their eldest, in 1887. The Freuds eventually had six children, the Ranks only one.

In the spring of 1923, Rank's daughter was almost four years old; he was 39, a prolific contributor to the literature of psychoanalysis and to the movement, an analyst and a teacher of analysts. He was optimistically broadening Freud's work, with its grounding in biology and its many connections to art.

Though consonant with *The Development of Psychoanalysis*, Rank's *Trauma of Birth* is more theoretical and provocative. Appearing in German at the same time, *Development* was published in English in 1925, *Trauma* only in 1929.

Rank views birth as a traumatic separation, psychological as well as physical, that reechoes through life: in weaning and walking, forming and losing relationships, joining and separating from groups, and facing death. He credits Freud, in a footnote to the 1909 edition of *Dreams,* with the observation that birth is the first and definitive prototype of anxiety.[11] Rank points to difficult breathing as the physical trigger; though his emphasis is on psychological separation, he includes obstetrical difficulty as a factor. In Freudian fashion he cites cases in which patients reveal, through fear of animals, a conflicted wish to be back in the womb. The common childhood fear of small creatures that disappear into holes reflects ambivalence toward female genitals and the womb. Rank ends the preface saying that the purpose of his work "is to draw attention to this *biologically based law of the form that determines the content.* . . . This we owe to the instrument of investigation and to the way of thinking that Freud has given us in Psychoanalysis."

In chapter 1, "The Analytic Situation" (the same title as the second chapter of *Development*) Rank notes that patients nearing the end of treatment have recurrent dreams of mother and birth: "It is proved then, that the essential part of the work of analysis, the solving and freeing of the libido 'neurotically' fixed on the analyst, is really neither more nor less than allowing the patient to repeat with better success in the analysis the separation from the mother. . . . *The analysis finally turns out to be a belated accomplishment of the uncompleted mastery of the birth trauma*" (4–5).

Freud had not stated criteria for ending analysis, though in the Wolf Man case he recommended a time limit for obsessive-compulsive patients. As in *Development*, Rank suggests that the analyst set a time limit for the transference—mother fixation—to be resolved. During the end phase the patient "repeats automatically the new severance from the mother (substitute) figure, in the form of the reproduction of his own birth."[12] The biological trauma ends fetal bliss and inaugurates psychological personhood; by analogy, ending analysis does the same. Since Rank was never analyzed, his conclusion is based on his work as an analyst, observations of other analysts, and his own experience as husband and parent. Some of his text is strikingly feminist.

> It has been noticed, especially in recent times, that our whole mental outlook has given predominance to the man's point of view and totally neglected the woman's. . . . We tacitly represent sexual relations only from the man's point of view . . . from an insufficient understanding of woman's sexual life . . . expressing the primal repression that tries to degrade and deny woman both socially and intellectually on account of her original connection with the birth trauma. . . . We believe that we shall reinstate the high estimation of woman that was repressed simultaneously with the birth trauma, and we can do this by freeing her from the weight of the curse on her genitals. (36–37)

Love and fear of the powerful mother, says Rank, precedes and biologically grounds the Oedipus complex. After birth and weaning, castration fear is demoted to "the third most important repetition of the primal trauma of separation." Only then is the Oedipus complex amenable to dissolution, leading the patient to become independent of the internalized father and to reach full sexual and emotional maturity. "The primal taboo is the maternal genital which from the beginning onwards is invested with ambivalent feeling." In mythological terms, the freeing of Theseus from the Labyrinth, by means of a navel string, symbolizes the birth of "the hero, and his detachment from the ancient primal mother [*Urmutter*]." The primal repression is failure to accept one's own birth, "clinging to the mother." In response to a draft of *Trauma,* Ferenczi sent Rank a note: "Your presentation of the ideal Greek human being and his detachment from the primal mother in art is one of the most brilliant parts of your work."[13]

Birth trauma symbolizes the ego's discovery of itself and its separation first from the mother, and then, in therapy, from the analyst-midwife, who is a temporary assistant ego. Rank correlates psychological birth with consciousness of anxiety, the newborn's first emotional experience. In this is the prototype of all subsequent anxiety, including fear of death, the final separation. Conversely, sexual intercourse enables couples to recover prenatal bliss. Women can fully experience the mother in themselves by giving birth. Men invest more of themselves in cultural and artistic productions.

Toward the end of therapy the patient feels like a newborn. Helplessness in the face of loss and differentiation is converted by the skills of the analyst-midwife into the patient's self-creation, or autopoesis: giving birth, consciously, to one's self. By willing to be oneself within a relationship, by accepting and affirming one's difference and having it accepted by another, the patient discovers or recovers the creative ability to change.[14]

Having learned in the beginning and middle phases to bond with the analyst, the patient learns in the ending how to bear the trauma of loss as the price of selfhood. Physical and emotional separation from the therapist, "the *essential* part of the analytic work, is accomplished by a reproduction of the birth trauma, so that the patient loses his doctor and his own suffering at the same time, or, better expressed, must give up the doctor in order to lose his suffering."[15]

Noting Freud's comment that successful therapy exchanges neurotic misery for ordinary unhappiness, Rank states that Ferenczi's "active" therapy was not really new but had always been a silent part of analytic practice, which brought "an effect through volitional influence and a change resulting from it." Here is the seed of what Rank came to call "will therapy." By contrast, intellectual insight is a minor element, sometimes an impediment. "Even simple therapeutic action can be arrested by too much knowledge and too much insight." Insight, whether accurate or spurious, can block present feeling and engagement. One does not change the deepest unconscious, Rank pointed out: "The only result we can attain in psychoanalysis is a changed attitude of the ego to the unconscious."[16]

The analyst portrayed by Rank is not the "blank screen" that supposedly enhanced the power of transference. Though Freud counseled the stolid demeanor of the surgeon, he revealed feelings and opinions to analysands he liked, some of whom socialized with his family and one another. Ferenczi disclosed himself to a fault later on, ultimately doing "mutual analysis" with patients, which alienated Freud.

In *Trauma* Rank claims, "My analyses are some of the shortest in duration, lasting from four to eight months at the very longest" (6). Some therapists and obstetricians began recommending Caesarian section for prophylaxis.[17] Seeking medical confirmation, Rank went too far, allowing this idea to detract from his main thesis. Also, he contradicted himself on the importance of experience over knowledge: "It is technically possible to begin with the disclosure of the primal trauma, instead of giving the patient time automatically to repeat it at the end of the analysis. By this method one is able to sever the Gordian knot of the primal repression with one powerful cut" (213).

As Ferenczi and Rank point to a "new interpretation of life" in psychoanalysis, their experience, "reconceptualized," leads them to reinterpret therapy. For them, remembering is like a diary or a photograph, while emotional experience is living. They echo Kierkegaard's "Life can only be understood backwards; but it must be lived forwards." They anticipate Sartre's "Existence precedes essence." Such optimism counters the pessimism of Schopenhauer, whose idea of fate and powerful biological will against weak controlling intellect Thomas Mann found exactly duplicated in Freud's id versus ego.[18] Rank and Ferenczi imbibed more of Friedrich Nietzsche and Henri Bergson than did their mentor.

≈ Chapter 14 ≈

Under the Knife

June to December 1923

I already made the concessions to Rank that you consider right. I see that
one should leave him to his devices and would like best not to influence the work
[Trauma of Birth] at all anymore. His finding is great indeed, but he doesn't
grasp it yet, and can't put it into proper perspective. Put some pressure on him
to see that he certainly gets it done in the summer.
—Freud to Ferenczi, June 1, 1923

On June 14, Ferenczi wrote Freud that "Rank is highly pleased about the concessions. . . . I, too, think that his finding can still achieve undeniable significance. I wrote him that I see the *etiological primacy of the Oedipus complex in the neurosis* as unshaken." Ferenczi met Freud's shibboleth test.

On June 19, Freud's beloved Heinele, 4½-year-old son of his late daughter Sophie, died of tuberculosis. He had been living in Vienna with his Aunt Mathilde. This killed something in Freud, he said, so thenceforth he could form no new emotional attachments. "He meant the future to me and thus has taken the future away with him." Jones said it was the only time Freud was known to have wept. "I myself was aware of never having loved a human being, certainly never a child, so much. . . . I find this loss very hard to bear. I don't think I have ever experienced such grief; . . . everything has lost its meaning for me."[1]

Deeply bereaved, and with a painful mouth, Freud began his summer vacation in July with Minna, in Lavarone, in the Italian Dolomites. Martha, with daughters Anna and Mathilde (and husband), came later. Rank and Ferenczi, with spouses and Helene, 4, went to Klobenstein, in the Italian Tyrol.

Klobenstein, Hotel "Post" ¶July 13, 1923

Lieber Herr Professor,

After reading your painful, sad letter [missing], I was ashamed to have bothered you with my complaining. Please accept this expression of my feelings as a sign of my sympathy.

We came here two days ago. Still not completely rested, and not feeling quite at home, we nevertheless enjoy the beautiful, very warm days, which are especially good for the child. As for me, I'm unaccustomed to "doing nothing" or "vacation work." So I'm waiting until the 15th, when a woman patient will arrive; the Ferenczis come on the 17th. Then the division of our days will go beyond the punctual meals provided by Herr Bemelmans. I needn't say anything more about the hotel here, which you know well, except that so far even your son-in-law Robert hasn't found anything that deserves to be skipped; he even shows flashes of enthusiasm on occasion. Incidentally, I find your daughter [Mathilde] like him, well recovered and in a better mood.

We were saddened to hear that your sister-in-law's condition leaves something to be desired; we can only hope the summer will bring some improvement. Since you write nothing about your own condition, you are presumably in good health, as is to be hoped.

Sachs has come here, too; it seems he's jealous of the time I spend with Ferenczi and he wants to be the third in the group. We've made an honest effort to find lodgings for him here, but I'm not sure that will work out; in all honesty, I wouldn't regret failure in this respect; we wouldn't like to experience another "Seefeld."

I left my manuscript [Trauma] with Storfer in Vienna, and it depends on him when and where (Vienna or Leipzig) it'll be printed. Technical and other problems remain to be solved. Anyway, I've arranged that when typesetting begins, proofs will be sent to you directly. I ask that you send them on to me with your comments. Ferenczi will also read a proof copy here, and I'll use everything for the final version.

From the complete works, production of the large Lectures is starting in Leipzig, but you are not to be disturbed with the proofreading.

With cordial greetings to you and your sister-in-law from both of us. Yours, Rank

"I have never had a depression before," Freud wrote Ferenczi on July 18, "but this must be one now."

Rank was also preparing *Analysis of Neuroses in Dreams*. This 230-page book presents his work with a young woman in 150 sessions over six months, the longest psychoanalytic case history published to date. Rank documents her ambivalent strivings in the end phase for staying and leaving, as she navigates between dread and hope, regress and progress, the desire to stay embedded in the analytic womb and the will for autonomy. "The conflict is only understandable and therapeutically solvable as a reproduction of the birth trauma, the separation from the mother, which has to repeat itself in the severance from the emotional fixation on the analyst." With the anguished dissolution of the transference, "the patient feels herself newborn, i.e., a reborn child."[2]

Besides his own writing, Rank prepared Freud's essays for sale separately. Freud wanted his writings to appear in theme-based anthologies released by the Verlag, so Rank also compiled *Studies on Literature and Art*. Also the Verlag brought out works on *Technique* and on *Metapsychology*. Anna Freud and A. J. Storfer joined Rank in editing *Collected Works*, in 10 volumes. Despite paper shortages and inflation, the Verlag released six more titles, including Freud's *Ego and Id*; Groddeck's *Book of the It*, and Reik's *One's Own and the Other God*.

Ferenczi, completing his book *Thalassa: A Theory of Genitality*, wrote Freud on July 25: "Rank's work has the effect of being a wet nurse in this; I'd like— also on account of the historically correct sequence—for my work to appear with his, if not before it." In *Thalassa*, named for a Greek sea goddess, Ferenczi argues that human life begins with the trauma of birth and is determined by a longing for the "sea-life" whence humans emerged: "The child, frightened, crying, shaken by the traumatic experience of birth, soon becomes lulled in this sleeping state which creates in him a feeling... as though no such tremendous shock had occurred at all. Freud has said, indeed, that the human being is not completely born; he is not born in the full sense, seeing that through going nightly to bed he spends half his life in, as it were, the mother's womb" (73).

Klobenstein ¶July 26, 1923

Lieber Herr Professor,

Cordial thanks for your kind lines and good wishes [missing], which unfortunately have not yet really come true. So far I've not been feeling quite well here; I'm unable to approach any type of work, though I can still enjoy doing nothing. We're leading a terribly unnatural life, which doesn't get more natural despite close contact with nature. It's hard for me to endure this "conflict of nature": there's a bit of every-thing, but nothing is complete.

News from the closer and wider world makes its way here sparsely. Of greatest interest for you is probably the fact that there is an Australian Journal of Psychology and Philosophy, of which two volumes, with strong analytical contents, have arrived. The editor is a Mr. Francis Anderson, a professor of philosophy in Sydney.

Before leaving I wrote Mrs. Riviere officially from the Verlag to convey your opin-ion. The letters must have crossed. Now she's written somewhat bitterly that she's taking note of this "information." She feels that things aren't looking good for her as Jones's Press has no money. By the way, Sachs discovered, another volume of the [International] Journal has supposedly just appeared. It's clear to me, too, that noth-ing will become of the Press. We'll hear a lot about this in August.

Incidentally, the partial Committee, assembled here, eagerly awaits your decision on the stay in August, since the selection of Annenheim [Germany] would change for the better our pre-meeting place and so, greatly, the summer plans of all of us. On the other hand, we're disturbed and worried about the meaning of [Dr.] Hajek's appearance this summer; hopefully just a special precaution. Please send some sooth-ing words about this soon in any case.

With deep regret we learned from Sachs of the latest passing in your family, and we express to you our sincere sympathy. [Theo, 18-year-old son of Mitzi, Freud's sister in Berlin, drowned.]

With all good wishes for the second portion of the summer, for you and your family, and cordial greetings to your sister-in-law and yourself.

Yours, Rank

Klobenstein, August 4, 1923

Lieber Herr Professor:

We're all glad you're free now, hopefully for September too, and that you feel so much better. If Lavarone is still as it was, you'll recall, this month should be more pleasant than last.

We hope so, too, but are still embroiled in plans: two venues could host the Com-mittee meetings, so we can't travel much, not knowing where we'll be during the second half of August. And we need to avoid Sachs: in the long run, he's just as hard to bear as the current stretch of cloudless (i.e., hot and dry) days.

My book is being typeset, and I hope you have the first galleys. If not, please advise me on a postcard: in that case, they were lost on the way from Gastein to Lavarone.

That would be a shame, for I'm eager to have your comments, but must finish typeset-
ting quickly if we are to be done before the demise of Germany [from soaring inflation].

The situation abroad is catastrophic for the Verlag: even after the latest key num-
ber of 30,000, the German book price vs. the Austrian price is 1700:7000, so it would
be best not to sell abroad. However, we should continue with production abroad as
long as possible, and that's what we're doing. (Gesamtausgabe [Collected Works] is
being typeset in Leipzig now.)

You presumably received the Zeitschrift, and the little book [Doestoevski] by
Neufeld. If you're missing anything, please make this known at the Verlag.

With best wishes for Lavarone to you and your dear ones, we greet you cordially.

Yours, Rank

Where is your sister-in-law, and how is she?

Klobenstein ¶August 10, 1923

Lieber Herr Professor:

Your kind invitation for the 8th crossed with an inquiry (postcard) from me; your
letter answers some of my questions.

Whether we come to Lavarone depends on so many intricate and personally com-
plicated questions, going in all directions, that I can't say right now—all the less since
my wife has been touring the Dolomites the last few days and is not expected back
until Monday. Perhaps on Monday I'd ask by telegram that the kind proprietor of
your hotel prepare for an invasion. Everything else you write about Lavarone sounds
better than here, where between 8:00 a.m. and 8:00 p.m. one actually can't go out due
to the heat, but can't do anything else sensible either.

Disregarding the place of the international meeting, which is not yet firm, Fe-
renczi's plans also play a role in our decisions; he wants to go to Karersee [Carezza,
Italy], but then would like the international meeting to be held there, so I'd have to go
to and from Lavarone again.

Ferenczi is doing his job of leaving me in peace most efficiently: he's working every
single day by himself—much more than I—so in a few days he'll finish the book he's
been delaying for so many years [Thalassa]. I only have the satisfaction of helping,
through my work, to surmount this difficult birth trauma as well.

Many thanks for your comments on my galleys. The core problem that you empha-
size I've intentionally saved for the end (penultimate section: "Psychoanalytic Knowl-
edge"). I really don't know whether I've got a clear solution, but it will be discussed, and
as stated, as the core of the whole thing.

The Verlag manages to continue operations, as you hopefully can see for yourself, despite all the shortages and dangers.

The third volume of Imago *is almost ready, and the Ferenczi issue [fiftieth birthday; Zeitschrift, no. 2 (1923)] will be ready for the Committee meeting.*

With cordial greetings to you and your dear family. Yours, Rank

P.S. I again request your sister-in-law's address; we'd like to ask about her condition.

P.S. 2. Children and Men: Responding to a Verlag announcement in Der Tag, a four-year-old girl appeared at the Verlag—alone—with 17,000 crowns in her hand to buy The Ego and the Id. *And the same day a certain Wachmann (Press—public prosecutor?) came in asking for Groddeck's* Book of the It.

Klobenstein, August 14, 1923

Lieber Herr Professor,

Your last news was such that I wanted very much to come to see you, even without your kind invitation. Meanwhile my wife returned yesterday evening from her Dolomites tour, and only today are we ready to discuss all our plans—on which, by the way, we've been working steadily since spring. In any case, I saw that we couldn't extricate ourselves from the Ferenczis without hurting their feelings, and since I didn't know whether it would be pleasant for you and your family if we came accompanied as usual, we had to abandon the plan for now, with heavy heart.

Today I made one last attempt to free up a few days to visit you myself during a tourist excursion, but this plan had to be abandoned since Ferenczi insisted on coming along—which we both think would create bad blood in the rest of the Committee, especially with Abraham and Sachs, who are also staying in the area.

So I have been "checkmated" here—literally and figuratively [matt also means "exhausted"]—where the heat's so oppressive one can't take a step outside during the day. With deep inner resistance to this entire "mad rush," I have finally declared myself agreeable to the following:

1. The first meeting will be at San Cristoforo on the 26th; from there, the Committee will come to Lavarone on the 29th to visit you.

2. Until then, I'll be practically interned here (at least that's how I feel), except I'll go a few days early to wander in the Dolomites; those few days are my summer recuperation time.

3. Meanwhile my wife and child (and Mrs. Ferenczi) will presumably go to Old Prague, where Urbantschitsch insists on taking us; I'll go there from Lavarone to pick them up.

4. Then I'd like to go to Vienna forthwith, where I'm due the first week of September (analyses!).

You can imagine how sorry my wife and I are that we can't visit you and your family, but the circumstances have become so intolerable that I can't budge without hitting barriers somewhere.

With cordial greetings from both of us to you and your dear family. Yours, Rank

*P.S. I just received, with appreciation, your postcard of the 13th (yesterday) concerning corrections for the galleys [*Trauma*].*

On August 16, New York analyst A. A. Brill visited Freud in Lavarone, and the next day Ferenczi and Rank in Klobenstein. Brill, who was Jewish, had a rival in Horace Frink, a Gentile, for leadership of American psychoanalysis. Freud had analyzed Frink and viewed his wealthy new wife as a likely contributor to the cause. Brill told Ferenczi that Jones had sent him a letter denouncing Rank as "a swindling Jew."

Klobenstein ¶August 20, 1923

Lieber Herr Professor,

We were glad to hear that Brill found you healthy and happy. Otherwise, his visit was anything but pleasant. Beyond his news about Jones, he tried to convince us to take his side in his conflict with Frink, but immediately took to his heels, as is his wont, when he noticed that I don't entirely trust him either. I'll tell you about the entire remarkable episode when the opportunity arises.

I do regret that the mood in the Committee, already extremely tense, has been worsened further by Jones's behavior; I don't know what stand to take with him. In any case, considering the separation between Press and Verlag, I'd like to convince him that it'd be appropriate for him to pass on to Eitingon his business concerns with the Verlag. Whether we can defend ourselves against him in other ways as well, I can't judge alone.

Predictably, in the end we're still stuck here. I won't go to San Cristoforo until the 25th, and would like to meet Eitingon that day since he'll be playing an important role in mediating the various conflicts. I got a telegram from him, but couldn't make out the sender location (only Villa Imperiale), so I haven't been able to tell him my plans.

After Lavarone, and a quick tour of the Dolomites, I'll pick up my family here, and, as I said, I'll be in Vienna during the first week of September, since Verlag business is also pressing.

We plan to transfer production [Collected Works] right back to Vienna since in Germany high wages are likely to exceed world parity.

Today vacation begins. Up to now I was conducting an analysis; it doesn't concern me since I feel breaking off will be therapeutic; yet this was certainly one cause of my general dissatisfaction this summer. Now I very much look forward to seeing you and your family, I hope that your plans for Rome still remain firm.

With cordial greetings, Yours, Rank

On August 21, Ferenczi wrote Freud that he "revised with Rank—about five times—the 'joint work' [*Development*], about which we'd still like to talk to you." He reports that Rank read his theory of genitality [*Thalassa*] manuscript and would give it to Freud on request. "I hope the Committee meeting will conclude peacefully; Eitingon's presence, especially, will contribute much to it. I also hope we'll restore complete understanding between Rank and Abraham. With Jones things are more difficult, since personal factors also figure in there. But we think it's not yet time to act more energetically against him, although we want to call him to account for certain things."

On August 26, the Committee met without the Professor, at San Cristoforo, 2,000 feet below Freud's holiday residence at Lavarone. Until that day only Rank knew Freud's true diagnosis: malignant epithelioma. Felix Deutsch and Anna, visiting Freud, joined the Committee for supper. Dr. Deutsch had seen a malignant growth that required more surgery. Fearing that his patient would not consent, might even commit suicide, Deutsch reassured Freud but shared the hard facts with Anna and the Committee.

Jones wrote his wife, Katherine, that night, "The chief news is that F. has real cancer, slowly growing & may last for years. He doesn't know it & it is a most deadly secret. . . . We have spent the whole day thrashing out the Rank-Jones affaire. Very painful, but I hope our relations will now be better. . . . I expect Ferenczi will hardly speak to me for Brill has just been there & told him I had said R was a swindling Jew (strongly exaggerated)." Ferenczi later reflected on how difficult it was to persuade Abraham that Jones's anti-Semitism was incompatible with being on the Committee. Jones had written Brill in April: "Between ourselves, Rank has been somewhat deteriorating of late and has not been behaving quite straight. Also his general way of conducting business was distinctly Oriental."[3]

On August 28 Jones described the Committee to his wife as "hours talking & shouting till I thought I was in Bedlam." The others said he was wrong and neurotic in regard to Rank. "A Jewish family council sitting on one sinner must be a great affair, but picture it when the whole five insist on analyzing him on the spot & all together!" He was almost forced to resign from the Committee and was on probation, ordered to resume his analysis with Ferenczi in Budapest.[4] Jones wrote about the events in his Freud biography: "It appears that I had made some critical remarks about Rank—I cannot remember now to whom—and he at once brought up this unfriendliness on my part. I apologized for having hurt his feelings, but he refused to accept this and demanded that I be expelled from the Committee. This the others naturally would not allow, Abraham in particular defending me, and there was a very painful scene with Rank in uncontrollable anger and myself in puzzled silence."[5] Jones dropped the following paragraph from his final text:

> As was to be expected in such circumstances, he added the accusation of my
> being anti-Semitic, and my comment that Jews would be happy if they had to
> do with gentiles less so made no difference. He quoted a sentence of mine in a
> letter I had written to Brill, which had presumably reached him via Freud, in
> which I was said to have complained of "Rank's Semitic behavior." Fortunately
> I had kept a copy of the letter, in which the fatal word had not occurred and I
> was able to prove later that this was a rather malicious addition of Brill's. But
> even Freud when we met shook his head and agreed that my marrying a Jewish
> wife was a suspicious circumstance! Against such accusations, springing from
> such emotional depths, it is useless to protest.[6]

On September 12 Jones wrote to thank Freud for handling the Committee crisis so well. Though claiming he had been unfairly treated, Jones acknowledged some fault: "You shall see that the help you gave me will bear good fruit, for I am not going to be content with the present unsatisfactory state of my psychology."

The Committee knew that Freud planned to take Anna to his beloved Rome for two weeks. They, with her consent, supported the plan. Back in Vienna in September, Freud was told the truth about his cancer. While in Rome, Freud received a newspaper clipping from the United States stating that he had a fatal illness. He wrote to Eitingon on September 11: "I read that I am slowly dying, no longer working and that all my pupils are going to my spiritual son Dr. Otto Rank."

Prof. Dr. Freud Berggasse 19 Vienna IX ¶September 26, 1923

Lieber Herr Doktor

Today at the meeting of [Drs.] Hajek, Pichler, and Deutsch it was decided I should undergo another operation in the next few days. I'm promised renewed energy in about four weeks. This new development necessitates additions to our last discussion. But on Friday evening the Lévy's are coming from Budapest. Therefore I'm writing this letter. Two further remarks:

1) The newspaper advertisements on the cover of the joint edition of Beyond/ Group Psy/ and Ego/Id are too tasteless. I'd be glad if you got rid of them.

2) Over time, your briefcase has become essential to me, but now it needs repairs and new stuffing. Our attempts to obtain similar blotter paper have been unsuccessful, so please reveal to Anna the secret of the origin of this precious material so that she can have it produced during my convalescence. Don't deal with it yourself.

Perhaps I'll see you very soon. Cordially yours, Freud

Freud wrote Jones the same day, "Now I hope you will drop the affair and I'll do whatever I can to influence Rank in the sense of kindness and tolerance.... Another practical item. I have made up my mind to make my nephew Bernays my agent in America and let him mind the American rights of my books." And to Eitingon: "A second operation is needed: partial resection of the upper jaw, since my dear neoplasm emerged there. The operation will be done by Prof. Pichler, the greatest expert in these matters." Freud underwent two operations: October 4, to remove and examine enlarged glands that showed no metastases, and October 11 for the major resection. The best prosthesis was still inadequate and "eating, smoking, talking could be carried on only with great effort and pain.... Freud's physical state, which varied from severe discomfort to real torment, persisted more or less constantly over the next 16 years." Freud allowed only Anna to perform the daily chore of removing, cleaning, and reinserting the prosthesis. "He made a pact with her at the beginning that no sentiment was to be displayed; all that was necessary had to performed in a cool matter-of-fact fashion with the absence of emotion characteristic of a surgeon."[7]

On October 22 Jones wrote Freud: "It has been an inexpressible joy to receive the excellent report of your progress—the brilliant success of the operation, the excellent prognosis.... And now you have the joy of convalescing, every day being an improvement on the last and leading back to your wonted energy and life-interests. How good to know that!" He then raised one problem: the American rights. "As it is a critical and urgent matter I propose to send Mrs. Riviere to Vienna to discuss with you both as soon as your health permits."

Vienna ¶October 25, 1923 [hand delivered]

Lieber Herr Professor,

I've taken the liberty of enclosing a letter that arrived today from Jones. Should you not wish for this visit, please inform Jones or Mrs. Riviere directly by telegram so as to avoid delay.

Today you also returned to me the previous letter from Jones. I would like to know whether I should answer it in your name—and what I should say—or whether you're leaving it up to me to answer in the name of the Verlag so you can discuss your own affairs in a later discussion between yourself and the Press.

Finally, may I remind you that the title page for "Five Lectures" hasn't come back to the Verlag; we don't know whether this means you're in agreement or you overlooked the request.

With best greetings. Yours, Rank

P.S. I'm very glad to know that you are back at home; I also hope to have a chance to see you soon.

Prof. Dr. Freud Berggasse 19 Vienna IX ¶October 25, 1923

Lieber Herr Doktor,

I was just starting to write to you when Paula brought me the letter you wrote today. It concerns the same affair, for today, through a special envoy, Jones also presented me with the threat. It would be simpler to discuss this in person, which can be arranged if you say it's essential, but now I feel so weak and in need of isolation that I'd prefer to spare myself such an encounter.

The outrageous positive pronouncements Jones dedicates to my condition in his letter are in stark contrast with my actual state. It is actually refreshing to recall that in his private comments on the topic, e.g. to Money-Kyrle or to Mrs. Riviere, he refrains from such effusiveness.

Concerning the matter itself, I think there's very little to say. I certainly can't risk the English members saying my hesitation has blown out the light of life for the Press. I'll have to give in, although I don't believe a word of the whole affair. I suppose things will go as they did with your translation proposals. We shall do without; we shall have no benefit from this—neither money, nor publicity, nor good nor bad translations.

If you share my view, I authorize you to write Jones that I'm leaving the American rights with the Press until the end of 1925. If in my opinion, and possibly in yours, the Press has accomplished nothing by then, I'll reclaim these rights.

Please give Jones this answer only if you agree completely. Otherwise, please let me know your comments, and I'll write to you via Anna. Tomorrow we'll send the telegram declaring the trip unnecessary. ["Visit inconvenient reception impossible no danger for Press."]

When Dr. Meyer is with you, please let me know his address and tell him he'll be getting back three books he suddenly sent me for absolutely no logical reason.

In the current confusion I have really misplaced the list of titles you wrote about. Please send it to me again. With cordial thanks for all the signs of interest and all the expressions of restraint, Yours, Freud

Dr. Otto Rank ¶October 26, 1923

Lieber Herr Professor,

It's very hard for me to agree with the position you take in your letter about the Press business. Of course it'd be simpler to discuss this with you, but I believe your subjective happiness is more important. Anyway, the whole situation is not as pressing as Jones suddenly makes it out to be. For me, it's simply a question of how I answer him; perhaps I should briefly tell you how things would have been had you expressed no opinion now. Thus you will best be able see where the difficulties lie for me. I would inform Jones:

1) It's not only the Press that wants to survive, but the Verlag and the movement too. Thus far, the Press has only hindered both. Recently American publishers (Jelliffe, Brentano's, and others) through your nephew have contacted the Verlag in order to get the American translation rights. If they agree to our physical and intellectual conditions (translation, etc.), the Verlag sees no reason not to take advantage of this source of income—for itself and to promote the movement. The Press could also participate in free competition.

In his long letter to me, Jones mentions contracts the Verlag has made with the Press. I don't know what he means, beyond your books, for no other contracts were signed, although at the time (about one year ago), Rickman apparently sent his drafts to all the authors (Abraham, Ferenczi, Reik, me, etc.).

As for the contracts concerning your books, for example, to this day it's been impossible to get from the Press the Lectures *contract, and of course there's even less of a trace of money. Thus the Verlag is free to accept any translation proposal from an*

American publisher, and will do this to the maximum—without worrying about the Press, i.e., its grumblings, which don't mean a thing.

2) As an author, I repeat my earlier stand: in no way am I bound to the Press, and I have the right to make decisions about English translations freely, for I've already been harmed enough by the Press and by Jones, who has blocked me from acquiring American translations, yet has <u>not</u> published the works in English himself. (The Artist is being translated, and I have two separate translation proposals for The Incest Theme.*)*

3) As for the other Verlag authors, I can't be responsible for them since the rights are shared. If an author should ask, I couldn't honestly advise him against my own feelings. If the author preferred the Press for some reason, the Verlag would have no objections, but would insist on dealing with the Press in a purely businesslike manner, i.e., demanding appropriate payment and compliance with a specific schedule.

4) Practically, though, the situation is such that the Press and—as I know very well—all the other publishers are mainly interested in your works. Thus if the Verlag wishes to propagate translations of other authors in America, it would also have to offer the publisher in question one or another of your books, or raise that possibility. (That's always been the case, even with German publishers.)

For the Verlag it's irrelevant whether you grant all the American rights for your books to the Press or to your nephew: in neither case would the Verlag retain any discretionary rights with which to reward other publishers.

As the Verlag director I am, to an extent, disinterested, but perhaps in a better position to be objective. Yet I'm sure that the decision must be made in favor of your nephew. Whether you'll give the Press a chance is still up to you: the Verlag and I will make no further decisions about this.

[The last page is missing.]

On October 28, Ferenczi wrote Freud to ask about some passages in *Ego and Id.* "This not easy reading is becoming especially interesting to me by virtue of the fact that in several places I think I have found the actual theoretical foundation for several practical-technical suggestions which Rank and I made in our joint work."

Internationale Psychoanalytische Verlag Vienna IX ¶October 29, 1923
Lieber Herr Professor:

Since taking a position on your suggestion in the matter of the Press is not as simple as saying yes or no, and since corresponding about this also seems too complex, I sent the enclosed temporary message to Jones today [missing]. I'd suggest you hold your final decision about this until we can discuss this unpleasant affair again for the umpteenth time.

Nor do I want you to be disturbed by this in any way during your convalescence, when you require tranquility, since I don't consider this whole matter as urgent as Jones portrays it in his letter.

My standpoint is that the Verlag will no longer delay the gallows for the Press any further—to the detriment of the Verlag itself.

With best greetings. Yours, Rank

P.S. Today I got a letter from Eitingon, who's delaying his Vienna visit until Christmas. On the other hand, Sachs announces he'll arrive Wednesday for a few days.

Please don't think that any news about your condition is escaping from me. I've been even more circumspect than usual, for I've had bad experiences with the reports I was obliged to deliver to the Committee [at San Cristoforo].

With most cordial wishes and greetings. Yours, Rank

On October 30 Freud amended his will, thinking that his worsening condition, with impaired speech and hearing, would keep him from earning sufficient income as a practicing analyst. "He asked that his children renounce their share in their 'anyhow modest inheritance' in favor of their mother, and that Anna's dowry be increased to £ 2000."[8]

Vienna Internationale Psychoanalytische Verlag ¶November 5, 1923 [typed]
Lieber Herr Professor:

About preparing your American publication, the remaining manuscript of which I think was sent off today, I'd like to make a suggestion:

That we begin this month with typesetting the first issue of the new, combined journals. For the first issue, I'd write a brief editorial foreword justifying the new arrangement and the new tasks the journal envisions for itself. I've been thinking of this foreword as very brief—2 pages at most—and it just occurred to me that we could insert, as the first contribution in the first issue, the historical article on psychoanaly-

sis that you just wrote, just as Imago opened with the article "The Development and Goals of Psychoanalysis." We'd of course explain the original purpose of the article to account for any peculiarities in form, since purpose may determine form.

Since you might not immediately approve this, let me justify the new arrangement further: the journal would then show that it's aimed not only at psychoanalysts—as the publication of the Association, it clearly is aimed at them—but also at wider circles of the public, to acquaint them with psychoanalysis; in so doing, and to increase their understanding of progress, it will convey the historical development and previous events of psychoanalysis. If this came about through you, it would benefit the entire undertaking, and I'd like to say that I'd have asked you to write such an article, had it not already been available. Please comment as soon as possible since, as stated, we'd like to start typesetting the issue this month. In any case, I recommend that you convey to the American, to whom you wanted to write about the release of Gesammelte Werke, that you retain the German rights for this article. (If we print it in the journal or elsewhere, we would, of course, cite the source.)

In conclusion, a few more details:

1.) Mr. Fagg submitted his article to me at your instigation, as he says, but he does not say whether he permits translation. Has he written you about this?

2.) I enclose a brief excerpt from the report on Ego and Id presented to the Berlin group by Sachs and Rado. Sachs asks whether it would be good for the authors to revise the report for the journal, in which case the omitted portions would of course be incorporated. I enclose this so you can decide.

3.) Please let me know the amount I borrowed from you (about four weeks ago in the Sanatorium [Auersperg]. It was seven pounds and an amount in dollars; I would like to ask you again about the dollar amount, since, in connection with the $20 something doesn't add up correctly. This is for my private information only.

4.) I enclose two letters that arrived today (Berlin, Budapest).

5.) Today you'll receive final galleys of Abraham's new book. If you can, please examine especially the second part (begins with galley 31); this is the work that Abraham presented to us, but much simplified and less schematized. You might convey your comments to the author, since he could perhaps make use of them before page proofs are done.

With cordial greetings. Respectfully yours, Rank

In early November, Committee members exchanged sharp letters over Ferenczi's charge that Jones had plagiarized a paper of his on autosuggestion. Abraham offered an Oedipal analysis of the problem: "You, dear Ernest, will probably remember our talk [at San Cristoforo] on your secret jealousy of Sándor and Otto as the favored oldest and the favored youngest son. In the end it is against the father and we all know that I tend to interpret both in-cidents as a result of the same affect."[9]

On November 12 Freud underwent surgery to excise malignant tissue found in a recent biopsy. Five days later he chose to undergo Steinach's reju-venation operation: ligation of the spermatic ducts, to increase testosterone secretion. There were no injectable sex hormones then, cancer was associ-ated with aging, so it was hoped that vasectomy would reduce chances of recurrence.[10]

On November 20, the day before Freud was due to go home, Rank visited him at the Sanatorium Auersperg. Freud recounted a dream about David Lloyd George (L.G.), British Prime Minister, 1916–22, a great orator called by his detractors "The Liar from Wales." Rank wrote an interpretation that night and a longer and clearer version the next day (underlined words are in English).[11]

Dr. Otto Rank Vienna ¶November 21, 1923

Lieber Herr Professor:

Last night an interpretation occurred to me of the "witty dream" you told me today. I'll take the liberty of sharing it with you, as I think it will amuse you. If, in this, I fall into what you regard as the deplorable error of psychoanalytic misuse, I'll comfort myself with the fact that you also do so in a dream by identifying yourself with L.G. (yes, he speaks about ego and id in the dream).

You dream the night before you return home from the sanatorium, specifically after the day (19th) when you wanted to start working again. In the dream you've already begun your work, and say to yourself: I've been silent long enough (like L.G.), and now I want to return to public life and my work—which, however, means to speak, and indeed to speak English (conducting analyses), in which the pronunciation is harder for us German speakers. Yet you know English as well as the great English orator. You even make jokes and puns in English.

That is, in the dream [see note for original wordplay in German] L.G. does this in your place, all the more in that he breaks one of your ground rules, namely, he mis-uses analysis in the service of politics. This means: "It's high time I return to work, and speak, for others do not understand me, but 'translate,' i.e. interpret me badly (the I and the It), and misuse psychoanalysis for their personal interests. The others understand nothing (nothing) or less than nothing (over-nothing)." (This is reminis-

cent of the progression: nothing, nothing, nothing at all!) Here, though, one notices that the "pun" relates to German: the Ich and the N-Ich-T, which presumably signifies the doubt: Will I be able to speak in English or not; will the others "understand" me or not? In the dream this question is resolved by the ego, which wants this, but not yet by the id (the organic!), which remains undiscussed. (The entire dream, with its character of a thought process, emanates more from the ego and the superego.)[12]

Perhaps this interpretation of the present ego-layer will provoke you to discover the position of psychology toward it—if that's possible—and I hope the deeper layers will reveal as decisive a will to heal as the ego-layer's will to work.

Cordially yours, Rank

[The letter of the night before ended]: "Of course that's only one meaning, the present meaning, of the dream—a meaning emanating from your ego and superego. What the id has to say about this is presumably harder to discover since the entire dream has more the character of a thought process [...]. But perhaps this interpretation will provoke you to think about this further. Here I mean "provoke" in a double sense, i.e. also in the sense of completing it, and I hope that even the deepest layers will reveal as decisive a will for recovery as the first level."

Freud concluded *The Ego and the Id*: "The id, to which we finally come back, has no means of showing the ego either love or hate. It cannot say what it wants; it has achieved no unified will. Eros and the death instinct struggle within it" (*S.E.,* 19:59).

On November 26, Freud replied to Rank's invitation to continue the dream interpretation, perhaps referring to the Frau Doni dream, which Rank had interpreted in 1905 (App. B). Now, spinning out Rank's puns regarding the *Über-Ich*, the murderous "super-ego," Freud looks via the text into Rank's own, perhaps guilty, unconscious. Freud's shorthand for dream, *Tr,* is shown as "dm."

Prof. Dr. Freud Berggasse 19 Vienna IX ¶November 26, 1923

Lieber Dr.

It's been a long time since you tried to interpret one of my dreams in an unusual, powerful analytic way. Since then much has changed; you have grown immensely and know so much more about me and the result is different. Your work gives me the opportunity to check where your assumption links to one of my associations, and, finally, I can focus on the interesting question of the standing of the superego.

I can't confirm everything you write (like a Sadger patient after enlightenment), but also have nothing to contradict. You correctly grasped the date and sequence of the dm.—it does concern an ideal return to the appointment for the 19th, from which I was kept by the [Steinach] operation. This operation will be abolished, as it were, with my imminent return home. It didn't happen, I was always at home, can start working as planned. Beyond this situation, two direct drm-causes are possible: a) I read in the newspaper about L.G.'s reappearance. b) Your letter about the special Dutch issue of the Zeitschrift *[1924, for G. Jelgersma, Leyden professor], as will be clear later, or even about the use of J's work. Both happened at once.*

There's no doubt about L.G.'s turning out to be me or disparaging others because they understand nothing, nor about the fact that the joke was actually conceived in German: I, nothing, over-nothing [Ich, nichts, über-nichts]. In the dm., in fact, only the nothing *was clear. The* over-nothing *was just interpolation.*

Now comes the question: against whom is the dm. directed? Directed mainly at no [sic] a certain person? The association refuses to answer, saying only Bonar Law [Conservative P.M. after L.G., who had throat cancer, could no longer speak, resigned in May after only seven months, and died Oct. 30 at age 65, three weeks before Freud's dream]. Yet instead we have the fact that the dm. was told to certain persons. Anna and Dr. Deutsch. It must, therefore, mean something for these persons. Now what I read in the newspaper said that LG was accompanied by his wife and daughter. Wife and daughter—that was decisive for the dm.-formation, they were my nurses, without whom I would not have survived those hard days. Thus it is clearly a dream of loving recognition for my women. My enmity, on the other hand, must apply to men. Emotionally I very much depended on Prof. Pichler; with the second operation came a disappointment, a loosening of the homosex. attachment. Back to the women! Dr. Deutsch is personally involved very little now. Why should I have related the dm. to him—and with hostile intent? A vague suspicion indicates this was a known way of sharing the dream with you. Maybe.

The criticism of Jelgersma is clearer to me. Remember that his merit was acknowledging the dm. and how much misunderstanding and presumption thereby! Yet he is to have an honorary issue of the poor Zeitschrift, *ill-treated by you and Storfer, the* Zeitschriften *which now attain in effect the place of women! Thus the affect shown in conversation with you later makes it quite probable that you (and Storfer) are also hidden behind the figure of Bonar Law.*

And the question about the superego? Does it act so forcefully too, showing such a brutal will to recover? Oh no, that would not be its way at all. There's only one association, the decisive "to L.G., Liar from Wales," *i.e., now the superego only says to the dm.: "Good, you old swindler and boaster! That's not true at all!"*

And now comes a second surprising association that leaves no further doubt about the behavior of the superego. LG's name is David, and it occurs to me now that Loe always called her Herbert "Davy" [his nickname] because she wanted a father surrogate (his father's name really was David). So this means: Watch out! The young man and the old interchanged. You [du] are not David, you're the boastful giant Goliath, who another, a young David, will slay. And now everything falls into place that you [Sie, i.e., Rank] are the feared David who with a Trauma of Birth *succeeds in devaluing my work.*

Having changed David back into Goliath, the superego no longer objects to the identification with LG, and may be silent. That's as far as I can extend your interpretation. I hope to see you soon. I've not yet been operated on again, am really pain-free and medicine-free.

Cordially yours, Freud

In *The Ego and the Id,* Freud wrote, in terms reminiscent of Groddeck, the father of psychosomatic medicine, that physical as well as mental illness is unconscious self-punishment: "In the end we come to see that we are dealing with what may be called a 'moral' factor, a sense of guilt, which is finding its satisfaction in the illness and refuses to give up the punishment of suffering. We shall be right in regarding this disheartening explanation as final. But as far as the patient is concerned this sense of guilt is dumb; it does not tell him he is guilty; he does not feel guilty, he feels ill" (*S.E.* 17:48–49).

Dr. Otto Rank ¶December 1, 1923

Lieber Herr Professor:

*Unfortunately I couldn't see you today, so I take the liberty of sending you the title page of my book [*Trauma*], asking you to officially approve, before publication, the dedication on the inside page, which I believe you tacitly accepted at the time.*

Please give the proofs, which I enclose, back to Pauli [Paula Fichtl, Freud's housekeeper], who awaits them. They should be sent off today express if the book is to be ready by Christmas.

With cordial thanks. Respectfully yours, Rank

December 1, 1923

Lieber Herr Doctor:

I gladly accept your dedication with the assurance of my most cordial thanks. If you could put it more modestly, it would be all right with me. Handicapped as I am, I enjoy enormously your admirable productivity. That means for me too: "Non omnis moriar" *[Horace: "I shall not completely die"].*

Yours, Freud

P.S. I'm free Sunday morning, and would like to see you on Tuesday at the latest.

In December 1923, Fritz Wittels, an early acolyte, published the first Freud biography. He wrote that Freud had "become an emperor . . . a despot who will not tolerate the slightest deviation from his doctrines." He was hard on Adler and Jung while hoping that Rank, "Freud's Eckermann," was keeping good notes of his intimate talks with Freud.[13]

Prof. Dr. Freud Berggasse 19 Vienna IX ¶December 29, 1923

Lieber Herr Doktor:

Regarding his book a correspondence with Wittels developed (open for your review) in which he's behaved in a very conciliatory way until asking that I reconcile with Stekel, who strongly wishes it, or that I at least tone down the reference in History of the Psa. Movement *[1914] ("initially so commendable, later became completely misguided") soon to be re-published. My judgment and opinions toward both of them haven't changed. But if a more peaceful atmosphere and avoiding scandal can be had through such concession, I think one shouldn't fail to do it.*

So please let me know whether it's still possible to make changes in the text of History. *If so, I'd like to insert the following words in place of those on page 17, section 4: "Stekel, initially so very commendable, influenced by my works, but whose subsequent development could only meet with my dissatisfaction."*

Don't despise my readiness to make peace. Perhaps it's related to my prosthesis.

I have confident hopes of seeing you and Ferenczi before the end of this year.

Oli and [wife] Henny left today. Cordially yours, Freud

Having courageously survived a year of difficult surgeries, Freud shows a capacity for compromise in the name of peace with a lesser critic than Adler or Jung. His endorsement of *Trauma of Birth* and warm exchanges with Rank suggest that the two were as close as ever, the son analyzing and blessing the father, who jokes uneasily about patricide.

≈ Chapter 15 ≈

Crisis

January to April 1924

I wish to thank Otto warmly for sending his remarkable book on birth traumas.
And hope also to see the book he wrote with Sándor (of which there are several copies
in England). Without pretending to have assimilated all its contents as yet,
I am sure that we could all corroborate many of his views at once, e.g., the close
connection between psychoanalytic treatment and repetition of pregnancy
and birth. Knowing the importance of "zum Beispiel" [for example],
we will remember Professor's analogy of cure and birth.
—Jones to Committee, Rundbrief, January 15, 1924

Within months of this endorsement, Abraham and Jones would declare that Ferenczi and Rank broke a Committee rule requiring members to have the group's approval before publishing.

The Vienna Psychoanalytic Society met on Wednesday, January 2, to hear Sándor Ferenczi present on the *Development* book, coauthored with Otto Rank. There was no time for private conversation afterwards, so Ferenczi questioned Freud by letter (Jan. 20) about his referring to Rank as a "co-conspirator" that evening. Though it seemed facetious, Ferenczi wondered if Freud's strong support had waned. Freud replied on January 22: "I am not completely in agreement with your joint work, although there is much in it that I value. I have discussed some of it critically with Rank, but on the whole I would prefer to hold off so that all of you won't be disturbed in your production. In this fashion I want to make my still being present in old age harmless. Your lecture was very strange; it didn't treat the book you wrote to-

181

gether at all, but rather your own thing, active therapy, as though you wanted to place it in opposition to the Rankian birth trauma. A derailment in the long-abandoned tracks of the brother complex."

[Typed by Anna Freud] ¶January 30, 1924

Lieber Herr Doktor,

Your interim Rundbrief was as it had to be. I share your hope that through it the "affairs" have come to an end for a while.

In the other point you are certainly correct. I noted with satisfaction that the relevant formulation does occur in your collaborative work. My comment arose from our critical discussion before the book had attained its definitive form.

All of us felt poorly today (Wednesday), so two of us missed the meeting of the Association. I am expecting you, if not necessary sooner, Wednesday evening.

Cordially yours, Freud

Ferenczi answered Freud on January 30 with a 10-page letter claiming he had never before heard a word of dissatisfaction from Freud, that the whole time he and Rank worked on the book Freud had been supportive, that Rank had not prepared him for Freud's ambivalence, and that "we did not deviate from psychoanalytic ground by a hair's breadth." Ferenczi justified their emphasis on experience over knowledge, active versus passive technique, therapeutic over scientific priorities: "What we attempted was only to use the knowledge already gleaned more energetically in technique, for once." He admitted some brother envy in response to Freud's last point, "*but only as a reaction, as conscious defense against the influence of this* [brother] *complex.*" The end-setting mandate came entirely from Rank, Ferenczi pointed out. As for Freud's aging and frailty, "You should not . . . leave us to our own devices. . . . Indeed we cannot do without your help." He then suggested a meeting: Freud, Rank, and himself.[1]

In a long letter to Ferenczi (Feb. 4) Freud admitted to liking the book less: "It has its birth defect in that it emphasized 'experience' in the manner of a slogan." He thinks the work could lead away from psychoanalysis on "a path for traveling salesmen"—a stern warning. Freud needs time to digest new thinking and wouldn't delay colleagues' work because they want everything approved. It seems "out of the question to me that either you or Rank, in your independent excursions, would ever abandon the ground of analysis."

If you make a mistake you'll probably notice it, "or I will take the liberty of telling you so, as soon as I know it for sure myself." He continues:

Things are more difficult for me with Rank than with you; he is also personally much more sensitive. At first, his birth trauma made me distrustful. In the first joy of discovery he seemed ready to see the primal motif of neurosis in birth, so that I told him, jokingly: With a finding like that, someone else would make himself independent. Later he moderated himself, his trauma impressed me greatly, I resolved to look out for it in the analyses, and now, after four weeks of fresh work, I have become quite skeptical again.... The strongest impression I have is that it is not possible in a short time to penetrate such deep layers and bring about lasting psychic changes. But perhaps I am really already vieux jeu *[over the hill].... Rank does not have the gift for flatteringly convincing presentation, which, e.g., is such a hallmark of your works, and he is, unfortunately, uncouth and not very skillful in all literary matters.*

Freud hoped Ferenczi could keep the Committee together, but declined the proposal to meet with him and Rank. Freud told Ferenczi of an "unpleasant" letter from Eitingon reporting Abraham's agitation about the two controversial books. Eitingon praised *Development* as a "great accomplishment" that showed how some analysts lost perspective as they plumb the depths, not only missing important current issues but even "a feeling for the most decisive point on the long path." He expressed doubts about *Trauma*, citing Archimedes: "It seems improbable that for removing an immense burden, for completely lifting the world of pathology from its current state, a lever as short as possible, indeed one reduced to a mere handle, is the most appropriate instrument." Both books exploded like a bomb in the Committee: Abraham, who was to become president of the International Psychoanalytical Association in April, with Rank as secretary, "is dismayed by Rank's aviator-like move forward." Eitingon asked Freud to present an overview of the two books, with a co-report given by "a 'more conservative' member—Abraham, for example." A symposium on the relation of psychoanalytic technique to theory was already planned for Salzburg. The Berliners expected Ferenczi and Rank to deliver the first report, Sachs the co-report.[2]

Eitingon's mention of "conservative" members may be the first acknowledgment of a political or philosophical division in the Committee. Freud, though wavering, was closer to the southern members than to the northern, personally and ideologically.

Freud answered Eitingon's challenge on February 7. He knew the two books upset the Berliners but expressed surprise at how much it bothered Abraham and at Eitingon's taking it so seriously. "How deeply wounded he must feel to make such an unjustified and impossible demand—that before publication the Committee be informed of the content of the works of its members!" Wondering if Eitingon heard that directly from Abraham, he said, "I can hardly believe it." Freud was not ready to take a stand, not wanting his authority to inhibit colleagues' work. Nor must he approve all their work, "provided, of course, that these works do not leave our common ground, and that is certainly to be expected neither of Rank nor of Ferenczi." He recalled making some remarks to Sachs that were critical of *Trauma*, perhaps suggesting that it "arose in opposition to me. Yet the fact that I accepted the dedication" proves otherwise. Without making a final judgment Freud, in agreement with Rank, would write a statement for the next Rundbrief that could even be shown to IPA members outside the Committee.[3]

Jones's biography omits Freud's thoughtful position on the new books and claims—despite Freud's reaction and contradicted by his own letter (see epigraph, above)—that members promised to have their publications vetted by the Committee.

Dr. Otto Rank Wien, I, Grünangergasse 3–5 Telephon 73-309 ¶February 7, 1924
Lieber Herr Professor!

I enclose the two Rundbriefe received today from Berlin and London, but they contain no points connected with our topic of yesterday. On the other hand, three things occurred to me subsequently—which I'd like to share with you:

1) According to Eitingon's letter and in my opinion, it's far more important that the other analysts (especially the Berliners) be informed that you don't regard the new proposals as heresies—not just the Committee, which of course knows that. Eitingon's proposal was not that you should write to Abraham, but that you should write a sort of report ("to all," as it were). Eitingon feels it's not only the Committee that is threatened, but also the Association and the Congress. Because I have the impression that such a "report" is not the way you'll choose, I'd propose, as a possible suggestion, that you compose the letter in such a way that it could be used (at least partially) by Abraham (and perhaps by other presidents) to bring this to the attention of the members. I also feel that a good way to spare the emotions within the Committee would be for you to say that you've heard various things from various sides and that you're making the Rundbrief available to the members of the Committee as presidents of the local groups, etc.

*2) As an indication of your personal orientation to my own work (*Trauma of Birth)*, you might note your acceptance of the dedication, which certainly excludes any objections on your part a priori.*

3) Eitingon's comment about the failure to announce my work is a distortion. I recall precisely that a few days after San Cristoforo, where we (Ferenczi and I) reported to the Committee on our collaboration, Eitingon told me that Abraham was very irritated at not having known about it earlier. At the time, we were both in agreement that the actual reason for his quasi-exclusion from the [prize] competition was that you had appointed him referee.

I thought these subsequent ideas for your information could be of use to you as you compose the Rundbrief. [The points were made by Freud, Feb. 15.]

With cordial greetings. Yours, Rank

Ferenczi answered Freud, hoping that "in the end the favorable impression will win out." He argues that shortening analysis is a goal, while some others—including Abraham—lengthen the process in a way that benefits neither patient nor research. It was no surprise that Abraham took offense. "I challenge his right to construe purely matter-of-fact scientific suggestions, made in a moderate tone, as a personal insult." His own theme of active therapy preceded that of birth trauma, which Rank elaborated after the second revision of *Development*, "as a consequence of the work itself, so to speak."

The setting of a date in each case only gave Rank the opportunity, in the patients' reactions, to discover the repetition of birth in the analysis. To include this after the fact in the joint work would have been impermissible and (since Rank alone discovered the idea) also unjust. In my striving to give illustrations to the work, I did, to be sure, also make references to the "trauma of birth" in Vienna [VPS, Jan. 2] after the fact, but I couldn't do otherwise, since my cases were already also under the influence of the Rankian idea.

...I, myself, can no longer dispense with elucidating and tracing back to the trauma of birth, indeed, the material has already forced me to form certain ideas about the relation of this trauma to the traumatic power of the Oedipus complex....The dan-

ger of getting onto the "path for traveling salesmen" is not present; you, too, consider the eventuality that Rank and I could slide off analytic ground to be out of the question....Every word of the joint work speaks about and in favor of psychoanalysis.[4]

Ferenczi thought it possible still to "paste the Committee together" for useful work if not amicability. His long letter probably did not reach Vienna before Freud sent his Rundbrief of February 15, which repeats some points made to Eitingon and continues:

The condition for our fruitful collaboration is only this: that no one leave the common ground of psychoanalytic assumptions—and of this we can be sure for each and every member of the Committee. Furthermore, there is another factor, not unfamiliar to you, which renders me particularly unsuited for the function of a despotic, always watchful censor. It is not easy for me to feel my way into unfamiliar thought processes; in general, I must wait until I have found access to them by following my own winding paths. If you always wish to wait with a new idea until I can grant it my approval, it runs the risk of becoming quite old while you wait.

My position with respect to the two books under discussion is the following. I consider the collaboration to be a correction of my conception of the role of repetition or action in analysis. I had feared them, and considered these occurrences (you now call them experiences) as undesirable failures. R. and F. point to the inevitability and the useful application of this experience. Otherwise, the book can be acknowledged as a refreshing and subversive operation upon our current analytical practices. In my opinion, the book has the fault of being incomplete, i.e., it does not explain the changes in the technique dear to the authors, but only hints at them. Of course, many dangers are connected with this departure from our "classical technique."...Ferenczi's active therapy is a dangerous temptation for ambitious beginners, and there is essentially no way to keep them from such temptations.

...In my illness I learned that a shaved beard takes six weeks to grow again. Three months after surgery I still suffer from changes in the scars. Thus I can hardly believe that in a slightly longer time—4–5 months—one can penetrate into the deep layers of the unconscious and effect lasting changes in the psyche....

Now to the second and much more interesting book, Rank's Trauma of Birth....I consider this work very significant....We have long known and appreciated the womb fantasy, but [with Rank] it...shows us the biological background of the Oedipus complex. To recapitulate in my own words: a drive seeking to reestablish the earlier existence must be connected with the trauma of birth. One could call it the drive for happiness, with the understanding that the notion of happiness most often applies in an erotic sense.

Going beyond neurosis, Rank enters the general human realm and shows how people change the exterior world in the service of this drive, while the neurotic spares himself this effort by getting back to the womb through his fantasy in the shortest way available. If one adds to Rank's view Ferenczi's idea that a man represents himself in his genitals, one gains for the first time a derivation of the normal sexual drive that fits in with our world view.

…Here Rank deviates from me. He refuses to enter into questions of phylogenesis and allows anxiety, opposed to incest, directly to recapitulate birth anxiety so that neurotic regression in itself is obstructed by the natural process of birth. Indeed, this birth anxiety would be transferred to the father, but he would be only an excuse for it. Basically, the orientation toward the mother's body or genitals should be an ambivalent one from the outset. Here lies the contradiction. I find it very difficult to decide here.…Indeed, every drive, as a compulsion toward reestablishment of an old condition, presupposes a trauma as the reason for the change. Thus there could only be ambivalent drives—that is, drives accompanied by anxiety. Of course there is much more to say about the details, and I hope that the thought invoked by Rank will become the object of numerous and fruitful discussions. No coup or revolution in conflict with our secure findings presents itself, but rather an interesting addition whose value should generally be recognized among outsiders.

…I value the works highly…and recommend all analysts not to form a too hasty opinion of the questions raised, least of all a negative one.[5]

Not having read this Rundbrief in advance, Rank responded to Freud in detail, challenging him with a combination of energy and tact.

Vienna, February 15, 1924

Lieber Herr Professor!

Allow me to respond to your kind invitation to comment on your Rundbrief, which I mailed out today. I find it very appropriate in its goal to preserve peace in the Committee, and greatly appreciate it as an expression of your personal orientation to us both. So, even more, I feel free to admit that your objective orientation to my work disappoints me somewhat. Not that I thought even for a moment that you should protect me and my work from our colleagues. You should and could only state your judgment, but it is precisely this that disappoints, as I got the impression that it was not wholly free of misunderstandings. Since my heartfelt wish is that you not misunderstand me—far more important than recognition by psychoanalytic colleagues, from most of whom I never expected much understanding of my work—please let me say how I feel misunderstood.

In your effort to provide the colleagues with a bridge to understanding and acceptance, you refer first to the old, familiar fantasy of the womb, to which I assign only a special position. Now the demonstration of the womb reality—if I may say so—is essential to my concept. But from this misunderstanding, you then speak of the "fantasized" return to the womb, whereas in my view, both in neurotic symptoms and in the sexual act, much more than that is involved, i.e., a partial realization.

I see another contradiction in that you honor the drive to return to the womb with a new name [Glückstrieb, happiness drive], while elsewhere you habitually see something old and familiar: on one hand, in accord with Ferenczi's genital theory, the sex drive, which wants nothing other than return to mother; on the other hand, given your own concept of the drive—as a tendency to reestablish a prior state—you see the essence of the drive itself, i.e., the libido. Finally, you leave open the question of whether there are only ambivalent drives!

I'd like to discuss the inhibition of incest-striving (return to mother) less in connection with drive theory, which is of course still uncertain and to be created, and more in the context of practical experience. To me, every simple case of impotence has shown the critical factor to be overwhelming anxiety toward the maternal genital, not paternal prohibition (I mean in all social forms). Nor can I understand how you can maintain your own discovery of birth anxiety as source and model of every anxiety, and your recognition of Ferenczi's genital theory, without also accepting the consequence I've drawn—not simply through logic, of course, but verified through experience.

I hope to be spared the misunderstanding that I present my work as something completely new and independent. On the contrary, I emphatically claim extensive correlations and significant connections with your own observations. Thus birth anxiety takes first place, conceptually. As I've said, there is no contradiction with your drive theory, but rather, ideal correspondence (reestablishment of prior state); and methodologically, too, I cite in my favor your proper analytic view that individual explanatory means should be exhausted before adducing phylogenetic points of view.

But also in therapy, where you seem to follow me least, I simply assume the need for end-setting, a concept you introduced; this ties in with your result in "History of an Infantile Neurosis."[6] There, based on the [Wolf Man's] experience of rebirth in the end phase of analysis, you arrive at a series of questions that till now resisted solu-

tion, but which, I can say without exaggeration, have become coherent and solvable through my approach, without contradicting your assumptions. With this I see un-ambiguous proof that the birth experience occurred spontaneously in your patients as the final cure, just as with mine. Based on analytic experience, not speculation, I can only understand this experience as generalizable psychoanalytically and thus generally human. Therapeutically, I believe that with this finding I've made progress in that something, indeed something new and significant, can now be understood and used therapeutically. I don't put such great value on shortening analysis as might seem. This shortening proves a welcome gain from new insight. And it is precisely the analogy you use [surgery] that affords the best way to present the distinction in our perfected technique. We by no means fail to recognize the enormous importance of analysis as research method. What we criticized in our joint work was just that any analytical therapist could, as researcher, over-extend his analyses, causing them to fail therapeutically. I don't mean that therapeutic analysis is a healing or regen-erative process, as you suggest in your analogy, but a surgical intervention that can, indeed must, be done more quickly so the patient is not brought down by the opera-tion. Anyway, this surgical incision is only possible if one knows ahead or can quickly determine the site of the ailment. The rest hardly matters, i.e. the depth of the root, is only a question of technique. I believe you'll agree that the trauma of birth, the earliest maternal tie, and everything up to weaning- and sexual trauma belong to the deepest layers we can penetrate. And I can assure you that in every analysis this is possible within the first month, without harm to the patient—moreover, easing and hastening resolution of all conflicts, neurotic and actual.

Finally, may I point out that your objection that we still have too much to learn before trusting our hypotheses in therapy was already invalidated by Ferenczi in his presentation here, in his comment that it's precisely this technique that gives us wholly new insights into the mechanism of neurosis-formation and the process of cure, and, on the other hand, has also presented a whole series of new problems, so one certainly cannot describe it as scientifically fruitless.

Of course much more could be said and—especially—discussed, but I'd be the last to press you to do so before you have sufficient impressions from experience to allow the best possible judgment. But I hope my comments may clarify existing misunder-standings and help avoid future ones.

Cordial greetings; with gratitude, as always.

Yours, Rank

Dr. Otto Rank Wien Grünangergasse 3-5 ¶February 21, 1924 (Thursday)
Lieber Herr Professor,

I've been in bed since Saturday with angina. Today is the first day I feel better. I'm sure I won't be able to work before Monday. Enclosed is a card from Budapest and a Rundbrief from Jones that came today. His "criticism" arises from the same feelings of resentment harbored by Abraham, and apparently directed toward Development: *that we had a secret within the Committee.*

I hope you can now enjoy the use of your new prosthesis without disturbance.

With cordial greetings, Yours, Rank

[Tuesday] February 26, 1924
Lieber Herr Doktor:

I hope you've recovered on schedule and will again be participating. Given the current situation with my ability to speak and the resulting mood—in the last two weeks we made no progress with the prosthesis—it's not likely that I'll attend the meeting of the Society on Wednesday. In that case, though, by [Wednesday] March 5 I would have seen you too infrequently, given that the situation presents us with much to consider. So I inquire whether you should come for dinner before and work afterwards.

Cordially yours, Freud

That day Abraham sent Freud a denunciation of Ferenczi and Rank. He saw in both books "manifestations of a scientific regression that correspond, down to the smallest detail, with the symptoms of Jung's renunciation of Psa." He remembered warning Freud about Jung at the Salzburg Congress of 1908; Freud dismissed it then as jealousy. Abraham foresaw the disintegration of the Committee and a damaging effect on psychoanalysis resulting from the two books. He would make a Committee meeting before the IPA Congress a priority.

Dr. Otto Rank Wien Grünangergasse 3-5 ¶February 26, 1924
Dear Professor!

After staying in bed for eight days I'm halfway back to normal routine, i.e. I conduct analyses in the morning and rest in the afternoon. On Wednesday Deutsch wants to try to let me go out for the first time, and if nothing stops me, I'll be there.

Whether I'll be able to go out again this week depends on my success the first time; I'll take the liberty of contacting you by phone. Perhaps we could make an appointment for Sunday morning. However, I'd appreciate seeing you before March 5 evening, when the discussion of my book postponed from last week takes place. On the other hand, in the March 1 Rundbrief we have to answer the question as to the meeting of the Congress.

Please allow me to ask you again later in the week when I can come. In the meantime you will hopefully be in complete possession of the new prosthesis!

With cordial greetings. Yours, Rank

Freud answered Abraham's challenge at length on March 4, stating with reassurance that although he is closer to Rank and Ferenczi geographically, Abraham's standing in friendship and esteem is no lower. He admits to a similar apprehension, recalling his own jocular comment that anyone else would "set up on his own" with Rank's innovation—but he stresses "anyone else," noting that Jung had strong "neurotic and selfish motives . . . his crooked character did not compensate me for his lopsided theories." Ferenczi and Rank are different, their motives good, they may fall into error as happens in scientific work. Assuming the extreme, that they conclude the birth trauma takes precedence over the Oedipus complex, then "physiological chance" (how traumatic was the birth, or how sensitive the newborn) would establish etiology. "What further damage would ensue? We could remain under the same roof with the greatest calmness, and after a few years' work it would become evident whether one side had exaggerated a valuable finding or the other had underrated it." Freud agrees to meet for Committee discussion on Saturday before the Salzburg Congress, though he is tired and will neither read a paper nor attend a meal there.

In response, March 8, Abraham specifies that he can accept a new finding arrived at legitimately. "My doubts are not directed at the results achieved by Sándor and Otto but against the *paths* they took. These seem to me to lead away from psa. Any criticisms will relate *solely* to this."

Having learned of Abraham's attack from Rank, Ferenczi wrote Freud on March 18 with a copy to Rank. He accused Abraham of "boundless ambition and jealousy. For only these passions could blind him in such a way that he—against all reason—could slander the joint work and *The Trauma of Birth* as garbage publications. He did not summon the courage to appear openly in opposition to us." That, along with his behavior at San Cristoforo—siding with Jones and downplaying his anti-Semitism—doomed the Committee. About the IPA presidency: only Eitingon—besides Freud—would be impartial.

Freud answered Ferenczi on March 20: "My trust in you and Rank is unqualified. It would be sad if, after one has lived together for 15 to 17 years, one could still find oneself deceived. But you attach too much importance to the fact that I agree with you in all particulars and Rank is terribly uncouth, puts people against him, does not behave with the cheerful superiority that would serve him so well, as the one who is nearest to me in so many respects. His accomplishments were inestimable; his person would be irreplaceable. Now, when he is preparing to go to America for half a year—certainly no secret to you—I am concerned that his health may not be up to the exertions that await him there."

Freud was unsure that he would still be alive when Rank returned. "I know, gone is gone, lost is lost. I have survived the Committee, which was supposed to be my successor; perhaps I will also survive the International Association. Let us hope psychoanalysis survives me." He would not interfere with Abraham's installment as IPA president, which had been promised; the Committee could decide otherwise. "To deny it to him now would be equivalent to a disciplinary action, which I don't believe I am justified in, despite the fact that he is wrong in his hostility toward both of you." He continued: "Yesterday evening I had a long scientific discussion with Rank and admitted to him that I made regress rather than progress in my estimation of your joint work and the Birth Trauma. . . . I also find that Rank's inept presentation, which I had already objected to in the first draft, bears much of the blame for the misrepresentations and suspicions of the Berliners. But he said he couldn't do it any other way." He castigates Rank for the "monomaniacal" presentation, the failure to integrate previous knowledge; hence, he is being judged for brazenness, for pushing ahead with a new technique to shorten analysis, which sounds like suggestion or hypnosis. "With Rank, I see, fortunately, only one similarity to the blessed Jung: being blinded by one's own first experiences, when one begins to practice analysis. . . . Otherwise I don't want to compare either the persons or the findings. Jung was a bad guy." Freud said that Ferenczi could show the letter to Rank, who knew that Freud's paper on the dissolution of the Oedipus complex, the first written after *Trauma,* would not be published for the time being—in draft, it contained some criticism of Rank's theory.

Lieber Sándor

Yesterday afternoon I got your express letter of the 18th; in my conversation yes-terday with the Professor, it lent me a certain degree of security, which I very much needed, and which we will probably continue to need in the hard battles that surely await us. (The Professor hadn't yet received your letter in the evening, but I told him that your views are known to me.)

Today I can tell you only briefly the results of the rather penetrating conversation, which, however, ended in a completely friendly spirit; I hope we'll soon have a chance for a discussion—already much needed.

First: The Professor got a new letter from A[braham] with nothing special, i.e. nothing substantive, only a request to await the detailed justification of the viewpoint he'll present in Salzburg. (A. gave up plans to come to Vienna.) The letter contains the assurance that he'll seize every opportunity to bring about a rapprochement. A letter of Sachs enclosed responded to Professor's comment on our behalf by saying that he too doesn't believe we want to replace the earlier viewpoint with our own, but if that is indeed the case, he'd consider it just as incompatible with psychoanalysis as Jung's or Adler's path.

Second: When I gave my opinion of these goings-on, the Professor conceded that Sachs is insincere and Abraham is decidedly unfriendly, but said he didn't believe their comments were as personal as we take them to be.

Third: The Professor directly accepted our conclusion that the Committee has ceased to exist, and in response to my clear request he also promised to open the meet-ing in Salzburg with this pronouncement. I said that before going into any discussion about this divisive topic we'll openly reveal all the personal conflicts and emotions. For my participation in the scientific discussion I reserved the right to appear in person, completely freely, as a private citizen.

Fourth: The Prof. objected to this last remark: he found it too brusque and believed it would place me in the wrong from the start. He also said he couldn't agree with us about the presidency. I defended our view, but didn't go further since you and I must first discuss this. This seems most crucial: any inflexibility by the Prof. about this point could lead to the breakup of the Association. Prof. seems to know this very well, for he said in summary that he'd certainly prefer not to attend the Congress, were it not for the fact that he wants to dispel, if possible, our opponents' pleasure in the demise of the Association.

In this situation, which you can see is most critical, a special problem for our planned counterattack may occur: it's not at all certain we can rely on Eitingon, who'd be our only candidate. I don't just mean "we personally," but in general, for Eitingon has disappeared, as it were. He hasn't communicated with anyone for weeks (including the Professor), and in Berlin there are only obscure rumors that his condition has deteriorated. Could you try writing him (registered mail)? (I assume that until the end of the month his address is Hotel de la Reine, Ospedaletti [Italy].)

Fifth: After discussing these personal questions, the Professor himself directed the discussion to objective matters and surprised me with the revelation that he is writing a small article in which he critically addresses The Trauma of Birth. He wants to leave it up to me whether and when this article will be published since he feels that it "would be interpreted" by analysts "as a statement against me, but mitigated by our personal relations." This predicted assessment really does characterize the article itself, which the Professor in part read and in part described to me. It's titled "The Dissolution of the Oedipus Complex"—ambivalence appears in the title's ambiguity—and shows that in development the Oedipus complex is not repressed, but destroyed, specifically by the castration complex, in whose place I attempted to place the trauma of birth—a step he can't agree with. He draws his objections to Trauma of Birth from the areas where they're hardest to contradict (etiological statistics of difficult births; perceptual and recollective abilities during the birth process, etc.). He gives the impression that he rejects it wholly, which he admitted when I made a remark to that effect. He said now he doesn't consider correct even the few points that first impressed him. To my question as to why he doesn't say this openly, he said his judgment is not really final, that he only wants to discuss the objections, and he considers its application to cultural adaptation attractive and valuable, etc. In response to my asking how that could be brought into harmony with rejection of the whole, he was evasive. The most peculiar thing about this article is that although my book apparently led him to the idea of the dissolution of the Oedipus complex, he doesn't even mention my discussion of sexual trauma, nor, especially, my attempt to explain why the Oedipus complex is destined to dissolution in the first place (see page 44 of my book), although the various possible opinions on this topic form the main content of the book. When I pointed this out to him, he said that my opinion on this was quite interesting. That was all.

At several points in the course of the debate it was clear that the Professor still has not read my book, and concerning the question as to the etiological significance of the birth trauma for the neuroses, toward which most of his criticism is directed, he finally had to admit to me that he had only read half of it. He has [...].

Given the opinion of the Prof., who wants to remain favorably disposed to us both, as he again emphasized, you can imagine the resistance we'll get from the others *when—inevitably—they learn or guess his position. In view of this I'm less ready than ever to make any concessions, personal or factual.*

Sixth: *And now to the other business and private matters.*

1) Immediately after the Congress I'll go direct from Salzburg to Cherbourg, where I board ship April 27. More details on America in person.

2) The translation of Development *was so bad that I sent it back to Miss Herford. The book is now being translated by the woman I previously mentioned [Caroline Newton]. I will look it over and take it along to America, where I'll have it published. As for your plans for translation, feel free to have whatever you wish translated: I hope to find publishers for it over there. In any case, I would advise you not to engage Miss Herford.*

3) The announced patients cannot have already appeared. (Anyway, I cannot guarantee that they will do so at all.)

4) We'll leave for Salzburg Friday morning the 19th; we assume you two will travel with us. A room there will be reserved. In any case, the two of you should come to Vienna as soon as possible—sooner the better, given that trains could be crowded during Easter Week. We think it goes without saying that you'd be our guests in Vienna. However, Tola asks me to tell you that in lieu of the uncomfortable lodgings in our home, she'll take the liberty of getting more comfortable lodgings nearby. Tola will write Gizella about this directly, so please don't involve yourself in this. I await your speedy reply.

Cordial greetings. Yours, [Otto]

P.S. The little that I can still do to "prepare" the Viennese members will occur in a course "on the technique of dream interpretation in psychoanalysis" that I am teaching here now, and in which the most important practicing analysts are participating. ([Eduardo] Weiss from Trieste has scheduled private technical sessions with me for the next few days.) What do you say about the takeover [of the program] by all the speakers from Berlin?

In his own words, Prof. tested my ideas on technique by giving all his current patients, most of whom have been in analysis with him for about two years, my book to read; he then had them tell him about their impressions. While writing this I still can't believe it's possible, but there's no doubt about it.

Berggasse 19 ¶March 23, 1924 [Sunday]

Lieber Herr Doktor

I'm firmly convinced that my critical comments last Wednesday [Mar. 19] have made little impression on you. That happens when one is under the spell of a new idea. Then it's really for the best if one is left alone. If only Ferenczi wouldn't always place such a high value on full agreement with me! I'm certainly not pressuring you. In God's name, let's just disagree.

Eitingon wants to come on April 13 and then go with us to Salzburg. You can discuss the current factional issues with him, too. A way has occurred to me for us to publish my article on Oedipus (in the Zeitschrift *[10.3: 245–52] and in Collected Works without provoking the unwanted impression. I'll add some material that occurred to me, and will conclude with the comment that your* Trauma of Birth *necessitates discussion that now strikes me as premature, or something similar. The article is complete; when typed by Anna it will be available to you.*

Since catching a cold I've been so tired that I won't be attending the next meeting of the Society. Therefore I'm firmly resolved to hand over to you the presidency [VPS]— preferably before the Congress so you can appear there in your new role. It makes no difference if the Society suspends official meetings until your return in October.

With cordial greetings, Yours, Freud

On March 24 Ferenczi answered Freud's letter of March 20. He recalled Professor's initial high praise for Rank's book. Ferenczi supports Rank's emphasis on the analytic situation and "the extension of activity to giving notice *every time.*" Assuming the timing was right, "I saw from this measure the most *remarkable* and, for myself, *the most surprising* effect." Rank assured him that birth/separation was not the entire determinant of the etiology of the neuroses, but Ferenczi found it compelling in his own work on genitality. The Oedipus complex, at the social level, reawakened the earlier conflict "between the longing for the womb and the fear of the womb." He defends Rank wholeheartedly, calling "frivolous" the rush to judgment by Abraham, Jones, Sándor Radó, and others. He finds Freud's position "vacillating and contradictory" but hopes it leaves the way open for "a favorable decision." Ferenczi writes that both he and Rank would oppose Abraham as president, favoring Eitingon or a "colorless" figure from outside the Committee.

Dr. Otto Rank Wien I, Grünangergasse 3–5 ¶March 25, 1924
Lieber Herr Professor!

I believe—completely apart from my personal feelings for you—that you underestimate the high respect in which I hold you as creator of psychoanalysis and my teacher, if you think your criticism has made so little impression on me. If it seemed so, it's probably due to the fact that sometimes I had the impression that your criticism—material viewpoints aside—has from the start not been altogether well-meaning. Otherwise you'd certainly not have neglected to mention aspects of the book you repeatedly stated were valuable, given that you so bluntly say how you see its weak points.

Apart from that, another factual matter disturbed me. Since you discuss in detail the possible explanations for the dissolution of the Oedipus complex in the body of the article, and then shed critical light on my viewpoint in an addendum, I think it would have been appropriate at least to adduce my attempt to clarify the dissolution of the Oedipus complex (page 44: "Sexual Trauma").

From such signs, underscored by your saying that I have "pique" against the Oedipus complex (rather than the castration complex), I sensed a not wholly unprejudiced opinion on your part, an opinion I openly confess has affected me painfully, especially since I think that it keeps you from freely investigating things in analysis, where they can really be seen.

I hope, dear Professor, that you won't take offense at the liberty I've taken, but I see in it not only the prerequisite for any personal relations, but also the best means of coming to an understanding.

As for your second suggestion, I don't know whether you're correct in attending only to your own position, and not that of the whole Vienna group, which will probably be very disappointed and will stop at nothing to turn you from your intention. Then there is also the practical difficulty that as of May I'll no longer be in Vienna, when the Society still normally meets.

With cordial greetings. Yours, Rank

On March 26 Freud sent Ferenczi a long letter typed by Anna, mostly recapitulation. Freud's admiration for *Trauma* has slipped toward 33 percent. Rank "doesn't say expressly anywhere, I believe, that he wants to put the trauma etiologically in the place of the Oedipus complex, but everybody senses this." Nevertheless, Freud will reprimand Abraham for his harshness. Another conflict simmered since Rank threatened to stop referring patients to Berlin because one of his analysands had been interrogated critically about Rank's technique.[7] A consolation prize for Rank: presidency of the Vienna Psychoanalytic Society, as Freud steps down.

On March 30 Sándor sent a long letter to Otto, enclosing Freud's of March 20 and expressing confidence that the disputes would quiet down in the year or two between this Congress and the next.[8] In early April Freud bowed out of the Salzburg IPA Congress due to influenza. Rank and Ferenczi had declined to be part of the program after a spat with Jones.

On April 3, Otto wrote Ferenczi, copy to Eitingon, that Freud would not attend the IPA Congress. There would be no point in having a Committee meeting in his absence. Rank said he wouldn't oppose the nomination of Abraham as president, and thanked Max for agreeing to be secretary in his stead. He mentioned Freud's intent to appoint him president of the VPS, at which he had already presided pro tempore. He said the Committee was finished, and thought the Congress might even be canceled because of Freud's absence.

This same week Jones indicated he was ready to abandon Freud in order to save psychoanalysis. In a letter to Abraham (in English) on April 8, Ernest sympathized with Karl "having also to undergo my experience being unfairly treated by one's best-loved friend [Prof.]. . . . It is not hard to make every allowance for him when one considers all the factors, age, illness, and the insidious propaganda nearer home." Jones says the motive behind *Trauma of Birth* is "flight from the Oedipus complex," which "Otto conceals from Prof and displaces onto us." The book was "secretly published," and, besides dropping out of the Congress symposium, Otto ignored their questions for weeks, stopped the Rundbriefe and made a "Jung-like decision to go to America without letting any of us know." Jones continues:

I will not sacrifice my intellectual convictions for friendship with any man on earth, not even Prof himself. It would be a strange irony if we lost some of Freud's intimate friendship through too great loyalty to his work, but it may possibly prove to be so. We may have to choose between Psa and personal considerations, in which case you may be sure I for one shall have no doubt.

The real tragedy is this. I fear that Prof, with his clear mind, cannot be altogether blind to the unconscious tendency in Otto. Ten years ago he would surely have put his work before all else; but now, old, ill, and tied by the strongest claims of affection (which Otto has fully justified in the past), he can hardly face the possibility of having once more to go through the Jung situation and this time much nearer home, with someone who perhaps means more to him than his own sons.

Jones thought that emotional issues were the real reason Freud would not attend the Congress. "You may show this letter to Hanns." Jones does not mention this letter in his Freud biography, where he claimed that Rank was never personally close to Freud.[9]

On April 9 Rank wrote Freud that because of a cold he could not meet as planned, but arrangements were in order for the early arrival of Sándor and

Max. He was pleased at a letter from Ferenczi (cc: Freud) declaring the end of the Committee and the Rundbriefe.

Professor Dr. Freud Berggasse 19 ¶April 10, 1924

Lieber Herr Doktor:

I'm very sorry, especially in connection with your travel plans, that you're ill again; I hope you won't go before receiving [medical] permission.

This week, though, I won't leave. The stay in Semmering certainly did me some good, and since we leave Vienna on the 17th, we can omit next weekend.

If you are on your feet by next Sunday and have no other plans, it would be easy for me to see you. Otherwise, of course, any evening next week before the guests arrive.

Ferenczi's announcement is quite suitable. Abraham will be very surprised about this cancellation. Unfortunately, he is very uninsightful. He wrote me that he hopes my "little ailment" will soon be surmounted and won't prevent my coming to Salzburg and perhaps making a presentation. He just won't believe I'm dealing with a new, reduced level of life and work.

I must thank you in person for your work on the beautiful edition of Collected Works.

With most cordial greetings for your swift recovery, Yours, Freud

P.S. I hope your dear wife has taken note of the cancellation for us, and for the acceptance by Tausk, Lou Salomé, and Ossipow. [Re: Rank's birthday]

On the same day, more forcefully than Ferenczi, Rank announced in a Rundbrief the obituary of the Committee: We have "definitively buried" it, he wrote. "The Professor conceded to me that the most instrumental thing would be to open the planned Salzburg Committee meeting with the statement that the Committee no longer exists."

At the time of the Eighth International Psychoanalytical Association Congress there were, worldwide, 263 members, of whom only 10 had attended the First Congress in Salzburg, in 1908: Abraham, Eitingon, Federn, Ferenczi, Freud, Hitschmann, Jekels, Jones, Rank, and Sadger.

Rank turned 40 on April 22; Helene and Felix Deutsch had a party for him. He hurried from the Congress a day early to set sail for America. Freud reassured Abraham on May 4: "I believe [the birth trauma theory] will *fall flat* if it is not criticized too sharply and Rank, whom I value because of his gifts, his great service to our cause, and also for personal reasons, will have learned a valuable lesson."

≈ Chapter 16 ≈

New York

May to October 1924

His first visit to the United States brought Otto Rank to the American Psychoanalytic Association (APA) as Freud's emissary. He left his wife and 5-year-old Helene for six months, counting on New York analysts who met him in Vienna to refer patients and set up lectures. He spoke at the New York Academy of Medicine's Neurological Society, Columbia University, and the New School for Social Research to as many as 150 in the audience. He was guest of honor at dinner parties hosted by *Psychoanalytic Review* editor Smith Ely Jelliffe and by Adolf Stern, secretary of the APA. He addressed the New York Psychoanalytic Society, and, on June 3, in Atlantic City, became an honorary member of the APA, speaking on the trauma of birth in its importance for psychoanalytic therapy. The audience that day included psychiatrists Karl Menninger, A. A. Brill, and William Alanson White and psychologist Jessie Taft, who became Rank's patient, friend, translator, and first biographer.

Dr. Otto Rank 117 West 58 St New York ¶May 11, 1924

Lieber Herr Professor,

After a week here that seems like three months to me, I finally have time to write you. Of course the nicest part was the crossing—without seasickness. Not getting seasick in New York itself is actually the hard part. You know yourself how ugly the city is, how horrible life here is, and how insufferable the people are. So it's really a comfort to me that I can work the whole day. Otherwise I couldn't endure life in this city, which really isn't arranged for living. I work from 9 A.M. to 6 P.M. with an hour break. At 6

P.M. I go to Central Park, near where I live. Not only are there squirrels, but also a small zoo with interesting animals (chimpanzees, seals, and the most extraordinary birds). That's my main recreation now. The reception I got here was very warm, and I believe sincere, but working with the people who were in Vienna before is very difficult and touchy, as you can imagine (Blumgart, Stern, Ash): they're terribly jealous of me and each other, and if I succeed in cleaning out the analytical Augean stables here, I'll have performed a real Herculean task. But mostly I doubt that is humanly possible.

From Frink, who knows I'm here, I've heard nothing. I won't be able to visit your nephew and relatives until next week, as this week I had to move into my own apartment. (For personal reasons I couldn't accept an invitation.) I can afford it, though, since I take no less than twenty dollars [per analytic hour].

Dear Professor, I'd be very happy to hear from you soon—especially whether the recuperation at Easter brought the hoped for success.

With most cordial greetings to you and yours, Yours, Rank

New York ¶May 17, 1924 Mr. Ed. Bernays [Freud's nephew]
9 East 46th Street New York

My dear Mr. Bernays,

I was so busy when I first came, getting settled, and since I have become so much occupied with my work that I have not yet been able to see you. I would like very much to meet for a chat. I am afraid this is possible only after 7 o'clock in the evenings, during the week or on Sundays. But it is possible next week, that I could see you for a short time between 11.30 and 12.15 on Thursday, Friday or Saturday. If this time is convenient to you would you kindly phone, and my Secretary will make an appointment for you.

Yours very sincerely, Dr. Otto Rank

[letterhead] Edward Bernays ¶May 19, 1924

My dear Sir [Dr. Otto Rank],

Mr. Bernays wishes me to say in reply to your note of May 17th, that on request of Professor Freud he was glad to render Dr. Rank the slight service of securing rooms for him on the day of his arrival.

He does not understand the tenor of Dr. Rank's letter. He certainly has no reason to request an interview with Dr. Rank in the manner suggested.

Yours very truly,

Eva H. Marks Secretary to Edward L. Bernays

Prof. Dr. Freud Wien, IX Berggasse 19 ¶May 23, 1924

Lieber Herr Doktor,

Your first letter has arrived. I'm very glad that you weren't seasick. Then the trip across the dirty ocean is a pleasure. I'm amused at the perfect match between your impressions and mine of 15 years ago. Nowhere is one so overwhelmed by the senselessness of human striving as there, where one no longer recognizes as a life-purpose even the enthusiastic gratification of natural animal needs. It's a deranged, anal, Adlerish mess.

I'm also very glad you have found the only sensible way to behave that suits your stay among these uncivilized beings: selling your services as dearly as possible.

It's nice that you've gotten nearly all my patients, whose analysis I recall with no satisfaction at all. It often seemed to me that analysis suits Americans like a white shirt suits a raven.

As for what's happening here in the Society, there's no need for you to learn of it from me. I'm still keeping my distance. Sachs offered to come to Vienna to help with Imago. I've exchanged some comments on editorial matters with Ferenczi. A manuscript by the sophist [Fritz] Kunkel has just arrived—a chapter of a book affectionately dedicated to me, as it were—and a manuscript by Hollós: "Analysis of a Premature-Born." I've not yet read the latter; it might be interesting for your theory of the birth trauma.

In Semmering my health was not shining, but has slowly improved since then. Those who value objective indicators will note that my physician only wants to see me every three weeks, and gave me permission to go to Switzerland in July–August. I stick to the subjective side: I'm dissatisfied and skeptical.

Perhaps you have heard that on the occasion of my birthday I became an honorary citizen of the city of Vienna. Still, not much has changed in this city since then. The horrible economic crisis and worries about the outcome of "restoration" still remain.

I was visited by Romain Rolland, and the day before yesterday by Alb[recht] Schaeffer, author of Josef Montfort. He was actually a disappointment. He looks like one of Hitler's boys, and is now far from analysis again.

Give my greetings to all the squirrels, and feed them for me with the nuts for the monkeys. The only zoo really worth seeing is in The Bronx.

Cordially yours, Freud

P.S. I've written another little essay: "Loss of Reality in Neurosis and Psychosis."

Adolph Hitler, 35, was tried for his role in the November Munich *Putsch* early in 1924. He had sympathetic judges and his speeches in court were

widely published in the press. Convicted and sentenced to five years for trea-
son with his secretary, Rudolph Hess, he served less than nine months in a
comfortable setting that allowed many visitors, while he dictated *Mein Kampf*
(1925) to Hess.

S. Ferenczi Budapest, May 25, 1924

Lieber Otto,

*The only news I've (indirectly) heard from or about you was a nice letter from your
wife in which she told us that she, too, heard from you only in telegrams, from which
she learns you're deeply involved in your work over there. So, I won't wait for letters
from you, but will share with you events since you left Salzburg.*

*Everyone, included the Viennese, seemed insulted that you departed before the
Congress ended. In his comic speech at the banquet, the sarcastic Hitschmann made
some satirical references to the "hero" Otto, who, it was to be hoped, would now be rescued from the water and successfully survive the trauma of birth. He also spoke about
the "genital theory"—and in a very tasteless manner.*

*Jones's banquet speech seemed positively like a eulogy for the Professor—very tact-
less. At the end he made a toast to Abraham and the Professor together. Abraham
responded by toasting Jones and the Professor. They've played their cards well! In
his private conversations with me, Abraham always referred to formal and objective
errors in your book, but clearly he was trying to demonstrate his peaceful intentions.
He even asked me to tell the Professor about this.*

*In my report to the Professor, I tried to be objective. Here's the sentence in his answer
that relates to you: "The Berliners (the afternoon of discussion) went so far in their
gentilezza [kindness] to accept Rank's confusion of physiological treatment with
psychology." Responding, I wrote the Professor that he underestimates the scientific
seriousness of the Berliners if he thinks they made their remarks out of gentilezza
(they are just as responsible as anyone involved in this confusion). The Professor supposedly looks very bad (reports Dr. Urbantschitsch). In his letters he complains of local
problems, not due to recurrence, but to the prosthesis....*

*Urbantschitsch, who's with us now, wants to set up a psychoanalytic consultation
center for teaching and other pursuits in Vienna (when he returns home). He'd like to
invite Bernfeld, Aichhorn, and Anna Freud as coworkers. His great plans for founding this seem to have been dashed in the financial crisis of Vienna.*

*I tried to calm Miss [Caroline] Newton, who told me in Salzburg about her dif-
ficulties with you—probably to be interpreted as afterpains of suggestion. A few weeks
later I received a letter from her asking whether in principle I'd be inclined to partici-*

pate in founding the American polyclinic and keep the project afloat for 2–3 years. She asked me to inform you as well. I didn't reject the proposal, but let my answer depend on news from you.

We've repeated our invitation to Tola and little Helene to come to Budapest (at Pentecost)....

Jones wrote to Pat[ricia] (Cole), whom he analyzed for two years (and I analyzed for one month). She's been away from England for a long time. She'd like to settle not in London, but in a provincial city. She's only thinking about this because she came to me. N.B.: She is the oldest and relatively the best analyst in London. She rejects his request with indignation and characterizes it as pure "Welsh" deceitfulness....

My wife sends her greetings, as does your old Sándor

P.S. A few days after Salzburg, Glover arrived with his wife and three English members in Budapest, where we received them cordially. In your honor, we permitted Róheim to make a presentation in English (strongly influenced by the genital theory and the birth trauma). I availed myself of the opportunity to enlighten Glover concerning certain misunderstandings relating to Dr. Freud and to the birth trauma.

Róheim, who has very serious conflicts with his father, on whom he depends financially, would appreciate it very much if you could find a position for him over there. He's willing to accept anything, e.g. working for an American publisher. It would of course be nicer for him if an anthropologist or ethnologist took an interest in him. Please think about this seriously.

Now I really have nothing more to say. Sándor

Prof. Dr. Freud Wien, IX Berggasse 19 ¶June 20, 1924

Lieber Herr Doktor,

I'll answer your two letters [one missing] briefly since I think it's important to answer as soon as possible to eliminate certain possibilities. So I'll limit myself to two points: your relation to my relatives, and the American rights.

On the first point, I can't understand how Edward could respond so impolitely. Perhaps your letter was really contrary to American form, but otherwise he is a good fellow; he should certainly have known that a foreigner in New York could not easily master that formal language. That you are perceived by these people as an apostate or opponent is an idea that I must attribute to your pessimistic attitude. First of all, they know nothing of the events that led, for example, to the mistrust among the Berliners, and secondly, they should have arrived at a completely different expectation from my letters. In brief, I cannot explain it, and will write directly to my nephew for an explanation.

The second matter is equally obscure to me. To your communication I can add the following. A few days ago Rickman told me he had heard from Glover that they had found a publisher, a friend of Strachey—I've forgotten the name—who supposedly is ready to acquire your publications, provided the American rights to my books are sold to him also. Of course that entailed the request that I approve this sale. My decided answer was that you alone now control the American rights, and that I have no intention of changing this. After getting your letter reporting that Jones had already sold these rights, I presented the matter to Rickman, asking him to explain the contradiction. He thought Jones was just bluffing so you'd make no contracts in America in the meantime. We were united in condemning this behavior. I see from your letter that you're not sure whether you understood Jones correctly. In any case, I'll send you a cable tomorrow assuring you that nothing has changed, and I'll write to Jones today to re-emphasize my decision. I'll put in your hands whether or not to grant the rights to Jones' buyer. Act according to your best insight.

I hope to see your wife and daughter this week and say farewell to them. My condition is not bad, the prosthesis is in order, but there are torments enough. We gave up plans to go to Switzerland, and seek a place to spend the summer at a comfortably close distance.

With cordial wishes and awaiting your personal news, Yours, Freud

Soon after arriving in New York, Otto, who had a surfeit of patients and lectures, encouraged Sándor to join him. Ferenczi, also an honorary member of the APA, planned a fall arrival. By June 30 Rank backtracked, and his "SITUATION UNCERTAIN" cable led Ferenczi to give up the plan.

Prof. Dr. Freud Wien, IX Berggasse 19 ¶June 29, 1924

Lieber Herr Doktor,

I enclose Jones's answer to my question concerning the supposed sale of the American rights. It is so insincere and tortuous that I'm doubly glad I dumped the whole thing into your hands. Proceed as you wish.

I'm experiencing quite a lot of discomfort, but managing. In the second week of July we'll move into the Villa Schüler, near the south train station in Semmering.

One more request. Can you order a book for me that supposedly just appeared in America? It's called History of Assyria, *by Olmstead. Hopefully this presents no difficulty for you. It's possible the book has appeared in England, in which case you need do nothing else.*

Cordial greetings. Yours, Freud

Dr. Otto Rank 117 W 58th St New York ¶July 11, 1924

Lieber Herr Professor,

Mr. Edward Bernays had a note sent to me today informing me that Boni and Liveright want to publish your American lectures in book form, and that you've referred them to me. I'll write B. & L. today that I must first get an agreement with you, but it seems very unlikely that you'll give them publication rights for $75.00, the sum your nephew mentioned in the letter. Now to the matter itself:

1.) In this affair, I can figure only as your representative, and will gladly do so if you wish; in my opinion, the Verlag has nothing to do with this.

2.) The rights are held either by Deuticke, who published the lectures in German, or (more likely) by Stanley Hall and the American Journal of Psychology, *where these lectures were first published. (I think it's correct that the 5 lectures appeared first in English, and Clark University, by inviting you, acquired the publication rights.) In any case, please tell me who you think has publication rights in America or if you think you have the right to decide this.*

3.) After this is resolved one way or another comes the question in which I could represent you: the honorarium. Putting it mildly, I find the $75 for the publication rights shameless. If you give me a free hand, I'd demand at least $1000—taking the risk that B&L might not publish it. But if you care mainly that the 5 lectures appear here in book form, and care less about the honorarium, please let me know your limit. Anyway, I think that up to a certain point this is a question of prestige; I don't think you should let them have this "cheaply."

This is the attitude I myself adopt toward various publishing contracts here; I gladly reject any publication offer presented merely as an honor if some American publisher wishes to make money from translations of my works. Quite frankly this is my position here now, and I'm not allowing any literary ambition to swell in my breast. Perhaps it's absolutely my position here, as I notice I'm not making anything but money, and have no other interests. Since arriving here, I have neither read nor written a single line—and even writing a letter is hard for me, as you can see.

I'm glad to contemplate your upcoming vacation, and hope that you will have a really fine and beautiful summer.

With cordial greetings to your family and yourself. Yours, Rank

Dr. Otto Rank 117 W 58th St New York ¶July 17, 1924

Lieber Herr Professor,

I was glad to get the book you wanted, just recently published by Scribner's; I'll have it sent today by Brentano's.

Re Jones: The sad thing is that, just like you, I'm glad to have nothing to do with him, but at the moment I can't take another step in this whole business without coming into contact with him. His last letter, a few days ago, reduces my role in the whole matter to my selling books here for the former "Press." He wants to grant me no other rights, but I'd prefer to decline the honor of being a "traveling salesman" for Jones. Regrettably, then, for the time being there is absolutely no possibility of doing anything for you or for the Verlag.

I hope you're enjoying the vacation, and cordially greet you and your family. Yours, Rank

Prof. Dr. Freud Villa Schüler Semmering ¶July 23, 1924

Lieber Herr Doktor

I owe it to Boni and Liveright that I heard from you again. Concerning this, I'll say only that I accepted each of your decisions, and that I can bear it easily should nothing come of it. You're certainly correct in putting prestige before other things, but I think you're intoxicated with money if you demand $1000; $300, even $250, would be appropriate, and still strike B&L as extravagant and impossible. My nephew hinted that the publisher wants to take something else to add to the Five Lectures. This must be stopped. Deuticke has no rights to this book, which was printed simultaneously or even beforehand in the American Journal of Psychology. If it were Europe, where a journal's rights expire after three years at most, there'd be no doubt as to my sole rights. I know nothing about authors' rights in America. Do they exist? One should ask.

I'm very glad Edward B[ernays] approached you again, in fact, following my cable. Though an American through and through, he's a good fellow. It's too bad you haven't gotten along better with him. To my reproaches he gave a detailed report on your transgressions of form, which makes further mediation difficult for me. I urged him to consider the things that may have been involved on your side, and assured him that you didn't intend any disrespect.

The day before yesterday I received a letter from T. Burrow, who seeks information from me, as he's disturbed by your birth theory. I'll answer in a mollifying fashion. Otherwise, he had no connection with me, and was, I believe, a Jungian; according to Uncle Max's report, he seems to be an incurable fool. But the issue itself has gotten my attention. In the months since our separation, I've receded further from agreeing with your innovations. In my cases after the two I completed I've seen nothing that coincides with your innovations; indeed, I've seen nothing I didn't know already. The final birth fantasy still seems to me to signify the child one gives the father analytically. I'm often very concerned about you. The elimination of the father in your theory strikes me as revealing much too much the influence of personal factors in your life—factors I believe I'm familiar with. This increases my suspicion that you wouldn't have written this book if you'd undergone analysis yourself. Thus I'd request urgently that you not become fixated, and that you leave open a way back.

My condition is perhaps quite good, but still ambiguous to me. I have so many troubles that I never experience a comfortable mood or any security. Others must be thinking in a similar way, for rumors were circulating in Vienna about a worsening of my condition, which Neues Wiener Journal—unasked—published and denied. I've dismissed Deutsch as my physician. Meanwhile I'm enjoying my beautiful current surroundings in these mountain heights, and am again writing a history of P/A for Grote's collection of "self-portrayals."

Many cordial greetings. Yours, Freud

Prof. Dr. Freud Semmering ¶August 6, 1924

Lieber Herr Doktor,

I enclose the two letters from Jones and from Boni and Liveright. Since you left the decision up to me, I'm prepared to allow the Five Lectures to be published by the two swindlers, and accept 75 dollars for them. Please deposit the money for me and deduct the cost of the book on Assyrian history, for which I cordially thank you. I'd have much preferred that the lectures appear alone as a special publication. Of course that doesn't seem to be the case, but we'll let it go.

We're having bad weather up here, but are otherwise quite comfortable. Lampl is here now. Abraham says he'll arrive on the 10th, and Eitingon will arrive on the 25th.

May the New York summer be easy for you! Cordially yours, Freud

On August 6 Freud wrote Ferenczi about Rank: "It is hard to make a judgment, since he is so discreet and uncommunicative. Something is happening with him under the influence of the ambitious little woman [Tola]. His letters to me are rare, brief, and ill-tempered." Ferenczi agreed with Freud's view of Rank, but cautioned, "His wife's influence seems to me rather to be favorable; she endeavors to moderate her husband" (Aug. 14).

Dr. Otto Rank New York ¶August 9, 1924

Lieber Herr Professor

Regarding your unambiguous rejection of my conception, the indirect reproach you express to me for not writing gives me occasion to tell you today what I wished to save until my return. All the more so, since I have the impression that for various reasons you want to know where you actually stand with me, in order to clear up the situation—which I also desire, since I consider it intolerable in its current form.

Now, the fact is that I've had exactly the same experience as you: indeed, for the whole time of my work here, which is highly varied and intensive, by the day and the hour I've found nothing but confirmation and completion of my conception, which, by the way, is confirmed here by many others, too. As it happened, just in the last few days I had another chance to see how the fantasy of giving the father a child can't be solved analytically and made therapeutically fruitful except by tracing it back to the mother and one's own birth. Further, I certainly don't understand why you place so much value on the final birth theory, which is, therapeutically and theoretically, far less important than the basic idea that the libido of transference is a purely maternal one and that the anxiety underlying all symptoms was originally associated with the mother's genitals, and only secondarily transferred to the father. If you interpret the phenomenon of transference starting with the father, then you get homosexual fixation in a man and heterosexual fixation in a woman as the result of analysis—which actually holds for all the cases that come to me from other analysts. The analysts among these patients have felt this both subjectively and objectively: subjectively, since they have lost nothing of their neurosis, and objectively, since they were unable to cure their own patients with this technique. This is attributable not to the people here, who are no better or worse than those in Europe, but to the shortcomings of method and technique. When people saw that their work gets easier and they achieve better results with the modifications I introduced, they praised me as a savior. I'm not so blinded as not to see a good portion of these successes are determined by complexes, but what remains is a portion of truth and reality that one cannot banish from the world by closing one's eyes. I have the definite impression that you don't wish to see certain things or that you can't see them, for sometimes your objections sound as though you hadn't read or heard what I actually said. (I'll just remind you that I once pointed out to you that you imputed something to Ferenczi and me that we had never maintained: it was precisely the opposite.) Now again you're saying that I eliminated the father. That's not so, of course, and cannot be: it would be nonsense. I've only attempted to assign him the correct place.

Here you apparently bring in personal relations between you and me where they don't belong. In this connection I was struck by the fact that you of all people claim that, had I been analyzed, I'd never have supported this conception. The only question is, wouldn't that have been very regrettable? After everything I've seen of results with analyzed analysts I can only characterize that as fortunate. And you know as well as I do, first of all, that the accusation that an insight derives from a complex means very little, and secondly, that it says nothing about the value or veracity of this insight. All the less so, since even psa. has shown that the very greatest achievements result from complexes and overcoming them. As I write this, it's painful to me that through a scientific divergence that one would think could be seriously discussed, a discordant note has come into our personal relationship. To some extent, that's probably inevitable in all human relations. Yet I think I hear from your letter that your personal feelings for me may be the same as always. Thus I regret even more so that objectively you cannot do me justice.

For example, I'm convinced you have an incorrect idea of how I practice psa. technique. I've given up no part of it, only added something I certainly consider very important, and which others, too, already consider indispensable for an understanding of the cases and for a therapeutic influence on them. I don't know to what extent I can still hope to show you on some occasion, through cases, what I can achieve. Anyway, my therapeutic achievements are more and better than when you yourself were speaking very highly of them.

Nor do I know the extent to which your judgment of, or prejudice against, my conception was influenced by certain rabble-rousers who seem to have the irresistible need to cast themselves from time to time as saviors of psa. or of your own person— without seeing that in so doing they only give rein to their childish envy. The latest plans and conspiracies I hear of in Berlin strike me as so stupid, and are so unworthy of a scientific movement, that I hope you won't pay much attention to them either. I'd like to know what anyone hopes to achieve through them. If there's a desire to drive me from my official positions, to which until now I was bound not by ambition but by duty and concern and work, this can be done without recourse to back-room politics— if you should wish it. If there is a desire to refute my conception, there's really no need to foment intrigue. The more light there is, the more pleasant it will be for me, as the profound ignorance of people like Abraham, among others, will be all the more apparent. Do you really believe, Professor, that an argument from someone like Abraham will impress me when I've lost faith even in your judgment in this matter? I think people are more interested in intrigue for its own sake than in attaining any definite goals. Yet this is precisely the point where I won't play along—if the cards for both sides are not laid out on the table. After my experiences with the defunct Committee, one can hardly expect me to become involved in a similar affair with concessions and compromises—supposedly in the interest of psa. but really in the personal interest of the participants, who certainly know how easily one can burn one's own fingers at the enjoyable spectacle of an auto-da-fé. Perhaps you'll tell me I'm mistaken—that Abraham is, on the contrary, ready for peace, etc. That's just the hypocrisy I'm fighting against: that sacrifices are supposedly being made in the interest of the cause, whereas they're of no use to anyone, but only destroy the movement in whose interest they were supposedly made. Let's not forget that the psa. movement as such is a fiction. The people who establish a movement are no fiction, and frankly, I am fed up with the people who are now occupied with establishing a psa. movement.

As you see, I'm stating my position toward the whole affair absolutely as frankly as I can, since in doing so I see the last hope of clarifying the situation as soon as possible, given that it has already become difficult for you as well, for when speaking with different people you have to take different positions toward my ideas. I also felt that you personally have a right to learn what I'm really thinking and feeling in this critical, and personally so painful, situation.

I was very glad to hear from you directly that you're satisfied with your condition. If one can trust the psychology of denial, this good condition will last a very long time.

Best wishes to your family and cordial greetings to you. Yours respectfully, Rank

The next day Rank wrote Ferenczi to explain why he withdrew the invitation to New York.

New York, August 10, 1924

Lieber Sándor,

I have the impression that you're making me a bit too responsible for the disappointment that not coming of course causes you. By describing the situation, I'd like to show that you're being unfair to me. If I've perhaps caused you disappointment, it happened in the firm belief that I was sparing you a greater one, which I think your coming here would have caused.

When I proposed that you come, I was influenced, as I said then, by two factors. At first I was fully occupied, and had a number of people on my waiting list. Secondly, I'd heard that some analysts here planned to invite Abraham. Both reasons have now disappeared. There's no talk now of inviting another analyst—Abraham is the last person one would think of inviting—and the swarm of patients, which people joked lined the whole length of Broadway, has shrunk so much that I'll have trouble filling my schedule next month. The usually very busy analysts have one to two patients now, and even Brill, the busiest, is here only three days a week. I know this is affected by the summer, but talking with analysts leads me to doubt autumn will be any better. I'd be unable to pass on or refer cases myself, so you'd depend on the others, who are themselves hungry fish that live on scraps from the big neurologists and psychiatrists. My own success here was unique and not to be repeated. I couldn't repeat it myself, for I had mainly analysts, who know what such an opportunity means, and who made great sacrifice to take advantage of it for themselves. Of course they want to be rid of me soon, having learned from me what they could, and that leaves little hope for acceptance of another stranger. Brill, with whom I spoke at length about your coming, is extremely jealous—even of younger colleagues, first and foremost you and me. His support of young colleagues is proverbial: he sends either poor patients or those with whom nothing can be done analytically (demented).

I've saved the life of psychoanalysis here, and perhaps thereby that of the entire international movement. The analysts here were mostly uncured and dissatisfied after their analysis with the Professor. As they and everyone else said, they came back worse than ever. Frink and others served as examples.... That was not the fault of the analysts, who simply repeated what the Professor had done with them. That is, they interpreted transference as a manifestation of the libido toward the father, whereby in male patients they produced a homosexual connection with the analyst, and in female patients a heterosexual fixation. Just as it used to be said that there was no virgin in Paris, in New York there is no patient (analyst or otherwise) who has not already undergone several analyses—including some in Europe.

When I came, the situation was as follows: psychiatrists with patients to refer didn't want to hear about psychoanalysis, but neither did the patients. The most dire aspect was that the analysts themselves were in despair: to an extent they criticized themselves, calling themselves ignorant, and to an extent they criticized the Professor and analysis in general. In analyzing them and showing them how one must analyze, I restored their trust in themselves and in psychoanalysis. They are extremely satisfied on both counts, so satisfied they think they need me no more (of course an inevitable aspect of their reaction against me as analyst, but which forces me to withdraw from here at least for a while, and would also make it difficult for you to get a foothold here). Now we have to wait and see what fruits my work will bear, and it's certainly possible that later one or even both of us can return....

Quite by accident I heard there are plans to render both of us harmless somehow. The leaders of this are of course Abraham, who's visiting the Professor in August,

and Radó, who has apparently taken on the role of your antagonist....In any case, I'll
undertake no further political actions, and will permit none to be perpetrated against
me. I am really tired of the whole thing....Yours, Otto

**Rank sent a note to Freud on August 14 introducing a neurologist visiting
Vienna. Freud replied promptly, before receiving Rank's of August 9.**

Semmering ¶August 25, 1924

Lieber Herr Doktor,

 I got a letter from you today, but it contains only an introduction for a superfluous
Dr. Wechsler. I notice that in the months you've been away, in situations critical for
us—for you and for me—you've shown no great need to let me know what is happening
in and with you. This worries me.

 Although I now see most events sub specie aeternitatis, *and cannot expend my*
full passion on them, I'm not indifferent to the changes in my relation to you. My
condition seems to indicate that I have, after all, some time left to live, and it is my
strong wish that during that time you not amount to a loss for me. You left Europe, as I
hear, in an agitated and suspicious frame of mind. The knowledge that I've somewhat
receded in my estimation of your work must have contributed further to your bad
mood. You probably overestimate the emotional significance of this theoretical differ-
ence, thinking that during your absence I've been accessible to influences hostile to you.
It's the intent of this letter to assure you that this is not the case. I'm not so accessible
to others, and others—Eitingon and Abraham visited me here for several days—are
equally sincere in recognizing your extraordinary achievements, and deeply regret the
curtness with which you are isolating yourself. There's no enmity against you, neither
among us nor among my family in New York. Before your return there is just enough
time to exchange letters. I'd like you to enlighten me and put my mind at ease about
your current condition.

 The difference of opinion concerning the birth trauma is not important to me. In
the course of time, if there is still enough time, either you'll convince and correct me, or
you'll correct yourself, separating what is a permanent new acquisition from what the
bias of the discoverer has done to it. I know you're not lacking praise for your inno-
vation, but you must consider also how few people are capable of judging, and how
strong are the efforts in most of them to be rid of the Oedipus complex where a path
seems to present itself. Even if there are many flaws, you shouldn't be ashamed of an
intellectually stimulating and rich production, which also brings its critics new and

valuable material. It mustn't be assumed that your work must disturb our established intimate relationship of many years.

To my cordial greetings I would add that I hope to see you soon. Yours, Freud

Semmering ¶August 27, 1924

Lieber Herr Doktor,

Had I waited just one more day I could have spared myself my last letter. I dare hope no repetition of this affair awaits us. But your letter was very painful to me. I didn't think you could write in such a way. There's no end to surprises. One can never be prepared for everything.

When you first mentioned The Trauma of Birth *to me, I made two comments, both of which I recall. (Perhaps my memory combines two things here.) The first was: "That's not the right presentation." You answered: "But I can't do it another way." Your presentation bears a large burden of responsibility for the critical reserve that arose in me toward your discovery after the first fascinating impression. The correct thing would have been to show how the innovation is founded on available facts you do not oppose, that is, on the libido theory, the Oedipus complex, and the role of the father. In your book, this is either completely omitted or touched on so superficially as to create the impression of residual indecision or of polite avoidance, while the consequence diverts one's thoughts to other matters—and with such failure in one's presentation those impressions are decisive. For example, you leave two paths open to me now, both leading to the same judgment—the way of observation and that of comparison with earlier opinions or, if you will, prejudices. My observations haven't yet enabled me to decide, but neither have they provided anything that would speak in your favor.*

In the last half a year I had six cases; five knew of your theory. Some had learned it from you. Of course I didn't suggest any contradiction. The result was that the analyses progressed as always, without any miraculous alleviation or acceleration. Your experiences are otherwise, but do you reject mine? We both know that experiences are ambiguous, and thus await further analysis.

The right to one's own opinion applies to me as well. I've attempted to respect it with each of my friends and followers so long as we could preserve common ground. When I was on good terms with Jung, he expressed the opinion that dementia praecox was of a toxic nature, and not to be explained by the libido theory. That didn't bother me. With Ferenczi's proposals on homosexuality, and with many aspects of his activity, I was and am not in agreement. I find that he overvalues full agreement with me, while I place no value on that. Even had you revealed that you couldn't believe in the primal horde or primal father, or that you held the separation into ego and id to be impractical, do you really believe that for that reason I'd have failed to invite you to dinner or that I'd have excluded you from intimacy on my part? Indeed, you were always very reserved in such critical opinions—probably too much so. And now you seem deeply troubled and irritated that I am inclined against your Trauma of Birth, *whereas you have my admission that it will never be easy for me to find my way into new thought processes that in some sense do not lie on my own path or to which my own path has not yet led me.*

The second path remains: comparison with earlier prejudices. There I have much to confess, e.g. my inability to understand how the magic formula of tracing the libido back to the mother is to produce the redeeming effect absent in other acts of analysis. According to our theory all object libido is originally narcissistic. This tracing back goes still further, and I have never been able to attribute to it a curative effect. By the way, can you always determine whether the libido has proceeded from the mother to another object, or whether the mother simply happened to be the first object (introduction of narcissism, which I am just now correcting), while the other components of the narcissistic libido turned to other objects? Those are all such dark and indeterminate things that a great amount of tolerance should be permitted in the interpretation.

We previously attributed the curative effect of analysis to overcoming resistance occurring when the repressed is converted to consciousness. The question as to whether that can be reconciled with the assumption that this effect derives from the success of the abreaction of the birth trauma requires a detailed discussion. The first impression is that the two ideas are incompatible. The entire topic is shrouded in an obscurity I have thus far been unsuccessful in penetrating. Your book has invoked it, but has done nothing to dispel it. Your treatment of anxiety seems full of contradictions. On the one hand, you claim that this anxiety is a beneficial construction as it forbids the desired regression. On the other hand, you claim that a desirable achievement of analysis is to eliminate this anxiety through abreaction of the birth trauma, thereby actually opening up the path to regression for the first time. Something is wrong here. I suspect that birth simply cannot be evaluated as a psychological trauma, probably because there is as yet no assignment of objects, but rather as a physiological trauma that could also be dealt with psychologically through restoration of the expression for an affect. I think you're opening the psychological account too early, but here I can't see clearly yet.

In a letter, even this long, one can only discuss aspects of the matter. I'd like to continue the discussion, dear Rank, over several winter evenings, when you're again in a condition to do so. But now comes the second pronouncement. I said then that with such a discovery another person would have made himself independent. I still hold fast to this qualification. Otherwise I'd have to declare the situation hopeless. There are nasty things in your letter. To ascribe "profound ignorance" to Abraham and to consider him a "forward rabble rouser"—that takes a disturbance of judgment that can be explained only by boundless affectivity, unconducive to overcoming complexes. An evil demon lets you say: "The psychoanalytic movement is only a 'fiction,'" and in so doing puts the words of the enemy in your mouth. An abstract thing can also be real, and therefore is no "fiction."

Your angrily bitter remark that you are glad you were not analyzed—otherwise you wouldn't have made your discovery, which is based on the existence of complexes—is unjustified. You overlook the danger that has already undone some people: that of taking what stirs within one and projecting it as a theory into science—that's not as good as overcoming it.

This exegesis is very painful to me, but parts of your letter sound as though you're determined, after over fifteen years of intimate collaboration, to break off your relation to us and our cause, thus giving in to the suspicion that initially outraged you so. If that's your serious intent, what can I do? What can I say to you that you don't already know and must have discovered for yourself in the last fifteen years? If my illness had progressed further, that would have spared you a certain, not easy, decision. Since I must apparently orient myself to living on, I stand before a situation I'd have rejected as unimaginable a short time ago. It's especially painful that I find the cause of this loss so insufficient. It's no comfort that I can't blame myself. My feelings for you have not been diminished by anything, and I can't give up hope that you'll come further toward calm self-reflection.

I'm in no hurry to post this letter, and will first ask your wife when you're due back.

Cordially yours, Freud

Enclosing Rank's hurtful letter of August 9, Freud wrote Ferenczi the same day: "We must be prepared for the worst outcome. . . . Rank hasn't officially declared his withdrawal. But it is as good as if it were written in the letter." If it happens, he hoped Ferenczi would take over editorship of the journals; Anna would assist. "Aside from you, only Eitingon will learn of Rank's letter and my intentions."[1]

The summer's flood of ink fills dozens of pages in recently published volumes of Freud letters, especially to Ferenczi. Freud recalled Rank through the years as "tenderly concerned, obliging, discreet, absolutely dependable, just as prepared to accept suggestions as he was uninhibited in working up his own ideas, on my side in all contentious matters, without inner compulsion," but "now, who is the real Rank, the one I have known for 15 [actually 18] years, or the one whom Jones has wanted to show me for years?" (Aug. 29.) Ferenczi and Freud both found Rank's latest book *Analysis of Neuroses in Dreams* (1924) "unpalatably written" and "unreadable," respectively.[2]

Ferenczi defended his appreciation for Rank's work but conceded that his friend had gone too far. He agreed, if needed, to take over Rank's Verlag responsibilities. Hoping "Rank's invaluable collaboration for the cause could be saved," Ferenczi wrote, "I feel very imperfectly suited to replace him!" Noting Freud's promise that Anna Freud, Siegfried Bernfeld, and A. J. Storfer would assist, he added, "you see that three to four people are needed to represent him alone (incompletely)" (Sept. 1). Freud responded, "I only fear Rank's stiffening in his bitterness, to put it straight-out: his neurosis, which has become manifest." While agreeing to suspend criticism, Freud justified his transition from positive to negative judgment and complained that "Rank's inclination to reduce everything to intrigues and personal motives is very regrettable" (Sept. 4).

Two days later he commented on a draft letter by Ferenczi to Rank, which had "a few outstanding spots and shows some omissions," such as "your reaction to the advantage of not being analyzed, a regrettable admission of the alienation from analysis that already exists with him." (Freud defended Rank on Dec. 15, 1922 against a suggestion that he be analyzed.) Freud's letter to Ferenczi continued:

He is in a discoverer paranoia, overpowered by his production, completely like Adler in his time, but if on the strength of that he makes himself independent, he won't have the same luck for his theory contradicts the common sense of the laity, who found themselves flattered by Adler's striving for power....If he comes to his senses it will naturally be high time to remind him of his extraordinary services and his irreplaceability, and pardon all his aberrations. But I don't dare believe in that; from experience, once the devil is loose, he goes his way to the end. It grieves me greatly that Jones may be right after all.

Aligning with Freud, Ferenczi replied on September 9: "His opposition to you still can't be justified by such a discovery, no matter how great it is, and his state of mind requires a pathological evaluation. . . . His attitude toward you remains almost inexcusable." Freud, "boiling with rage," concluded on September 13 that Rank intended from the beginning "to establish himself on the basis of a new patent procedure that was kept secret, and requested your participation. I'm surprised you went so far along in this secret hum-bug. . . . I can only imagine that my apparently imminent demise uprooted him so, and that my recovery upset his calculations." Ferenczi (Sept. 21) fears Rank has gone too far, basking in exaggerated American praise. He is ready if need be to turn away from his friend, adding that Rank "was right to the extent that he better appreciated the neglected mother relation."

Dr. Otto Rank 117 W. 58th St New York ¶September 16, 1924

Lieber Herr Professor,

Reading your letter of August 25, I noted with regret that you haven't yet—or not at all?—received my detailed letter of August 9, which was written before Wechsler's.

Nevertheless, I'm glad your letter solves the most important problem for me, my personal relation to you, in a satisfactory manner. I, too, see no reason why a scientific difference of opinion should necessarily prove disturbing here, and I was glad to hear the same opinion from you.

Dealing with this difference of opinion itself does not seem to me to be as simple as you suggest. I have the impression that you don't want to be convinced, and from your standpoint, I can understand that very well. As for me, I shall work further, according to my experience and orientation, and undisturbed by agreement or criticism, for long ago I began applying to my critics as well your well-intentioned advice not to trust human judgment very far. Obviously, one can never please everyone. The only mea-sure is and remains whether one can be true to oneself. This is the case now, and if I have anything to be ashamed of, it could only be the reaction of some so-called friends and colleagues to this, my work.

And now I come to the third point, the discussion of which in your letter satisfied me least. I can't understand why you want to convince yourself that there is no enmity toward me, given that recently you yourself have provided so much proof of it. But I no longer care much how one person or another stands toward me. Everyone should and can find happiness in his own way, and I'd like to claim this right for myself too, especially concerning my intellectual company, which I'd like to seek out for myself, instead of being married to it through my relation to psychoanalysis. In this sense, many people should have understood the supposed gruffness with which I have with-drawn—rather than criticizing it.

I'll leave New York in September after a period of work that was satisfying in every way. But since my family's vacation was seriously disturbed by weather and illness, and since I really need some recuperation myself, we'll spend some time in the south, so I can't be in Vienna before the end of October. I also feel a much greater need for rest and freedom, and more than before I'm thinking about shifting many official burdens to nimbler shoulders; my absence has shown that this is entirely feasible.

I hope to find you as well as can be expected from your own pleasant description, and cordially greet you and your family in the meantime.

Yours, Rank

Freud shared this letter with Eitingon on September 27, writing that Rank was "coolly withdrawing"—Anna's expression. That he has money "will certainly not make him more pliable. Otherwise I'd be glad for this success of his." Freud sees profound "bitterness and alienation" in Rank's claim that Freud does not want to be convinced. To Freud it is outrageous that Rank "has told no one 1) what he actually teaches, or 2) what he does technically. You knew that . . . I was, on the contrary, very ready to be convinced by him (but of what?). After this letter one might as well give him up."[3]

Abraham, who visited Freud during the summer, wrote him sympathetically, mostly avoiding controversy. Jones, unfazed by criticism of his handling of the American publishing rights, wrote Freud on August 12 that Frink had had a breakdown and was an inpatient. As to Rank's success in New York, "he has three things to offer that Americans most desire: the latest novelty, quick results, and a schematic system which evades the laborious fight with the repressed infantile." Jones heard that the Budapest group was using Ferenczi's ideas "to feed their own resistances." He regarded the VPS as unstable and the Dutch and Swiss groups as unimportant, so "that leaves us with Berlin and London as the only staunch defenders of psychoanalysis."

Freud replied to Jones (Sept. 25) with contempt for Americans, who were good for money, nothing else. "My attempt at giving them a chief in the person of Frink, which has so sadly miscarried, is the last thing I will ever do for them." He attributed Frink's breakdown to a failed attack on Brill. Freud was disappointed that Angelika Bijur, Frink's former patient and second wife, did not provide some of her "millions" to the Verlag. (Freud encouraged the divorces and the new marriage; Mr. Bijur threatened to publish an ad in the *New York Times* criticizing Freud, but became ill and died.)[4] Jones, in a long letter (Sept. 29) tells Freud of Brill's recent stay with him in London. They had not met for 11 years; Jones found him "much improved . . . a gifted analyst," though they were not in agreement on some aspects of technique. "He and Oberndorf are the only two who are uninfluenced by Rank's theories.

Many other members, including most of those who were with you in Vienna, evidently find them a valuable outlet for their resistances and are having analysis with Rank.... [Rank's] disparaging remarks about both your person and your work are the most painful, though the most comprehensible." Rank's "manifest neurosis," visible to him as early as 1913, had now "gradually returned in the form of a neurotic character," a "denial of the Oedipus complex" and "a regression of the hostility from the brother (myself) ... to the father"—evidently Freud. He castigates Rank for publishing his birth trauma paper in the *Psychoanalytic Review*, "the refuge of all malcontents," and the English language rival to his *Journal*.[5]

Freud told Eitingon (Oct. 7) news of Rank's behavior in New York and reports that Ferenczi "has parted with him in all the essentials." Freud will postpone the leadership change at the VPS by having Federn be his proxy. "Anna spits fire when Rank's name is mentioned. I remain cool, but I must admit that this is a nasty turn of events."

Dr. Otto Rank Meran [Italy] Pension Tannheim ¶October 10, 1924
Lieber Herr Professor,

After a pleasant journey I arrived here in the beginning of the week, where I found my family in good health, although our little one still needs further recuperation. Given this, and my own need for rest after the hard work of the last few months, we decided to stay another 14 days, so I can't arrive in Vienna before month's end. I'll delay answering your last long letter until then, since I also hope to clear up various problems at hand in a personal discussion.

I look forward to finding you in good health, and in the meantime send you and your family the best greetings.

Respectfully yours, Rank

In a note dated October 21 from Italy, Rank proposed meeting Freud on arrival in Vienna, Sunday, October 26. Freud agreed, confiding to Jones (Oct. 23): "I nourish no illusions on the result of this interview." Freud and Rank had not seen each other for six months.

≈ Chapter 17 ≈

About-face

October to December 1924

I still retain a vivid impression regarding the quality of the several speakers. With one exception all seemed to me unimpressive, if not actually dull, until the slight, boyish figure of Rank appeared beside the speaker's desk. He was the very image of my idea of the scholarly German student and he spoke so quietly, so directly and simply, without circumlocution or apology, that despite the strong German accent I was able to follow his argument and I thought to myself, "Here is a man one could trust."
—Jessie Taft, on the APA annual meeting, New York

Psychologist Jessie Taft became Rank's staunch supporter and translator. Her description of his first American appearance points up his subdued, attractive, convincing manner.[1] He impressed many others, too, although reports from A. A. Brill and others indicate a change during the summer to flamboyant and hostile, as in his letters to Freud.

Anna Freud first met Rank around 1906, at age 10. Now 28, she wrote Max Eitingon about the harsh letter from Rank to her father, which he had also seen. "I no longer believe that suddenly Rank will wake up and be his former self; maybe he never was the one we seemed to see all those years? . . . How can one know anything at all about people, if they can be either way? . . . He is full of hidden, cheap meanness. This becomes clear knowing that the ones he speaks of are all Papa's former analysands."[2]

On October 20, Karl Abraham wrote Freud from Berlin, with sympathy and support for the impending meeting with Rank. He reassures Freud that they can handle a turnover of the Verlag directorate and that the Committee could be reestablished without Rank. He refers to the 1923 San Cristoforo meeting.[3]

> *Otto's efforts were directed towards blasting the Committee apart. We sat then in judgment over Ernest's incorrect behavior, because the continued existence of the Committee seemed in danger due to this behavior. The much graver danger lay in quite another quarter.*
>
> *With hindsight, I'd like to say that the neurotic process in Otto has been in the making over the course of several years. While he tried to compensate for his negative tendencies by over-conscientious work, his need for friendly togetherness with us others lessened and his arbitrary and tyrannical behaviour became more striking in many ways. Added to this, there has been an increased emphasis on money interests and, simultaneously, increased irritability and hostility. Thus, an undeniable regression to anal sadism. The disappearance of all friendly feelings towards you has recently become very clear. When I consider all this, I can also now only take an analytic point of view; I do not feel a trace of hostility towards Otto. My reaction is one of infinite regret that you have to suffer this trial, and particularly with Otto, and that Otto himself seems to have come—apparently unstoppably—onto a pathological track. I noticed together with Hanns and Max at our meeting that they were both strongly involved emotionally and for that reason reject any further getting together with Otto, whereas I finished with the emotional side long ago and can now only stress the psychological hopelessness.*

On October 26, Freud reported to Ferenczi about his three-hour meeting with Rank that afternoon: "The result was absolutely surprising, in no way understandable. He said it doesn't occur to him to want to separate from us and analysis; he holds fast to everything he has learned, only he has some things to add to it." Rank, fearing for his position after the attack from Berlin, went to America to look at prospects for a future there. He promises to give a full explanation at the meeting of the Vienna Psychoanalytic Society. As to the severe criticisms about him, he "doesn't want to admit that his book, his utterances, and his behavior were somehow able to justify this." Freud could not trust him now: "He still owes an answer to some questions and gets disconcerted. . . . I didn't spare him at all, and finally sent Anna to give him a going over. . . . So, on the whole, I don't understand the matter." Rank said he'd like to spend a few months in America again, but a permanent move was "far from his mind." Freud warned that an editor/publisher could hardly expect to work only six months a year in the office.

Ferenczi and Eitingon joined Freud and Rank in Vienna the last day of October. Rank resigned as Verlag director and *Zeitschrift* co-editor; he would continue to edit *Imago* with Sachs. Storfer would direct the Verlag, and Radó would edit the journal in Berlin, assisted by Eitingon and Ferenczi. Rank would sail to America before Christmas, for several months.

Freud conveyed all this to Jones on November 5: "As you see, an open breach has been avoided. Rank himself did not intend one, and a row is not in our interest either. But all more intimate relations with him have come to an end. We cannot explain his behavior; however, this much is certain: he discarded us all with great ease, and is preparing a new existence for himself independent of us." Freud regards Rank's accusation of bad treatment as a way of making his decision easier. Freud credits Jones with being mostly right in his predictions but postpones judgment on Rank's analytic technique, much of which remains a secret, something "not customary in scientific activity."

Jones replied, "I am as sorry I was right as you are yourself. . . . Bearing the brunt of his neurotic behavior in these last years forced me to think deeply about him. . . . My one hope was that you should never know, and my endeavours to prevent this cost me dearly in many ways. But I was throughout very fond of Rank. . . . I still wish him well in his future life, though I fear he has not chosen an easy path."[4]

Freud assured Jones that the Rank affair had not affected him deeply, for three reasons: "old age, which no longer takes losses so much to heart"; a relationship that "amortized itself" in the 15 years; and feeling "in absolutely no way to blame for this outcome." That same day, Ferenczi acknowledged that Jones was right about Rank in a Rundbrief reestablishing the Committee.

Writing Brill in New York, Freud repeated the latter two of his three points, adding, "No doubt the question is very complicated, with the personal and the scientific so much intertwined that to deal with these separately is impossible." He continued:

> I think you've found him out completely. It's the dollar that lures him. But there
> are other motives on top of that. Probably the shock of my serious illness and the fear
> resulting from it, the loss of his existence. Furthermore, the temptation of making dis-

coveries in analysis that is characteristic of all unanalyzed beginners. With Jung it was the same.

…He denied speaking against analysis or against me in New York.…As to the value of his theoretical and technical innovation, I confirm that your judgment on both agrees completely with that of our Berlin friends, Abraham, Eitingon, Sachs— and Jones as well.…He indeed behaves like someone who has invented a patent medicine with a secret formula.…About the personal conflict with him I also speak as little as possible. You are the first person to get a sincere letter from me about this.

Of course it very much pleased me that you forcefully took on the stupid boys [dumme Jungen] in the Society. Hopefully you'll keep your strong influence. I know you'll use it in the same way. Still, be more careful with this letter than on the last occasion with Frink. I assume Rank has begun a precarious undertaking and I'd not like him to say because of a misstep that I pursued him to America and am to blame for the collapse of his hopes. I think it's enough if you oppose him in your own name. If you are asked about me you can say that I see absolutely no way to judge the matter so long as Rank denies his technique and hides his theoretical deductions, and that we're all prepared for an objective test as soon as we know something.

…My health has perhaps not been restored to the extent that my good friends wish, but I exist and work to a certain extent. We must not forget that aging itself is an illness.

It's fine with me that you have reconciled with Jones.…

Cordial greetings, and, again, please handle this letter discreetly, seeing with your own eyes and doing only what is necessary. Your faithful Freud[5]

On November 19, Freud wrote Eitingon about his farewell with Rank, about to leave for New York. Rank was depressed and hardly spoke, "unable to pull himself together." Freud recounts the dramatic interview verbatim, to be shared with Ferenczi and the Berlin group. Freud told Rank:

"You have spread a great darkness over yourself; that cannot go on for half a year. A few days ago I got a letter from Brill describing events at the last Society meeting. In the end, he became angry with everyone and left. One after the other, the people you analyzed stood up and made declarations as a result of your stimulus; the one declared that there was no further need to analyze dreams; the other that we are now free of sexuality; the third expressed how nice it is that one need only interrupt the patient and direct him toward the birth trauma. That is supposedly what the people have learned from you."

He demurred, smiling, and said, "I can't help it if people use me to bring their defenses to light."

Then I avenged myself. I said, "Those are the same people you defended against me in your letter—the people about whom you said, 'They are seeing the successes of my analysis,' declaring that you were glad not to have been analyzed. The same people whose savior you celebrated yourself. Now we hear what the successes of your analysis are, and if they look like this, the overlap with the suspicions first expressed in Berlin is highly evident. You may say you have been misunderstood. Well, in six months it will be time to clarify such misunderstandings. When you come back we will both know what is going on with you."

He interjected, "Why did Brill, with whom I have of course spoken myself, pay attention to what they said? Why didn't he tell them what he had heard from me?"

I said: "Because he probably had not assumed that you were sincere with him." Then I let myself go. I said, "It isn't easy for me either, after 15 years of work and such friendly relations, to let you leave like this. But that can no longer be changed. You have told me that your efforts to establish a secure existence for yourself have led you to America. So you probably assumed that with my disappearance your existence is threatened. I believe you are wrong. The foreign patients would have continued to come to you, as my heir. But let's assume it were so. Then you could have explained this to me honestly; you would have traveled away with my approval and all my influence at your disposal. You did not do that; you had to add the invented claim that I've treated you poorly. On the one hand that honors your feelings, for it shows that the departure has not been easy for you, but it does not honor your health. You've had to let the neurosis assist in bringing about the solution."

He remained silent for some time, and then said: "Thank you for offering me another chance to speak with you."

I ended, saying: "We cannot hold back the reports on your book much longer. Their main point of view will presumably be that it's not possible to judge your theory until you've provided more complete information. If you do so, then at least one portion, the purely objective part, can be brought into order. As for the other portion, nothing can be done now. You had an excellent position here. You were loved and respected by all. The envy you complained about so much was certainly a sign of that. Now you leave here as a person one avoids. I don't know if you really needed that. But, vous l'avez voulu [it was your decision]."

Then I rose and bade him farewell with most appropriate polite words. He was so uncomfortable and ashamed that he wouldn't even bid farewell to my family, but asked me to extend best wishes to them. And I asked him to greet his wife for me, whom I will, of course, not be seeing so soon. Thus ended the encounter, and I must say I was mostly feeling terribly sorry for him. It often seemed as if he wanted to express something that would release him, that would free him, but the pride of the naughty child always kept the upper hand.

In response to the letter from Brill, which I sent to Ferenczi and will soon be in your hands, I gave an accurate depiction of the events here and of our current position toward Rank. I added the strict instruction that he make no indiscreet use of the letter, but wait to see what Rank does, and, if necessary, take up the fight against Rank in his own name. Of course I don't want Rank to say later that my vengeance followed him to America and prevented him from establishing himself. It won't work anyway: if he doesn't succeed, he'll surely blame me again.

On November 21, Anna told Eitingon how she felt on seeing Rank in October: "He seems uninvolved and sloppy, like a stubborn, poorly brought-up child. Papa reports after their last talk that he complains about his inability to work, and is unhappy. . . . If one could grab him and shake him hard (not just physically, of course) then everything would come out of him, perhaps much meanness and very bitterly but honest and real. Papa and I didn't do that. . . . But perhaps for that more warmth and affection were needed than any of us had left for Rank."

A week after Rank left, Freud wrote to Ferenczi (Nov. 28), "astonishingly, he returned from Paris," saying he hadn't parted well with Tola, but "in reality because he is in a deep depression."

Responding to Freud on December 2, Ferenczi had not yet seen the letter to Eitingon but knew that the session "went more miserably than our last discussion. The return from Paris might indicate the beginning of a neurotic depression." He filled in details about Toni Freund's estate, with which attorney Paul Rosenfeld, Rank's brother, was helping. In reply, December 4, Freud reported meeting with Rosenfeld, who "behaved very unsuspiciously." On December 7, Ferenczi told Freud that he had forwarded Brill's letter about Rank to Berlin and had written Brill about his own strong disapproval of Rank's behavior. He suggests that Anna be added to the Committee: she "gave us valuable help in the last, difficult negotiations with Rank."[6]

Anna accepted Committee membership—replacing Rank—enthusiastically. It came as a present for her twenty-ninth birthday. She "replaced the youngest of her father's filial order of six—she was once again the youngest of six, but by election, not by fate; and her acceptance in this group of knights . . . pleased her father as much as it pleased her."[7]

[Otto Rank] ¶December 12, 1924

Hochverehrter Herr Professor,

As you probably know, I didn't return to Vienna in good health. In fact, I turned back on the way; during the trip, everything that gave me an answer to the unresolved questions I'd been facing, with so little understanding, finally became clear to me.

I'd therefore request urgently that you grant me an opportunity to speak with you; at that time I'd hope at least to clear up everything you'd like to, and as far as possible, with your helpful understanding, to make amends for it.

Respectfully and thankfully yours, Rank

A new series of monthly Rundbriefe began on December 15. Ferenczi wrote a long one, distancing himself from Rank, denying that anything in *Development* went against psychoanalysis. "A really unified Committee that wants to be more than a formal body, is possible only when its members also relate to one another in a human fashion." Rejecting Ernest's claim "that *two* members of the earlier Committee published works that diverge from psychoanalysis," Ferenczi explained that *Development* was submitted for a prize, hence was kept secret, but was seen by Freud, whose suggestions for revision were followed.

Freud sent his Rundbrief, cosigned by Anna, telling that Helene Deutsch, back from Berlin (analyzed by Abraham after Freud), planned to start a training institute in Vienna with courses and trainee-patient-supervisor arrangements for control analysis of candidates—a model that became standard. "Jones is quite right when he wants to put the emphasis this time more on a group of people who share interests than forced personal intimacy. But the latter exists already and there is certainly nothing to be done about it." At the end: "Last but not least, in the Rank affair a surprising, for each of us pleasing, turn has taken place, about which individual members will be informed directly."[8]

Jones "had no clue" about Rank's "surprising turn" (Dec. 18): "My first thought was that he had given up analysis and accepted a position in a bank; my second is that he had decided to settle in America. But the latter would be more *erfreulich* [pleasing] to you than to me."

Dr. Otto Rank Wien, I Grünangergasse 3–5 Telephon 73-309 ¶Dec. 20, 1924
Liebe Freunde! [Dear Friends!]

After everything that has happened recently with me, and because of me, I feel the need to inform you, as persons directly or indirectly involved, of a change that has occurred in me and with me, and which, I hope, justifies me in addressing you in the old way as former common friends and co-workers—with the intention, first, of clarifying my situation, and to the extent that one or another of you was personally affected, of apologizing for this and putting it right.

Only after the most recent events in Vienna, about which you are presumably well informed, has my recent orientation and behavior toward the Professor become clear to me. Certain things apparently had to happen *before I could understand that my emotional reactions against the Professor and against you, to the extent that you represent for me the brothers who stand close to him, resulted from unconscious conflicts, an account of which I can give to myself and to you only now that I've overcome them.*

From a state I now recognize as neurotic, I've suddenly come to myself again. Not only have I recognized as the actual cause of the crisis the trauma of the Professor's critical illness, but I have been able to understand the type and mechanisms of my reaction as resulting from my childhood and family history—the Oedipus complex and the brother complex. Thus I've had to overcome conflicts in reality that I'd have been spared, had I undergone a timely analysis, yet I believe I've overcome them through this painful experience.

From analytical discussions with the Professor, in which I could explain my reactions in detail in terms of emotional factors, I can hope I've succeeded, first of all, in clearing up my personal situation, since the Professor found my explanations satisfactory and has forgiven me personally. In the future there will be opportunities for discussion, illumination, and approach in the scientific arena as well, where, after the elimination of my personal resistances, I'll be in a position to see things more objectively. Thus I firmly believe that I'll be able to put right absolutely as much as possible.

But before this can occur I'd ask each among you to understand my emotional remarks against him as resulting from this state—and to excuse them as reactions not to be interpreted personally. Here, as an exonerating factor, I emphasize that I never took these remarks beyond our inner circle, and that they thus appeared only in recent circulars and meetings of the Committee, and finally in two letters I sent the Professor from America this summer.

I feel especially obliged to make amends with Abraham, whose occasional critical remarks I obviously took as cause for stronger reaction, and against whose role as my accuser before the Professor I recently reacted with such force, resulting from my brother complex. I can only hope, dear Abraham, that my painfully gained insight into this situation, and my sincere regret concerning it, will allow you to forgive and forget the offense I directed toward you, resulting from that orientation.

As for Jones, I've certainly been at fault toward him in like manner, resulting from the same orientation, but I believe he has given me more causes—more emotionally colored on his side too. Nevertheless I would also ask you, dear Jones, to forgive me for injustices directed at you personally, and I hope that you too can move beyond still existing resistances to me far enough to recognize the sincerity of my regret and appreciate it accordingly.

As for Sachs: our old and intimate friendship has fortunately prevented you, dear Hanns, from being drawn into the series of brothers in a similarly emotional manner. Should you, however, have been unintentionally affected by any part of this, it occurred more as with a twin brother, and thus applied much more to myself, given that this motive of self punishment could perhaps also have played a role with the older brothers.

As for Ferenczi and Eitingon, who also held a special position for me, I accordingly wrote them separately, though in the same sense, since they personally offered me their kind assistance quite recently here in Vienna, and still wished to save me, as it were, while I was unable to understand this and was therefore unable to accept it.

I'd be glad to hear that my explanations have found the same analytic understanding among you as they have with the Professor, and that they will also give you the satisfaction I hope will be taken as the prerequisite for recommencing our collaboration in the not too distant future.

Best greetings, Otto

In this letter Rank uses the intimate (*du*) form, prefacing last names with "dear" [abbr. *l* for *lieber*], an informal but less intimate manner than writing Karl, Ernest, Hanns, Sándor, and Max. He abjectly apologizes, accepting—indeed quoting—Freud's explanations: a reaction to Freud's cancer; an Oedipus complex expressed as brother complex; a need for analysis. He had already won Freud over, so this was the necessary second step. That he finds fault with Jones makes the confession less abject and more credible. He was coming out of a depression.

Freud elaborated to Ferenczi (Dec. 21): "It was a satisfaction and a relief to me when he arrived one evening all broken up, in order to—confess, in the process of awakening from a condition that one can summarize hardly any other way than psychiatrically. Since then he's been almost completely free, once again his old self, or better than he was. What he opened up to me was a tragedy, which very easily could have had such an outcome. I don't have the right to give you all the explanations that I got. Perhaps he'll do that himself one day. Until then it wouldn't surprise me if a piece of distrust remained in all of you. Knowing everything, I've completely overcome it." Anna was convinced, too, as she told Eitingon (Dec. 24): "For many hours he poured out the story of recent months to Papa. . . . I talked with him only at the end; surprisingly he'd recovered his old face and personality again in every respect: even his voice and bearing as before. . . . Maybe something has shaken him the way we wanted to shake him and what possessed him has let go of him again. I've made peace with him. . . . Even though Papa thought himself finished with Rank, this change gave him great pleasure and happiness."

Ferenczi was glad, although, he told Freud, "a trace of distrust has remained in me. But by and large I am reassured by Rank's very honest sounding letter." He already had signaled Rank of critiques to come, in which he, too, would participate.[9] A "Dear Otto" letter from Eitingon, Sachs, and Abraham dated December 25, was welcoming of Rank's "promising turning point" but noted the "neurotic conditioning of your actions—which none of us doubted—in itself of course has nothing to do with exoneration from responsibility." They would look for the steps that follow his new insight to "return us to the old situation of friendship and trust." They wanted more of the history. Did his successes or failures in America play some role? They assumed Rank had "no plans to publish anything new in the near future, when you will be occupied with reviewing your earlier concepts." A separate letter from Eitington the next day emphasized: "In Abraham's case the will and inner readiness to reestablish our old relations in their full scope are the very greatest, and open up the best prospects. Let us now realize them!"

Dr. Otto Rank Wien, I Grünangergasse 3–5 ¶Dec. 30, 1924

Lieber Herr Professor,

I'm taking the liberty of sending you, for your information, the Berlin Rundbrief, which arrived today, and Eitingon's letter, which arrived earlier. I believe that despite the reservations in reacting, which were to be expected, I can be quite satisfied. Before writing again to the group I hope I can discuss with you the form in which I should go into individual questions.

Given my brother's serious condition, my plans haven't become firmer. The diag-

nosis is unfortunately the feared, unfavorable one [cancer]. There remains only the question of whether and when he will decide to undergo an operation. Perhaps I'll leave soon if my presence here is not urgently required. Hopefully I will know more by the end of the week, in which case I'll take the liberty of calling.

With best wishes for the New Year. Respectfully yours, Rank

The surprising about-face raises the question, Did Rank sincerely apologize as he recovered from an illness, or did he play to his colleagues? Rank acknowledged great anxiety about Freud's possible demise—a threat to his own professional survival. His flamboyant, sometimes arrogant behavior in New York and the needlessly provocative, strategically foolish, letters to Freud suggest a hypomanic episode followed by severe depression. Sympathetic to Rank, Jessie Taft observes, referring to Rank's adolescent diary and the letter to the Committee of December 24:

> From the time of the *Diaries,* Rank as in this letter has always understood his own manic-depressive swings, which for him were usually related to the periods of extreme creativity with the aftermath of exhaustion. The intimations of neurotic illness given by Jones in Volume II and reinforced in Volume III by a definite psychiatric diagnosis of "cyclothymia," which he finds to have been recognized by Freud also for a number of years previously, could have been no surprise to Rank who, after he had ceased to exist for Freud and Jones, managed to live for twelve years with a "psychosis" that seemed not to interrupt the creative drive, the therapeutic practice, or the teaching engagements, maintained to the time of his death in 1939.[10]

Rank's condition, now known as bipolar disorder, has a genetic as well as a psychological etiology. It is associated with bursts of excitement, creativity, overconfidence, and erratic behavior, coupled with phases of profound depression and emotional paralysis. Psychologist Kay Redfield Jamison, herself afflicted, includes among its notable sufferers William Blake, William James, John Ruskin, Robert Schumann, Mary Shelley, and Virginia Woolf.[11]

≈ Chapter 18 ≈

Reunion and Ending

1925–1926

I have honestly no feeling against Rank, and have never had any on personal grounds,
and am only too happy to think that he is regaining insight and may perhaps become
once more a friend and psa. collaborator. . . .
Rank has temporarily regained intellectual *insight into the situation. . . . In short,*
I distrust Rank profoundly, for I know well how unscrupulous he can be when it
suits him and when he has the power, and I feel that we have no guarantee for the
future. That he should once more have deceived Professor was inevitable and not
surprising. . . . The essential question is whether Rank's temporary regaining of
analytic insight is to be followed by our discarding the whole of ours.
—Jones to Abraham, December 24, 1924

J ones was more candid writing privately to Abraham than in the Rundbriefe. On January 3 he sent a letter to "Dear Otto," welcoming Rank's
gesture of friendship with caution:

As it is a long time since I have been able to write to you with the hope of securing an
objective understanding of what I want to say, I will at once seize this opportunity of
adding a few remarks of my own on the situation. The past cannot, unfortunately, be
wiped out by a mere word or even the best intentions alone....It was disappointing to
find I had increasingly to deal with your habit of secret taciturnity and your refusal to
consult together with me before making decisions in affairs for which actually I was
responsible....I was the only member of the whole Committee who refused to accept
the neurosis,...and insisted on treating you as normal and responsible for every-

thing.…A word from you of friendly cooperation would at any moment have been able to change the whole situation and immediately to restore our old relationship, for few things have ever given me more pain than the impairment of this. I can assure you that none of this impairment proceeded from my side, it being thoroughly against my will, and this will I hope be easy for me to prove now that you are more willing to listen.

Freud supported Rank in a letter to Jones on January 6: "He was really in a manic state when he caused all that trouble, and I saw him in the depression which resulted in the clarification and restoration of his former personality. . . . He paid dearly and suffered much." Freud would not share details of what he knew, but said Rank was on the way to "being cured and assured against a relapse." Relieved that Rank was no "apostate," Freud asked Jones to "forget the past and allow him fresh credit." Rank was about to leave for America to "try to repair the damage." Jones replied (Jan. 10), "I also share the purely intellectual reserve expressed by our Berlin friends and am bound indeed to be distinctly skeptical about the security of the future. This, however, in no way affects our attitude of willing helpfulness as well as of personal sympathy, so we all hope for the best."

Eitingon received additional information: Rank had become financially independent: "He made a gift of $1,000 to the Verlag. His wife is resisting a permanent move to America." Freud and Lou Andreas exchanged letters: she commiserated, faulting Rank for giving up his place as favorite son. If Rank charged $20 per hour in New York, in six months he easily earned over $10,000.[1] Rank addressed the committee:

Dr. Otto Rank Wien, I Grünangergasse 3–5 ¶January 7, 1925

Liebe Freunde!

I want to thank you warmly for the demonstration of friendship and trust—especially comforting in such difficult times—that your letters have brought me. Of course I understood very well that turning to you with my letter was only a first step, and that further steps and acts must now follow to convince you of the sincerity of the change that I have undergone. In any case I assure you that your friendly manner has really helped me keep on the path I've begun.

From discussions I've had with the Professor, the next and most important step is for me to embark as soon as possible on my planned voyage to America—though with quite different assumptions and conditions. Accordingly, I'll go this week. News from there indicates confusion in the minds of the analysts to which I greatly contributed, and I'll strive to bring people to their senses by setting things straight, elucidating in discussions and lectures, setting aside difficulties and resistances. So doing, I'll clarify my position scientifically. I'll retract, qualify, modify the rash, uncertain, or danger-ous and align what's new—to the extent possible—in the context of previous work. This essential effort will, I hope, give me material and perspective to construct my framework, which of course I'll publish. So, I impatiently look forward to getting the manuscript by Sachs, whose critical viewpoints I'd consider and use comprehensively. (For now, please address it to Vienna, whence it will be forwarded.)

The voyage to America gives occasion to answer and clarify—at least briefly—questions posed in the letter from Berlin. My turnaround came only after my depar-ture from Vienna; I returned from Paris in order to talk things out with the Professor. Here, purely personal, or, I should say, human motives were involved; my American achievements and plans were not directly related. In a purely psychological sense it was impossible for me to leave the Professor that way—to leave him in the lurch—as I could do the first time in a manic state that, as a direct reaction to his illness, was to spare me the grief over the loss. Finding him present again, I succumbed to the com-pulsion to recapitulate the whole process, but this time unsuccessfully, since my guilty conscience broke through in a depression, forcing me to return and express myself to the Professor. At November's end, wanting to go to New York, after breaking off rela-tions in Vienna, I was returning there with hopes of success; even if the situation had been as critical then as it was later—due to my trip being postponed—that could not have kept me from going, since I of course went to America the first time independent of the Association, and would have again.

I hope this explanation suffices for now, and I regret that the difficulties of last week don't permit me to consult personally with at least one of you. I'd already obtained a visa to Budapest, and I'd have accepted gladly the kind invitation to Berlin, but we must leave our discussion for later. I hope to be spared the discussion of details one cannot present even to one's circle of friends, entrusting them at most to one's analyst. The Professor, of course, is familiar with the situation in every detail, and I think that should do for all of you.

> *In the firm hope that the new year will see me among you again, and with the best wishes of friendship to you all, I remain, Yours, Otto*[2]

Freud gave Rank a letter to transmit to Brill, dated January 6. Freud writes: "An unexpected but very delightful thing happened. Rank has turned around, becoming his old self, and giving convincing proof that he again deserves our full confidence." Freud repeats what he told the Committee about Rank's sudden return from Paris, the depression, analysis, and (unspecified) insight. "Now is the time for us to show him the sympathy that he has earned by fifteen years of faithful work, and the tolerance that one who has recovered from an illness may claim." He assures Brill that Rank wants to undo the damage he caused, and would conduct seminars in New York with his analysands at no fee and, Freud hoped, with Brill present. "I still work 6 hours a day and with mixed feelings I trace the signs of rising popularity that now become visible in Europe as well."[3]

In 1925 the Verlag published Rank's monographs *The Double,* and *The Artist* (4th ed., with added essays). He was working on the *Incest Motif* (2nd ed.) as well as the compilation *Sexuality and Guilt* and the first volume of *Technik der Psychoanalyse*—all three published in 1926.

A candid reflection on Rank from a Freud analysand is that of New York psychiatrist Abram Kardiner. "[Rank] had a method to cut down neurosis at the main trunk instead of picking at leaves and twigs. We all flocked to him." The American analysts earned two to five dollars per session and were envious: "For a fellow who wore patches on his pants in Vienna, he was charging twenty dollars a visit." Besides would-be patients, stockbrokers telephoned Rank, who "got Americanized fast" but was "not a swindler." Kardiner's recollection includes errors—that Freud did not know about *Trauma of Birth* before publication and that Rank owned a Rolls Royce. Kardiner thought Rank "had bigger fish to fry, and no longer cared about Freud." Kardiner, never a Rankian, considered Rank to be "the most extraordinary catalytic agent that ever hit the psychoanalytic movement."[4]

Ferenczi's Rundbrief of January 17 expressed his need for more time before he could fully trust "prodigal son" Rank, though he expressed "joy about his conversion." On February 6 Ferenczi probed Freud with questions about Rank's theory and practice before and after the "analytical discussion" and his attitude toward his colleagues. Then he told in confidence—only to be shared with Anna—that Frau Rank had asked to be analyzed by him! Freud was pleased: "Then you'll learn everything from her and also understand my behavior against him" (Feb. 9).

Freud wrote Jones, February 11, that Rank's letters told of "making good progress in pacifying the analysts there and clarifying the situation for them."

[radiogram] ¶February 13, 1925 NEW YORK

PROFESSOR FREUD NINETEEN BERGGASSE VIENNA

= AFTER FAVORABLE COMPLETION ARRIVE LAST WEEK OF FEBRUARY

CORDIALLY = RANK

Anna, her father, and Eitingon referred to Rank's "Rosenfeld" face during his depression, and the reemergence of his familiar face afterwards.

On February 16 Jones wrote Brill: "I do not share Freud's optimism about Rank's recent change of front, particularly when he couples it with the diagnosis of manic-depressive. In fact I see no guarantee whatever for the future. At the same time it would be good news to hear that Rank is doing something to clear up the mess he made."

In his mid-February Rundbrief Freud expressed disappointment that Frink, whom he favored over Brill as leader of the American Psychoanalytic Association, was psychiatrically disabled. He discussed a complaint from Caroline Newton, who was not accepted in the New York Society despite being a member of the Vienna Psychoanalytic Society. Rank was on his way home, having completed his New York stay with good results, he wrote. En route Rank lectured in Paris at the Sorbonne and, with analyst René Laforgue, dined at the home of [Greek] Princess Marie Bonaparte, who became Freud's patient, trainee, and friend. Rank's brother, Paul Rosenfeld, stricken with cancer in December, had died earlier in February, at age 43.[5]

On March 3, Freud informed Eitingon that Rank was back, still depressed but able to do some work. A letter from Brill arrived that day "fully confirming Rank's report on his activity in America." Jones (Rundbrief, Mar. 13) complains of delays due to "severe neurotic inhibitions on Radó's part. Ever since the Congress, there has been a perpetual struggle between him and me." He also countered Ferenczi's "optimism about telepathy being used as objective proof of the contention of psychoanalysis. . . . Any mixture of the two subjects could have only one effect, that of delaying the assimilation of psychoanalysis." He is glad Freud decided to "sacrifice any interest he may have in telepathy" for the cause. Ferenczi had visited Rank and found "no trace of the taciturnity and obvious dishonesty" that the Committee addressed in November. "He has insight into the methodological errors of his work . . . with the good intention of allowing himself to be taught" (Mar. 15, Rundbrief).

Freud wrote: "Received, read and approved the report by Sachs on *Trauma of Birth*. I think it benefits Rank and gives him impetus that he needs to come out of his lethargic depression. He has, furthermore, the best intentions to bring all in order, get realigned and come to Berlin very soon if his one patient brought along from America—a melancholic—did not for now require his daily attendance."[6]

On Easter Sunday, Ferenczi wrote Freud that he was treating one of the patients Rank analyzed in New York: "I was able to catch a glimpse of his technique . . . not very favorable" but he would postpone judgment. "Rank doesn't write to me; I hear from Eitingon that Rank's depression persists." He notes a mixed review of *Development* in the latest *Zeitschrift* by Franz Alexander, fellow Hungarian, a training analyst in Berlin. He agrees with Alexander's comment that active therapy "allows the tendency to re-enact more play, in fact, occasionally provokes it." Ferenczi recalled that Freud favored a technique that "works *against* the patient's tendency toward reproduction," a point missed by Alexander. Freud had called it a "triumph" when something "the patient wishes to discharge in action is disposed of through the work of remembering." Freud praised Alexander's review to Ferenczi, although "he may have missed a nuance in my position vis-à-vis reproduction [reexperience]. Freud adds, "One still can't get started with Rank. He is apathetic, at the same time he avoids explaining his theory." Years later Alexander acknowledged *Development* as the source of the "corrective emotional experience" in therapy.[7]

Abraham's Rundbriefe, March and April, rail against Groddeck, the "wild analyst," whose recent lectures in Berlin included rambling personal, coarse free associations despite his wife's presence. Ferenczi answers: "I think, dear Karl, that you're handling the Groddeck case somewhat too rigidly, in contrast to your otherwise skilled diplomacy, praised by everyone. He is an original . . . and a respectable person to boot. . . . Cockiness is really only an exaggeration of courage, which he doesn't lack." Jones reported on his week in Paris. "The news about Rank, confirmed also by what I heard about him in Paris, is very regrettable, though not surprising. . . . We cannot treat him, either personally or scientifically, as responsible, so that our attitude can only remain friendly but pessimistic."[8]

Wednesday, April 29, 1925

Lieber Herr Professor,

*For the last few days I've been experiencing an acute inner crisis which unfortu-
nately hasn't waned enough for me to be able to discuss it. So, today I don't want to
bother you with my presence; I ask only that you excuse me for waiting so long before
telling you, but I'd been hoping until the last moment.*

*Hopefully next week I'll be enough improved to be able to see Eitingon. I've seen
Sachs, and thank you for that. My wife will remain away for fourteen more days.*

Best greetings. Yours, Rank

Prof. Dr. Freud Wien, IX Bergasse 19 ¶May 2, 1925

Lieber Herr Doktor

*I was very much saddened by your last letter. I understood, though, that the long
delayed conference will finally take place May 6, and now am sure that we will see
you there. No longer should you withdraw from your friends, who so much desire your
recovery.*

*On the simultaneous occasion of my 69th birthday, I would wish for a happy
countenance on your part, announcing the successful resolution of conflicts.*

Cordially yours, Freud

Ferenczi and Eitingon found Freud in good spirits on his sixty-ninth
birthday, physically recuperating and displaying "astonishing intellectual
freshness and productivity." They attended the VPS meeting, which showed
"a new and fresh spirit," with some younger members. Rank was reserved:
"He seemed so very dominated by his personal (neurotic) conflicts that, despite much effort, we were unsuccessful in moving him to a discussion about
scientific questions" (Ferenczi Rundbrief, May 16, no longer sent to Rank).
Freud confided to Eitingon that although Rank was less depressed, there
were "new complications" that made him unavailable as a co-worker and that
he hoped to go to New York in the fall. "Having ascertained the state of
things, I must agree with him that analysis would not be appropriate now.
Perhaps it will occur in time if, after surmounting the real problems, there
are neurotic remainders."[9]

Brill regained the presidency of the New York Society, which he would
head for 11 years, six of those also as head of the APA. Jones reflected, "it
was not easy to win new adherents; in 1925, for instance, there was only one

analyst west of New York, Lionel Blitzten in Chicago."[10] Blitzten was ana-lyzed by Rank and by Alexander, who later became a major influence in the United States.

Freud's June Rundbrief revealed: "Rank is out of his depression, we con-tinue our discussions, I believe, with good results. I'm able to demonstrate to him how his theory and his neurosis are strikingly complementary."

Dr. Otto Rank, Wien, I Grünangergasse 3–5 ¶June 15, 1925

Lieber Herr Professor,

Many thanks for the kind note. In any case, I will attend the meeting of the [Verlag] board on Wednesday. If it doesn't last too long, and if you have time for me afterwards, I'd be glad to stay. If this isn't possible, I'd ask you to set aside another evening for me. On Wednesday I'd also like to arrange the visit that includes my wife and child.

Respectfully yours, Rank

In answer to Ferenczi's report that anti-Jones sentiment was growing in England, Freud asks for restraint, not intervention. "Jones is making ample use of the general human right to have flaws, but we know his value too well not to be indulgent toward them." Freud thought it was hard to differentiate personal objections to Jones from resistances to psychoanalysis among Brit-ish society members (June 18). On June 20 Josef Breuer died, at age 84. Freud wrote condolences to the family and a *Zeitschrift* obituary.

Wien, Grünangergasse 3–5 Tel 73-309 ¶July 8, 1925

Lieber Herr Professor,

I take the liberty of disturbing your summer rest, today only, to tell you that the last few days I've begun work on the paper (Training Analysis), and that I've come far enough with the idea for the Congress presentation to let Eitingon know I'll do it (topic to be announced).

As soon as it takes on a more concrete form I'd like to discuss it with you. Please let me know, at your convenience, whether you prefer a specific day of the week (and at what time?) for my visit, so that I can work it into my schedule in a timely manner.

We plan to remain in Mödling until month's end, then go to Lido.

I hope you're feeling well now, and that you don't miss [oral surgeon] Pichler, in particular.

With best regards to your family, and cordial greetings to you. Yours, Rank

Freud was pleased with Rank's progress and his willingness to present "On the Genesis of Genitality" at the September International Psychoanalytical Association Congress in Homburg. Rank planned to visit Semmering [Freud] for a day: "I no longer find it doubtful that he will overcome his difficulties," Freud told Eitingon on July 16. On August 7, Freud summed up Rank's visit for Eitingon, who was frustrated trying to get information for the Homburg program: "He wants to address the problem of anxiety and libido to prepare the integration of his material within ours. He is again well, very energetic, clearly hypomanic, which he acknowledges. It's almost certain he won't ever return to the crooked paths, but equally certain that a return to health is inconceivable. Even the recovered Rank will differ from the previous one and will have a different relation to us. The abnormal phase ended, leaving certain changes. He's affluent now and independent and has created a new basis of existence over there. He's in no hurry to retract his theories; there, too, much has solidified. Anyway, criticism hasn't shed enough light on his innovations." Freud mentions his own work-in-progress on anxiety, written in response to Rank's theory. He described it to Ferenczi on August 14 as "a criticism of the Rankian theory on the basis of a modified concept of the problem of anxiety. . . . For a long time there was a question as to whether it shouldn't remain unwritten. But fate has willed otherwise."

Abraham, who was suffering from a lung infection, wanted Freud to endorse a film on psychoanalysis. Freud refused even to meet with Samuel Goldwyn or to consider an offer of $100,000. Yet some newspapers reported that he was actively involved. The project strained his relationship with Abraham and Sachs, who consulted with director G. W. Pabst. The (silent) movie *Geheimnisse einer Seele* (*Secrets of a Soul*) opened in Berlin in 1926 to great acclaim.[11]

Dr. Otto Rank Lido [Italy] ¶August 25, 1925

Lieber Herr Professor,

My stay nears its end and I'm glad to tell you that it was successful in several ways. I worked a lot—practically, theoretically, and mainly personally, i.e. on myself. In so doing, much has become clear to me that I'd like to relate to you if you can possibly meet next week.

I'll arrive in Vienna on the morning of the 28th and stay until September 1, when I leave for the Congress. Kindly let me know what day and hour would suit you best for my visit.

Things have gone very well for me here; my family will stay here until the 31st. We
hope you and yours also had a pleasant time.

With cordial greetings to you and your family. Yours thankfully, Rank

On August 27, Freud reassured Ferenczi, who feared that the critique of
Trauma would devalue active therapy: "My essay contains nothing about active therapy and concerns itself only with the theoretical side of Rankian
doctrine which, incidentally, comes off quite well, the relation to anxiety." He
faults the American press for their "fabricated news" and closes with a jibe at
America and religion: "The Statue of Liberty in New York harbor should be
replaced by a monkey holding up a bible."

Wien Grünangergasse 3–5 ¶August 31, 1925

Lieber Herr Professor,

Due to my hasty departure from Semmering, I couldn't convey to you the deep
sense not only of appreciation, but also of unfading closeness to you and your life's
work, that I am only now truly beginning to feel. But I probably wouldn't have been
able to tell you this even had I stayed longer, for such a thing can hardly be said with-
out becoming banal. Yet I know that this time you also understood, as in old times—yet
newly—and that means everything to me.

I'm sending you the presentation, which I've just finished typing, so that you can
see the benefit derived from our discussion; only now does all of this strike me as good
and usable.

I'm already looking forward to visiting you after the Congress; if you'll permit me,
I'd like to bring my wife along.

I greet you cordially, as in old times. Yours, Rank

At the Ninth Congress of the IPA, Bad Homburg, September 3–5, Anna
read her absent father's paper on differences between the sexes, and Ferenczi
spoke on contraindications to active therapy. Abraham presided despite his
illness and reported to Freud that Rank read a paper "at furious speed, so no
one could follow. . . . Added to this, the euphoric mood and another journey
to America . . . means a new manic phase." He and Rank had a good talk,
"which should certainly have a good effect on our future relationship." Ferenczi said "Rank's personal behavior was normal and friendly." Jones wrote
Freud, "he spoke to his old friends about scientific questions but evidently

had no personal feelings of friendliness to express." The apparent snub led Jones to write 32 years later: "He did not display any personal friendliness to any of us."[12]

On October 18, Freud told Ferenczi of a new patient from Paris, Princess [Greek lineage] Marie Bonaparte, referred by Dr. Laforgue. "She is not an aristocrat at all but a real person . . . knows and has a good opinion of [Henri] Bergson and can talk about very interesting things. Such people are most suited for my intention [as analyst] of being bothered only minimally. But there are evidently not many of that type."

Hotel Holley, Washington Square W., New York, N.Y. ¶October 23, 1925

Lieber Herr Professor,

I cabled you today that I hope to be at home for Christmas, and would like to try to explain to you why I believe this original intention of mine is the correct one.

Mainly, I feel relatively well, but am not happy; I miss my wife and child, and am homesick for Vienna, but I feel absolutely healthy. Since I saw you last, having decided to go, I've had no more feelings of anxiety or guilt, and on the hot ground of New York I feel quiet and secure. I've begun work, but am not fully occupied since I accept only people I just need to finish up or those I can start with, who can continue in Europe. "Consultations" also bring income: I see people a few times in order to determine whether they're suited for analysis, whether it should be more instructional or therapeutic, when, by whom, etc. Anyway, my activities cover the costs of trip and lodging, and I hope to either bring along some analyses or arrange them for spring and summer.

I haven't dealt with the other matter, as I wanted first to observe my reaction here, but I'm quite sure I'll be able to deal with it successfully. There should be no external difficulties, and I believe I've overcome the internal ones. My remaining conflict relates to the socially more important father side, and I believe the time has finally come to deal with this on the level of further scientific work you suggested at the time.

I feel that this, precisely, can't be done here. The external conditions for this work aren't appropriate, nor is my psychic constitution in this still "revolutionary" atmosphere. I can do it only in Vienna, where all conditions are favorable, and I can present things to you before I swallow them hot; I hope you'll still be willing to discuss them with me.

Finally, the most important thing bringing me back to Vienna for Christmas is my family. I feel it unfair to them to stay away from home longer than absolutely neces-

sary. I feel this is no longer so, as I manage to accept only people who might follow me
to Vienna later. Even if I'm a bit hasty with this, I think it's enough: everything else
seems unimportant next to the goal of making my wife and child happy and trying
to make good what they've had to suffer because of me. The first step, then, is to come
back as soon and as well as possible, after dealing with everything here—which can be
done in the next few weeks.

I hope you're well, and I'd be glad to have a few lines from you.

With cordial thanks. Yours, Rank

Hotel Holley Washington Square N.Y. ¶October 27, 1925
Lieber Herr Professor,
I'm glad to say that since my last letter I've made further and, I think, great prog-
ress addressing my inner journey.

Various signs, including my attitude to dealing with the conscious material, make
it clear that emotionally I'm still—or only—stuck in the brother complex, while the
father conflict has receded. It seems that the death there of my brother in the spring
summoned me back quite far into the childhood *conflict just as I was struggling to*
overcome it. Now everything seems favorable for resolving the brother complex and,
with that, for the final resolution. This shows my great desire to return to my old rela-
tionship to analysis and its champions, and I'd be grateful for your further help with
this, as I need it for my psychological healing, and it may be useful for analysis, too.

Just as it seems that in analysis insight comes only after the issue has been inter-
nally resolved or surmounted, I see clearly for the first time, with the brother crisis
seeming to fade away with this trip, what a powerful unconscious influence it had on
me. Not only on my attitude toward you, my colleagues, and my work—on which I'll
say more—but also with my personal concerns. Of course I did not doubt about being
able to deal with them, but I couldn't find the right way—now clear since I discovered—
again, I mean emotionally—that the man who'd played such a limited role in my life
was not my father but very clearly my brother, *who really played the role of father—*
not so much to me, but to my mother; taking my mother from me, so to speak, after she
was free from my father, and I wanted to take her after his death freed her from him.
Thus, in resolving this, I remained stuck in the brother complex, and now am able […]
brother, who eliminated the father and took the mother for himself.

Finally, to share an insight into my current psychological situation and mood, I'd
like to tell you what I dreamt last night after those issues became clear during the day.

I saw you sitting at a round table—the kind we also had at home—slicing and distributing pieces of a cake or dessert. Beside you stood Federn (or Hitschmann), for whom you put a piece on each plate, and he seemed to be passing the plates (to the other "children," who I didn't see); I didn't even see this one person clearly, but only knew he was there. While you cut up the cake, he told you I'd decided not to stay in America, but in Europe (as if, in so doing, he'd remind you not to forget me while slicing). In fact I got the next plate (from him), on which lay two small pieces; you added a third large one, while fixing your gaze on me. I seemed to understand what you wanted to say with this silent gaze, and so took the big piece to eat.

In the next scene I was at Brill's house, apparently invited to stay there, since I was wearing a comfortable dressing gown (without starched collar) and chatting with Brill (about my trip there), when Mrs. Brill unexpectedly entered. I excused myself for my faulty attire, said I hadn't expected her again, and thanked her for her visit. Then I was given cake there too; once again, there were two pieces, and I was just about to take the larger one when another woman came in and claimed that piece for herself. I gave it to her and comforted her and myself by saying that the piece I kept for myself was crispier (browner) and that I like it that way.

Current causes (which will simultaneously provide information on events here):

1.) Yesterday Mr. and Mrs. Liebman visited me, on advice of their old family doctor Stieglitz, since they were disturbed by news they had from you about their son. As parents, both, especially the husband, are rather neurotic but as good as gold; they care only about the welfare of their child. From the not very interesting discussion I'll mention now only what is relevant for the dream. They asked me, among other things, whether I would be ready to take on their son if you were to drop him (you will recall that Dr. Stieglitz recommended me when the boy was still in Pfister's care; the entire family very much respects Dr. Stieglitz's advice). I told them they should be glad you wanted to retain him for the time being—as long as possible—and that you'd be leaving to them the decision on his future, should you drop him. If you find he's unsuited for psychoanalysis, I couldn't help him either. If you drop him as per your "custom" (which I believe and hope is only an excuse for his parents), we'll let you decide whether to send him to me. I hope you'll find my actions here correct; in any case, I was satisfied with myself in this, a product of my wholly changed orientation. I probably would've acted no differently anyway, but would perhaps have regretted not being able to compete with you; this time, I handled the situation objectively and realistically.

2.) Today's the first meeting (this semester) of the psychoanalytic group here. I hesitated a bit as to whether I should first officially announce my presence here (to Brill, of course), so I'd likely be invited out of politeness, but decided not to, just wait calmly and see how things turn out. Given the new circumstances, one motive for going would *be to get along with these brothers too! But I think my decision was correct, for there were too many real reasons against my going. Thus, once again, I think by not going I acted more realistically, for at the meeting I might have tried, and been able, to play too much the superior role (thus not that of the brother—or that of the elder brother-father).*

Interpretation: *Both dreams seem to reveal this. They clearly show the childhood basis, for I recall hundreds of times throughout childhood when I argued or fought with my brother over the bigger or better piece. Federn and Hitschmann are older brothers to the extent that both had taken on your position as confidant and representative, a place I held later and hope to gain again. They are not visible—just you and I: the old situation of the favorite son, preferred by the mother (it can only be the mother who distributes the dessert). ([There is] a possible higher-level interpretation that you also represent the older brother: the silent gaze, which voluntarily leaves to me the mother, the biggest piece, and the position.)*

Brill is the president here, whom during my last visit here you made your confidant: thus the same situation here with respect to the upcoming meeting, which I apparently want to attend only as the elder brother's equal. The faulty attire is brother-identification, for my brother often went about the house like that (dressing gown, without starched collar). (Incidentally, in dream #1 I am probably also the elder brother, who usually got the bigger piece for himself.)

Regarding Mrs. Brill, a Christian, "my American woman" occurred to me. Now she strikes me as just as unpleasant a type as Mrs. Brill is in reality. This would correspond to the fact that I'm glad to relinquish my mother, who's unwelcome to my current ego, to my older brother (though to an extent I'm still the older brother, too); in the dreams, she belongs to him. The second woman—in the dream already a double of Mrs. Brill but apparently a nicer one—an Ideal Mother, claims the piece of cake, which I give to her. Insight 1: my wife—ideal mother, i.e. almost no mother, since she commands! 2. Through a detail-association about my real mother: You (specifically, she claims not the bigger piece, but the softer one, since she cannot chew very well; this is you, but also my own mother, who has had false teeth for years). (Here deeper associations with your castration [sic] and with anxiety about the mother.)

Here, in your interest and my wife's, the two positive elements in my life (beside the child), I renounce my mother and the brother-identification, and gladly take what is best for myself.

Overdetermination of the two dreams (Liebman-appearance): the pieces of cake represent "fat morsels"—patients—that you distribute to your students. But that leads again to your role as the caring mother, whom I feared losing due to your illness. Here the closing—we come full circle, to the starting point of the whole crisis.

Now briefly about my work here. Until now, as stated, I've accepted only five peo-
ple, or, putting it better, I could only take five as I've firmly decided to be in Vienna for
Christmas. This is more important to me than anything else, even if I don't advance
psychoanalysis more now. Otherwise, I haven't been able to work much, not due to
"resistance" as much as lack of concentration (the hours are irregular, like life in gen-
eral here) and of will.

On the other hand I got invited to lecture in Chicago and am considering it, since
with my shortened stay here I think it would be good to make myself and psycho-
analysis known in Chicago so perhaps people will come to Vienna from there, too.
And it wouldn't bother me much to take off a week or so here.

I hope this letter hasn't gotten too long. By the way, don't be afraid, dear Professor,
that I'll disturb you more, in writing or in person, with my analysis. I think I'm through
with it, unless something special and unexpected happens, but there's no reason for
that and I have no such worries. I think when I get to Vienna the time will be ripe for
a scientific discussion, which will be much less tiring and also, at least, more inspiring
than the analytical drudgery you have enough of all day long. It will also bring back,
at least for me, something of the good old times, whose disappearance I regret more
and more now.

I hope you go on feeling very well, and will have no problem cutting up the cake.
Please give my regards to your family, and be cordially greeted yourself.

Thankfully yours, Rank

In their Rundbrief, November 15, Freud and Anna said: "From Rank are
direct messages that he's fine in America, that he is determined to return
to Vienna at Christmas, and will try to regain his former position among
the analysts." Five days earlier she had written Eitingon, "I wonder how that
[Rank's optimistic effort] will work out, and believe it won't be easy. The
Society has forgotten him so quickly and completely. . . . Not one person took
the opportunity to ask what's going on with Rank. . . . But it was he himself
who kicked himself out with such energy."

New York ¶November 22, 1925

Lieber Herr Professor,

Cordial thanks for your kind letter [missing], which came at the right time: not
only did it arrive on Sunday morning, when I'm free to write, but it also connected
with my mood.

In the last few days I'd been thinking about writing to you today so before I come you'll know, more or less, how I'll be. I'm glad to say I think I'll return healthy! That's the main thing, with the sure feeling that if so, all else, whatever may come, will arrange itself for the better. I really feel that way now. I'm not leaving here disappointed, nor do I renounce anything here, nor do I expect too much in Vienna. Despite all this, or maybe because of it, I feel lighter and freer than for a long time, and quite self-sufficient and independent, too—especially psychologically.

I've resolved everything here to my satisfaction, and, I hope, to that of others, i.e. my wife and you; I think I've resolved everything in an objectively correct way, too. With my wife there were, as expected, no difficulties, as soon as I was ready to do without her and everything she stands for. Not only is she herself a highly respectable person, but she still loves me and for my sake is ready to deal with whatever I suggest. She's happy with the child, not with her husband—but with him she wasn't before! I hope, with current efforts, I've improved the relationship between us.

To wife and child I've found my way back well and good and am sure I can win my wife back, although this whole episode, especially the last part, was a hard trial for her. It's mainly for her sake and the child's that I'm returning now; I don't consider it a sacrifice, or a duty, to give up something here to come back, but rather, I have a strong urge to put an end to this unhealthy situation.

As for future professional prospects, I have no major worries; they were just a product of my general condition. Concerning America for now, I've done all I can for myself and for analysis, and as I see it, that's a lot. The chances for a position with a good future here remain the same, but can be realized only with preparation over many years that I can do just as well in Europe, while others, especially [Frankwood] Williams, can promote things here without me. What I've accomplished so far: a whole group of serious people working, a real force, is becoming supportive of psychoanaly-sis. If all goes as I predict and Williams plans, this will be the key to the development of psychoanalysis in America, perhaps in the world, for this center comprises not only psychiatrists, but also the huge territory of the "social workers" and the entire problem of education and instruction, social concerns, and character.

Besides Williams, whose analysis has gone very well and seems to end well, I have six of his close and more distant colleagues; some in analysis, and some I'm preparing for future analysis here or in Europe. Incidentally, three are coming to Vienna now to continue, two or three of them can't come until summer, others will follow. This work of building up a corps of colleagues I can do in Europe just as well as here, indeed, I must do it there—disregarding personal reasons—for financial reasons, since of course they can't pay much, but on the other hand are seriously interested and aren't afraid of the sacrifices this entails. So you see I've not given up on a future in America, but I'll let the way I decide or will have to decide in the future depend on how things develop, rather than on my own outbursts of temper. Of course my wife's view of these plans and possibilities plays a big role.

From this picture of the American situation you'll see I'm not associating any grandiose plans with Vienna. If you had this impression, it mostly expressed my mood at the time, hence was more psychological than real, or more simply: it was mainly the wish for your acceptance, we might say, in the old way—not as my old self, for I'm no longer my old self. It's not the position as such that I strive for, and I actually had doubts that seem to coincide with yours—namely, that as president I'd need to have some official contact with the other groups, i.e. with the presidents, which would reestablish a committee-like relation that hardly seems possible to me and, further-more, not even desirable. In this respect, objective differences of opinion might arise (I'm not speaking of scientific or personal ones)—regarding organization of the move-ment, etc. On the other hand, both for the Association and for me, it would be better if somehow—with one foot in America, so to speak, while directing the movement a bit further here—I could officially represent the Association. At some point I'd like to discuss with you these general questions of the movement. As far as I can see here, the great movement in which I'm now interested seems to be developing away from the official psychoanalytic organization, although Williams, who's a member of the Association and several committees, is working to maintain contacts. But the others don't make it easy, though they seem to want to join this great movement. This conflict is crass here, but I think it exists in Europe, too. The old groups have grown somewhat rigid and academic, if not "orthodox": I don't mean academically, but in feeling. Their viewpoint is too narrow since it's purely medical. The movement has passed them by, and will more and more if the organization doesn't find a connection with them soon. In the last few years, though, these groups seem to isolate themselves more and more from the great social movement, so I don't know whether it's worth a struggle for unification that seems unreachable.

But I hope, dear Professor, you won't misunderstand me; I think I see things quite objectively. Personally, I'd be glad to work with all who wish to work and not fight; I've influenced Williams, though he's quite independent, to try to work with the groups as long as possible. He described a meeting of his education committee where his sensible and mediating ideas were all accepted, but the members had an incurable emotional confusion. He may find it a stupid waste of precious time educating them. Maybe the movement will carry him along and force him to work independently.

Scientifically and personally, meanwhile, I've made more progress. The book, a section of which served as my Congress presentation, is now ready in draft form. Since there were various rumors circulating in the Verlag about that presentation, I've sent it to Psychoanalytic Review *for publication. On the other hand, some love for my old research area has once again awakened in me, influenced perhaps but not triggered by the interest of one of the largest publishing houses in translating my* Incest Theme. *I promised to complete the second edition soon, and a young assistant at the local psychiatric clinic, who is also about to become a member of the group here, has expressed interest in doing the translation (he's done good ones of Kretschmer and others). Thus I can reconnect with that area of research, and then return to the abandoned works of my early period if I have time.*

Finally something else to which, for the time being, I assign no great significance, but mention as something hopeful. My millionaire has been here for a few weeks, and is out of the depression that had oppressed him since 1920. He is, of course, somewhat manic, but feels very well, and has now made a series of decisive resolutions in a manner that suits him and his family—resolutions he'd warded off through the depression. Although that receded this summer (he left me in May), he doesn't want to admit that analysis helped him, but appreciates me personally. (He's correct: I couldn't help him much analytically, but got him on his feet again with "active therapy"—pulling him out of the fixations he had for decades.)

He visited me once, and tomorrow evening I'll see him again; if circumstances allow I won't fail to urge him to do something for psychoanalysis. (Just recently, he had his splendid seaside estate set up as a children's home.)

The other opportunity to help the Verlag, or at least one branch, Imago, *arose on the horizon in the form of a plan I was given to set up an American edition of* Imago! *Another millionaire—here they just seem to be waiting to donate their money—seems ready to finance this for several years. I said I'd support the plan with you and the Verlag, provided it could gain materially from this. I hope to hear details next week, but won't make any definitive decision before you have the details. I'm not doing this alone.*

While I'm rather alienated from the idea of the former Committee and have outgrown it, I'm happy with the reorganization you suggest. I glimpse a good omen, too, because the group you prefer doesn't have the pettiness of the other group (Abraham, Jones), and provides in Ferenczi scientific tolerance, in Eitingon social sensitivity, and in your daughter the non-medical-pedagogical. I think I'd work well with this group, personally and objectively, if the members are willing, and confidently hope I can win back your daughter's trust. Incidentally, it's good that I wrote to Ferenczi some time ago expressing hope that the old "prewar" relations between Vienna and Budapest might be restored with my return.

Despite all plans and perspectives for the future, I definitely intend to set up a permanent home for my family in Vienna, at least a new, larger and more comfortable apartment, and reside there at least for the time being.

On December 9 I board the giant steamer "Berengaria," arriving Cherbourg on December 15, meet my wife in Paris, where we'll have a few days just for ourselves before I return to Vienna during Christmas week.

I look forward to seeing you again healthy, and greet you cordially, as in old times. Yours, Rank

Freud and Ferenczi supported nonmedical analysts (e.g., Rank, Reik, Anna Freud, Joan Riviere, Caroline Newton); Jones straddled the line. Brill strongly opposed them. According to Ferenczi (Nov. 28), Brill spoke harshly "against lay analysis and the Europeans who don't turn away lay practitioners. He even threatened to break with you Herr Professor, if things continue this way." Brill claimed that Jones, whom he had recently visited, shared his opinion. Freud responded, "Brill's threat will not cause me to change my position on lay analysis. I won't cling to the Americans."[13]

Karl Abraham died on Christmas day. The persistent bronchial and lung problems may have been cancer. The Committee was bereft and the IPA without a president: "perhaps the greatest loss that could hit us," Freud wrote Jones on December 30. Ferenczi, in Berlin for the funeral, informs Freud (Jan. 14, 1926) of a preview showing there of the Pabst film, "to our displeasure." The audience included Jones and Sachs, who "is hiding more and more in the cloak of Abraham, who can't defend himself. I'm often reminded of your opinion that Sachs doesn't belong on the Committee."

Martin Freud recalls a visit to his grandmother's flat when his son Walter was about four (1925). Amalia's children, grandchildren, and great-grandchildren usually assembled on Sunday mornings. Little Walter, bored, wandered to the staircase and then out to the street, where he proudly helped a man crank up his truck. Hearing the engine start, and missing Walter, Martin and his sisters rushed outside to find his son triumphant, expecting applause. Instead he was carried upstairs, where he heard "a full and hostile account of his shocking exploit given to father by all the aunts, all talking at once." Grandfather Sigmund Freud was moved to "the severe form of anger usually shown by men who normally have excellent control of their tempers. . . . Neither my wife nor I found it pleasant." Freud said there was no sense "in becoming attached to a boy who must sooner or later kill himself in danger-ous episodes" and had "a few cutting remarks about parents who were unable to control their children."[14]

This episode took place while Rank, former mechanic and filial protégé, was finally separating. Grief-stricken at the loss of 4-year-old Heinele in 1920, Freud said then that he could never make such an emotional bond again.

1926. Rank's return should have been amicable, in light of his euphoric (perhaps hypomanic) letter from New York. He is little mentioned in the first months of 1926. "Due to a fever with otitis, Rank's wife has developed a semi-toxic emotional disturbance, which is improving nicely. It seems to be nothing serious—a result of long-repressed tensions. He was very fright-ened." She had some analytic sessions with Freud in January.[15]

Although Ferenczi was interested in the IPA presidency, Freud supported Eitingon, who was already Secretary—and more businesslike. Anna Freud became IPA secretary. Simmel and Rádo took over the Berlin Institute. When Freud had angina symptoms in February, Ferenczi proposed coming to Vienna to analyze him! Freud demurred, promising instead to refer pa-tients if Ferenczi made the move. Subsequently Freud was more emphatic, saying that one could not justify psychological intervention in a patient of 70 with "toxic etiology and anatomical findings."[16]

On April 13, Freud wrote Eitingon: "Yesterday Rank was here—for a final farewell. He is moving first to Paris . . . though America is probably in the more distant future." He continues:

On a slow, peaceful path, the daemon in him has now established what it originally wished to conquer violently through an attack of illness. In this context, the gain through illness is, in the form of material independence, very great. I admit I deceived myself greatly in the prognosis—a repeated fate; on the other hand, Abraham's pre-mature diagnosis certainly accelerated and favored its course. The fact that Rank is leaving before my birthday (and thus excluding himself from everything) is symp-tomatically interesting, but otherwise arouses no regret in me. . . . Theoretically Rank seems to be retracting nothing; our conversation about my book on anxiety revealed irreconcilable differences. Practically, he seems to be holding on to his technique. He

also indicated he's come much further in his insights although he correctly assesses his
own state as manic again.

Angered, Eitingon wanted to cancel publication of Rank's *Sexuality and Guilt* by the Verlag. Freud wrote (Apr. 19): "Your reaction against Rank was more violent than I intended to provoke. I think it should not depend on favor whether or not his small collection is published by the Verlag. We mustn't forget that it's the Verlag that he founded and directed for many years, and that he is even among its creditors." But Freud was surprised and provoked by Rank's next book, *Psychoanalytic Technique,* volume I, published by Deuticke. Ferenczi got word of Rank's departure from Eitingon, and asked Freud about it, who answered on April 23:

> *The fact that he can't find a proper place to live here certainly plays a part; also the*
> *need to conceal difficulties with his wife, the outcome of which can't be foreseen. The*
> *main thing, however, is that he's now carried out in a, so to speak, sober, cold way what*
> *he originally wanted to achieve in the stormy attack of illness: loosing himself from me*
> *and from all of us. What is ambiguous are the two facts, that he didn't want to give up*
> *anything of the theory in which his neurosis had precipitated itself, and that he also*
> *didn't take the smallest step to approach the Society here.*
>
> *I don't belong to those who demand that one has to manacle and sell oneself*
> *for eternity out of "gratitude." He received much as a gift and accomplished much*
> *in return, so we're even. But on his farewell visit I didn't see any occasion to express*
> *extreme tenderness, I was honest and hard. But we can make the sign of the cross over*
> *him. Abraham was right.*

On May 6, from Paris, where he was establishing a new practice, Rank sent a birthday gift to Freud: the works of Friedrich Nietzsche, 23 volumes bound in white leather. The gift pointed to the intellectual debt each man owed to the philosopher-psychologist Freud said he could not read because Nietzsche's writing was too rich with ideas that he could only approach gradually, scientifically. Then came Rank's last letter to Freud.

Paris 31 rue de Chazelles ¶May 23, 1926

Lieber Herr Professor,
> *I was very glad that our birthday present pleased you; I also heard from my wife*
> *how fine and festive everything was. My wife also informed me that she wants to visit*

you later. Of course I don't know what she told you, but perhaps afterward you can really understand me better. In any case, I thank you for your kind involvement in her destiny, which it is now clear will remain permanently tied to mine. We'll pass the summer together, and plan to set up a household in Paris in the autumn.

Simultaneously with this letter my new book [on psychoanalytic technique] is being sent to you. It will perhaps surprise you, though it's nothing more than the logical development of my concept. Unfortunately again incomplete, but since you're reserved with judgment you'll hopefully appreciate it in the context of the other portions, specifically of the underlying theoretical depiction, which I hope to produce in the course of this year, although for the foreseeable future I'll be occupied with analyses the entire day.

In the course of next month I'll come to Vienna to pick up my family for our vacation in Switzerland; I hope to be able to see you then.

With cordial greetings. Yours, Rank

They never met again. Having read part of the new book, Freud disparaged Rank's technique to Ferenczi (June 6): "Its main character is crafty perspicacity without critique, an unusable work attitude. He combines the worst errors of those who have fallen away from us; like Stekel, he acknowledges boundless arbitrariness in the interpretation of dreams, like Adler, he sees of all analytic reactions only one, the struggle for the undisturbed possession of the mother object; Adler, the striving to be superior to authority (of the father). Both occur naturally, they don't need to be discovered."

Freud wrote to Jones that Ferenczi stayed a week with him en route to New York, and they met with Dr. Frankwood Williams to enlighten him on "Rank's distortion of analysis." Jones wrote back about a visit from Dr. René Laforgue, who told him that Rank claimed to be on "most amicable terms" with Freud, citing the birthday present costing $300. In reply Freud said, "The conclusion would have been justified if I had given the present to him." No, the gift had other motives: "the oppressing feeling of owing so much to me, even in money, a reaction of gratitude, or rather against gratitude, a tendency to boast of his newly acquired riches and a self-destructive impulse to spend all he is earning. . . . I am not sure at all what the final result of his career may be, he does not belong to those easy-going scoundrels, to whom success in life is assured."[17]

Ending his chapter "Disunion," in the Freud biography, Jones wrote: "We are not concerned here with Rank's further career any more than with those of the earlier dissidents, Adler, Stekel and Jung." Noting some similarities between Rank and Jung in their divergence from Freud, Jones concluded: "Jung was not afflicted by any of the mental trouble that wrecked Rank and so was able to pursue an unusually fruitful and productive life."[18]

≈ Chapter 19 ≈

Willing, Feeling, Living

1926–1939

*The undischarged, unreleased, or traumatic experiences are not repressed into
the unconscious and there preserved, but rather are continued permanently
in actual living, resisted, carried through to an ending or worked over into
entirely new experiences. Here in actual experience . . . is contained not only the
whole present but also the whole past, and only here in the present are psychological
understanding and therapeutic effect to be obtained.*
—Rank, Will Therapy

Published two months before Rank moved to Paris, *Inhibitions, Symptoms,
and Anxiety* (1926: *S.E.,* 20) was Freud's answer to *The Trauma of Birth.*
Freud reverses his theory that anxiety derives from repressed sexuality,
declaring, instead, that anxiety precedes and leads to repression of sexuality.
"Rank's contention—which was originally my own—that the affect of anxiety
is a consequence of the event of birth and a repetition of the situation then
experienced, obliged me to review the problem of anxiety once more" (161).

But Freud rejects Rank's emphasis on the emotional pain of separation
from mother. Birth "is not experienced subjectively as a separation from the
mother, since the foetus, being a completely narcissistic creature, is totally
unaware of her existence as an object" (130). The first internalized object
in the infant's psyche is paternal, symbolized by the superego, heir to the
Oedipus complex.

For Freud, the emotional experience of loss and separation anxiety derives
from fear of castration, not from the child's love and fear of its mother, as
Rank argues. Freud claims, "At birth no object existed, and so no object could

be missed" (170). On the one hand, he recognizes the merit of Rank's "discovery of [the] extensive concatenation" between birth and physiological anxiety (151); on the other, he denies the traumatic emotional consequences of separation at birth: "It becomes impossible to shut one's eyes any longer to the far-fetched character of [Rank's] explanations" (136). As to the origin of emotional suffering, concedes Freud, "we are as much in the dark about this problem as we were at the start" (149). Despite overturning his theory of anxiety, Freud kept infantile sexuality and castration fear intact. Rank answered Freud's critique:

> We know too little about the newly born and its sensations to be able to draw hard-and-fast conclusions about it. But in spite of isolated observations of children and even child analyses, the same thing is true for the child in general, in whom hitherto too much of the adult, especially adult sexuality, has probably been projected. Freud's warning... holds also for his own assertion that the mother does not represent an object for the newly born.... For it is certain that the newborn child loses something as soon as it is born, indeed as soon as birth begins.... One might perhaps say that in parturition the ego finds its object and then loses it again, which possibly explains many peculiarities of our psychical life.[1]

In *Trauma of Birth*, Rank argues that the infant relates emotionally to its mother from birth as the first "good" and "bad" object. The newborn retains a feeling of *"primal ambivalence"* toward the "lost primal object, the mother," a powerful figure from the start of life. Ambivalence is strong and inevitable. Mother is loving and generous, but also inhibiting and beyond the infant's control, hence anxiety-provoking, "a dark threatening power, capable of deepest sympathy but also greatest severity."[2] For Freud, on the contrary, it is the omnipotent father who inhibits the infant, thereby forming the superego, and mother provokes anxiety only because she is a desired and paternally prohibited sex object. Freud saw the relationship between mother and son as conflict-free, "altogether the most perfect, the most free of ambivalence of all human relationships" (*S.E.*, 22:133).[3]

In Freud's Oedipal narrative, mother has no will, power, or identity of her own. Silhouetted against the powerful father, the mothers of Little Hans, Dora, the Rat Man, and the Wolf Man are not agents. Freud found little trace of will in the female psyche, which remained a mystery. "*Was will das*

Weib" (What does woman want?), he asked Marie Bonaparte in 1925. A year later: "The sexual life of women is a *dark continent.*"[4] Strikingly, nowhere does Freud consider mother to be a bar, or prohibition, against the incestuous desires of the little boy. Father is source of the superego, as Freud reminded the Committee in early 1924: "The incest prohibition—where does that come from? Its representative is apparently the father, reality, authority—which does not permit incest. . . . Here Rank deviates from me. . . . Basically, the orientation toward the mother's body or genitals should be an ambivalent one from the outset. Here lies the contradiction. . . . In analysis one will come up against the father again and again as the bearer of the prohibition" (Rundbrief, Feb. 14, 1924).

In May 1926, Rank published the first of a planned three-volume work, *Technik der Psychoanalyse (Technique of Psychoanalysis).*[5] Volume 1 was subtitled *The Analytic Situation.* "I have now for several years attempted systematically to trace back the analysis of the transference to the time before the development of the Oedipus complex," begins Rank, "and to use the experience of the pre-Oedipus situation in the analytic transference relationship as a therapeutic agent."[6]

With "the analytic situation," Rank underscores the here-and-now relationship between patient and analyst. As Ferenczi and he had proposed, "it is not intellectual knowledge but emotional experience in the analytic situation that forms the essential therapeutic factor in the cure." Relationship—not insight—is the basis of transformation. The effective therapist provides above all a meaningful human connection, not an exercise in historical reconstruction, no matter how ingeniously formulated. "When one asks the patient what ideas come to him now (here) his associations can relate only to the actual analytic situation, namely to the analyst, and must first be interpreted as such. Many associations to dreams are unintelligible without their relation to the analytic situation from which they emerge."[7]

Freud claimed that Rank avoided "the Oedipus," dismissing the father's importance in the child's emotional life. Rank answered, "I endeavor only to systematize the cause and, thereby, put things in their right place, as, for example, the importance of the father—which I value by no means slightly, but only in another way."[8] Like Ferenczi, Rank regarded love as the prime healing factor in psychotherapy. In the opening phase of therapy, "We give the patient the mother love sought for since his earliest childhood."[9] While necessary, love is not sufficient.

Regardless of the gender of patient or analyst, "The final aim of the psychoanalytic cure is only to be gained through identification of patient with analyst as father, instead of wanting him to be mother. But the presupposition for that final aim is solving the mother fixation. For the patient is compelled to reproduce in the analytic transference the primal mother-relation: namely, the union and the separation." The patient wants, at once, to hold on and to let go. During the end phase, the analyst artfully "leads the patient to his own ego." A servant-leader, the analyst plays the role of skilled midwife for the birth of individuality and self-realization.[10]

"Moreover, I find myself in the fortunate position of being able to refer to the '*History of an Infantile Neurosis*' [1918: *S.E., 17*] in which the [Wolf Man] likewise represented and comprehended the cure as a re-birth experience. . . . From the painfulness of these typical birth reactions, under which the separation in the end phase of my analysis took place, I inferred a 'trauma of birth.' This, I suppose, could not have been recognized earlier because it had suffered a much stronger repression than even manifestations of infantile sexuality."[11]

The longest and most important of Freud's case histories, *Infantile Neurosis* was written to refute Adler and Jung, who opposed the focus on infantile sexuality as the main cause of adult neurosis. Neither Adler nor Jung responded to it. Rank was the first to challenge Freud's Oedipal interpretation of the case.

Sergius Pankejeff, a wealthy Russian aristocrat, came to Freud in 1910 at age 23, suffering from obsessive-compulsive behavior and depression. The nickname "Wolf Man," which Freud never used in his case history, refers to a dream whose latent meaning explained the patient's neurosis.

> I dreamt that it was night and that I was lying in my bed. (My bed stood with its foot towards the window; in front of the window there was a row of old walnut trees. I knew it was winter when I had the dream, and night-time.) Suddenly the window opened of its own accord, and I was terrified to see that some white wolves were sitting on the big walnut tree in front of the window. There were six or seven of them. The wolves were quite white, and looked more like foxes or sheep-dogs, for they had big tails like foxes and they had their ears pricked like dogs when they pay attention to something. In great terror, evidently of being eaten up by the wolves, I screamed and woke up. (S.E., 17:29)

The recurring nightmare, supposedly first dreamt just before the patient's fourth birthday, led Freud to conclude the small boy had been traumatized by witnessing parental intercourse *"a tergo"* (from behind) several times before age two. From this dream of six or seven silent, immobile wolves—curiously, Pankejeff sketched only five in a drawing—Freud reconstructed a primal trauma: "He was able to see his mother's genitals as well as his father's organ; and he understood the process as well as its significance. . . . He received the impressions when he was one and a half; his understanding of them was deferred [until age four], but became possible at the time of the dream owing to his development, his sexual excitations, and his sexual researches" (37–38).

The wolf symbol was "merely a first father-surrogate" (32), threatening Pankejeff, near age four, with castration fear for Oedipal desires—whence originated his life-long neurosis. This "fear of his father was the strongest motive for his falling ill, and his ambivalent attitude towards every father-surrogate was the dominating feature of his life as well as of his behavior during the treatment" (32). Freud declared the therapy successfully ended on July 14, 1914, one year after he set a termination date—which later inspired Rank to invoke end-setting himself.

Remembering the primal scene was the turning point, after four and a half years of analysis. With Freud, healing was possible only by offering interpretation of repressed memories from infancy. Once accepted emotionally by the patient, insight into the Oedipus complex would prove curative. The analyst reveals the past in the present. Although Freud published the Wolf Man's case as successful in 1918, Pankejeff returned five years later to work with Freud, from November 1919 to February 1920 (122). Then Freud began collecting money to provide a yearly stipend to Pankejeff, who had lost his fortune during the Russian Revolution. Freud gave Pankejeff an autographed copy of the published case, and the patient felt he was one of Freud's great favorites—a kind of spiritual son.[12]

In volume 1 of *Technik*, Rank speculates that the Wolf Man's dream was provoked by ambivalent feelings of separation anxiety in the analytic situation, not recalled from childhood. The psychoanalytic couch represents the child's bed, with its foot toward the window through which trees were visible. The "six or seven wolves" might be Freud's six children or the "wolfish" analytic colleagues, including Rank himself, whose photographs adorn the office wall. "I am convinced that this patient knew that Freud had six children; he is the seventh who alone is saved . . . by Freud = the mother."[13]

According to Rank, the Wolf Man, jealous of Freud's children and clos-est disciples, dreams up a fantasy that he is the seventh child of Freud, a branch on the "genealogical tree of psychoanalysis," a member of the inner circle, and Freud's favorite patient. The dream pleases Freud, a tender—but intimidating—mother-surrogate whom Pankejeff must give up in the pain-ful process of ending analysis, no matter how anxious he feels about letting go and moving on. "Whether or not the anxiety relates only to the father, as Freud thinks, or also to the mother (birth anxiety; the dream is dreamt in expectation of a birthday) may be left an open question."[14]

On May 30, 1926, Ferenczi told Freud of his own first reactions to Rank's *Technik*. Acknowledging his close collaboration with Rank and respecting "some of his ideas," he announces, "I can finally free myself from him, since his character traits also force me to tear up *corum publico* [in public view] the all too brotherly commonality that we manifested publicly for a time."[15]

On June 6, Freud responded with a savage critique of Rank.

His demon is egging him on to a course where there is no stopping and no turning back. His whole behavior is evidently calculated to cut the tablecloth between us and him, and he must succeed....

He interprets the wolf-dream of my Russian (at age four) from the analytic situa-tion twenty years later! If that isn't an attempt at self-parody, then it can have only one purpose. One is given to understand that I was taken in by the patient and misperceived a recent product of transference as a report out of the past. (The fact that, instead of transference he always puts "analytic situation" is characteristic in and of itself!) ...how did [Rank] withdraw from the obligation to share his doubt with me and to ask me what I think about the possibility of such a deception?[16]

Freud told Ferenczi that he asked Pankejeff, then living in Vienna, to "care-fully share with me everything he can say about this dream," and reported to Eitingon that the Wolf Man recalled only two or three photographs on the wall when treatment began in early 1910. Having finished with his former protégé, Freud recounts Frau Rank's farewell visit.

She completely shares our point of view, and is quite unhappy about the [Technik] book, the proofs of which she didn't want to read. She feels he's trying to be "sent away." She says he tolerates no objections from her, and will never let himself be held back when he has an insight. The poor woman, who would like to stick with him—though she is finding it difficult to do so—must be sure of our discretion. I have great doubts as to how this marriage will end up. Rank's last connection to us is that of participation on the Verlag [Board]; this participation should be quietly dissolved.[17]

In his critique of *Technik*, Ferenczi breaks publicly with his best friend: "According to Rank's view, at the deepest instinctual level the biological attachment to the mother regularly dominates the analytic situation, whereas what Freud assigns to the analyst is in essentials the part of the father." Although Rank's view has "some value . . . it becomes worthless when it is carried to such violent extremes that the explanation of symptoms with reference to fear of the father, or rather castration (an explanation which is obvious and often the only one possible), is disdained or actually declared to be dangerous on the grounds that patients are thus 'driven ever deeper into their infantile fear of the father, from which in the end there is no therapeutic escape.' " Defending Freud's reconstruction of the primal scene, Ferenczi cites Pankejeff's recent personal testimony in order to "completely demolish Rank's hypothesis" that the dream was provoked by the anxious prospect of separating from Freud, subjectively experienced as a maternal-surrogate. Rank's "super-interpretation of the wolf dream . . . has shattered our confidence in the author's judgment in regard to psychoanalytic theory and technique."[18]

Freud was pleased: "I received your Rank critique, find it decisive enough, somewhat flatter on the point about the analysis of the wolf-dream than it would have turned out with me. In this I'm certainly laden with affect, of which you were able to sense only a reflection."[19]

From 1926 through 1934, Otto Rank lived and worked in Paris. Among his best-known patients were Anaïs Nin and Henry Miller. On her second visit to Rank, he asked Nin to leave her diary with him. "It is your last defense against analysis. . . . I do not want you to have a traffic island from which you will survey the analysis, keep control of it. I don't want you to analyze the analysis." Soon afterwards she said, "I talked to Rank as I talked to my journal. . . . I feel his sympathy, a far-reaching one. I can tell him everything." Two months later she thought about "the order and progression of our talks. The order made by reality. But since Rank does not believe in that literal sequence, I perceive a new order, which is the choice of events made by the salient impulse of memory—the relief created by a sense of the whole. . . . He has made me swim in life, rather than collect aquariums!" She recounts his subsequent affair with her and his reluctance to return to New York in 1934 without her. "He wanted to give me the ring Freud had given him. He wanted to cast off the father."[20]

Rank made trans-Atlantic voyages every year or two to keep up his practice and teach in the United States. In late 1926, he delivered a series of lectures in New York (in English) from his forthcoming book, *Grundzüge einer genetischen Psychologie* (*Basis of a Genetic Psychology*), planned as a three-volume work.[21]

"Genetic" does not refer to genes, but to psychosocial origin and the development of object relationships. Rank begins, "This book is a direct continuation, development, and extension of my new orientation in psychoanalytic theory and therapy. . . . However disconcerting it is that the founder of psychoanalysis—from whom my concept matured—has taken such an emotionally bitter attitude toward [*ToB*], I am neither disillusioned nor confused in continuing my subsequent work." Returning to a central theme: "I have now again . . . come up against the [maternal] object and the object relationship, which presupposes anxiety just as much as libido"—fear just as much as love. There is no lack of ambivalence in the mother-child relationship, even for the little boy.[22]

Rank criticizes Freud's unwillingness to go "behind" the Oedipus situation to the "primal object relationship" of the child with its powerful (or "bad") mother:

> [Freud] sees in the mother merely the coveted sex object, for the possession of which the child battles with the father. The "bad mother" he has never seen, but only the later displacement of her to the father, who therefore plays such an omnipotent part in his theory. The image of the bad mother, however, is present in Freud's estimation of woman, who is merely a passive and inferior object for him: in other words, "castrated." When he recently deprived woman even of a super-ego, which embraces the higher ethical and social abilities, he quite overlooked the enormous share the mother and the child's relation to her have on the development of the ego and its higher capabilities.[23]
>
> . . . The real formation of the ego takes place under the influence of the mother in the pre-Oedipal phase.[24]

In his chapter "The Genesis of the Object Relationship," Rank mentions that the small boy "must, so to speak, make his father bad, in order to keep his picture of the good mother clear."[25]

Volume I of *Genetische Psychologie* offers a theory of the genesis and development of object relationships—the ego and its relation to the super-ego—presaging major themes of the next half-century that were not associated with Rank because his name, by the late 1920s, had become anathema for certified psychoanalysts.[26]

> Above all, the genetic point of view compels us to consider the object relationship from the side of the ego. The construction and development of the ego takes place under the influence of the object relationship, and, in turn, the ego has influence on the object relationship. . . . The relation of the ego to the object is twofold . . . because of the child's original idea of the mother as both good (vouchsafing) and bad (depriving) object. . . . [The] new object relationship at the Oedipus stage differs from the primary relation to the mother in that now the two mother roles, the good and the bad, are divided up between the father and the mother. . . . The success of this division determines the kind and intensity of the child's later sexual and social relations. This is why the Oedipus complex has such an important bearing upon the later fate of the human being's object relationships. But that should not blind us to the fact that the Oedipus complex is only a transient phase of development and that its success or failure has been decisively determined beforehand by the original relationship to the mother. The Oedipus situation compels the child to project on to both sexes the ambivalent attitude that originally referred to the mother only. . . . Every object relationship nevertheless holds destructive elements within it, since the deposit of overcome and renounced ego phases always involves a breaking up and reorganization of the ego structure, which we know and fear as the destructive side of love.[27]

Angered by Rank's "anti-Oedipal" theorizing, Freud reacts to Rank's latest book in a letter to Eitingon, June 20, 1927: "Rank's *Genetische Psychologie 1* shows him in full mania, confused, incomprehensible, impudently aggressive. . . . Rank flirts with Jung, Adler, and Stekel; the unconscious is a mystical concept; the significance of sexuality has been very much overvalued; we know no more about the sexuality of the child than we do about the newborn, and anything that seems to show more was suggested to the child; the castration complex has never been experienced, and more such nonsense."

On July 2, to Eitingon, Freud calls Rank a "*Hochstaplernatur*"—impostor by nature. "I'm curious whether he has overcome his conflicts in this way. Probably. A cure—*ad pejus* [for the worse]. That can happen, too."[28]

In 1928, Rank published *Genetische Psychologie,* volume 2, devoted largely to emotions. He begins, "In [vol. 1], we examined the ego's development from the object relationship. Now we want to consider the force that keeps these processes going: the emotions." Rank argues that "the human emotional life is the center and real sphere of psychology . . . although psychoanalysis has contributed relatively little to understanding the emotional life. . . . [Moreover], in the psychoanalytic literature the word *feeling* is scarcely used, although in essence our whole emotional life rests on feelings and is directed by feelings." Drawing on language more akin to Martin Buber than Freud, Rank observes: "One could designate the feeling life as 'Thou-Psychology'— because it determines our relation to fellow men and, at the same time, to reality itself."[29]

> We see this clearly in the love feeling—which unites our I with the other, with the Thou, with men, with the world and does away with fear. What is unique in love is that—beyond the fact of uniting—it rebounds on the I. Not only, I love the other as my I, a part of my I, but the other also makes my I worthy of love. The love of the Thou thus places a value on one's own I. Love abolishes egoism, it merges the self in the other to find it again enriched in one's own I. This unique projection and introjection of feeling rests on the fact that one can really only love the one who accepts our own self as it is, indeed will not have it otherwise than it is, and whose self we accept as is.[30]

In 1929 and 1931 Rank published volumes 2 and 3 of *Technik.* Translated as *Will Therapy,* they present Rank's full elaboration of his work with Ferenczi in *Development*: a paradigm shift from offering intellectual understanding— insight into the infantile past—to jointly experiencing a feeling relationship.

Rank argues, "The only means of healing which psychotherapy has learned to use is itself a human being, the therapist, whose own psychology also must have a decided influence upon the treatment and its outcome." The analyst's emotions influence the analysand. "I have attempted to write a 'Philosophy of Helping.'" The aim of therapy, rather than to remember the

repressed past, is to help patients "learn to will" in the present. "The feeling of experience, purposefully and with intent, is made the central factor in
the therapeutic task, not merely endured as the troublesome, if unavoidable,
phenomenon of resistance."[31]

Following Nietzsche, who maintained the equivalence of willing and the
emotional life, Rank employs "will" and "counter-will" to capture the emotional give-and-take of the relationship—"an actual feeling experience"—
between patient and analyst.[32]

Franz Alexander, in a harsh review of *Development,* attacked Ferenczi and
Rank for valuing experience over transference in the analytic situation.
"Transference *is* experience in analysis," declared Alexander.[33] But to Rank,
using transference to reconstruct the past allows both therapist and patient
to escape the emotionally charged present. Psychiatrist Clara Thompson,
analysand of Ferenczi and analyst of Harry Stack Sullivan, recognized Rank's
breakthrough:

> Rank was the first to point out that in doing this the patient is led away from
> the living present, the area of real feeling. As he put it, it is always easier to
> talk about the past because it is not present. He and Ferenczi stress, for the
> first time, that not every attitude toward the analyst is transferred from the
> past, that there is some reaction to the analyst in his own right, and that it is
> actually anxiety-relieving and, therefore, stops the progress of the analysis, to
> point out to the patient, "You do not really feel this way about me, but about
> your father, etc." Thus, if the patient finally gets the courage to tell the analyst
> he looks like a pig, the whole issue may be conveniently buried by referring it
> to the past, saying, "That must be what you thought of your father." Two things
> may happen as a result—the analyst does not have to face the fact that he does
> look like a pig and the patient feels, "I got safely out of that one," but does not
> feel more secure thereby because he knows he really meant the analyst and not
> his father. From that day on he is likely to assume the analyst's feelings have to
> be protected.[34]

In minimizing the reality of the intersubjective relationship, says Rank,
Freud denies the energetic feeling of will experienced in the moment by both
parties. "Where Freud met the will of the other, he called it 'resistance' (to
his will)." Rank turns resistance, or counter-will, into a creative factor: the
"negative reaction of the patient represents the actual therapeutic value, the

expression of will as such." Vital to the differentiation of self from non-self, and to furthering individuation, resistance is "proof, however negative, of the strength of will on which therapeutic success ultimately depends."[35]

In the end phase, the therapist yields and the patient separates. Counter-will is transformed into will, for the patient's benefit. The therapist has to lose this inevitable will struggle in order to free the patient's creative power.

In the patient's "present experience we have . . . his whole reaction pattern, all his earlier ways of reacting plus the present." Freud "made the repression historical, that is, misplaced it into the childhood of the individual and then wanted to release it from there, while as a matter of fact the same tendency is working here and now."[36]

For Rank, there is no "container" in the mind called the unconscious. Instead of *Verdrängung* (repression), indicating unconscious repression of the past, Rank preferred *Verleugnung* (denial), a word capturing the patient's need or willingness to stay ill. All emotional life is grounded in the present: "The neurotic lives too much in the past [and] to that extent he actually does not live. He suffers . . . because he clings to [the past], wants to cling to it, in order to protect himself from experience, the emotional surrender to the present." But separating, no matter how anxiety-provoking, from outworn phases of life, including relationships and internalized others, is required for emotional maturity, just as much as connecting with others. Letting go of the past, or stepping outside the ruling ideology of one's unconscious values, assumptions, beliefs, and expectations, marks the most significant and painful experience of transformation in the here-and-now: "This, then, is the New, which the patient has never experienced before."[37]

Both constructive and destructive, willing is expressed in creation or lost in neurotic symptoms, that is, self-destruction. The neurotic wills himself or herself unfree, perverting the primal, creative life-force into its own denial. The neurotic is "a personality denying its own will, not accepting itself as an individual." Unable to affirm his or her own difference, the suffering person hurls a Big No—or, at best, a Big Maybe—at living. The patient is a "failed artist" whose creative energies have gone astray. Although a creative product, the neurosis is "negative willing." The neurotic denies himself or herself because of excessive guilt over separating and individuating—excessive anxiety over accepting his or her own "difference," a signature word that Rank equates with "the consciousness of living."[38]

What is "difference"? What is "the consciousness of living"? Human beings are thrown into the world at birth and thrown out at death. Just as we
forget that we are born to die, we forget that we are living. That which is conscious—including self-consciousness—is more mysterious than that which is
unconscious. This is also the meaning of Rank's frequently misunderstood
claim that "the whole of psychology becomes of necessity a psychology of
consciousness."[39]

Far from banishing the unconscious, which he refused to reify,[40] Rank is
alluding to the even more perplexing mystery of consciousness. Rank calls
"difference" the real problem, "a problem of the present, in other words, the
consciousness of living. The tendency to get free of it may be the strongest
psychic force in the individual, as it manifests itself in striving after happiness
and salvation."

Existentially, angst is a consequence of consciousness, or more correctly,
the self-consciousness of a person who is willing to affirm the time-limited
existence forced on him or her at birth by fate. "First comes the perception of difference from others as a consequence of becoming conscious of
self ... then interpretation of this difference as inferiority ... finally association of this psychological conflict with the biological sexual problem, the
difference of the sexes."[41] The difference between nonexistence and existence precedes and colors all other difference—whether it be sex, age, race,
intelligence, or nationality. Existence comes first.[42]

Not anti-intellectual or opposed to insight, Rank distinguishes between
the repressed hysteric Freud hoped to cure with insight and the hypercon-
scious neurotic who already has too much insight:

Today one sees such hysterias hardly at all ... but many more compulsion neurotics, woman as well as men and even more individuals who, without rep-
resenting a clinical type, suffer simply from self-consciousness, from a too
extreme introspectiveness. . . .

Becoming conscious helps the one, while the other is helped by ... the
emotional experience. The one suffers from knowing too little, the other from
knowing too much. . . . One must feed the former with truth, the latter with
illusions, that is to help heal his too complete and final disillusionment with
self. The tragedy is that neither can bear truth or illusion anymore because he
cannot bear himself as an individual different from others.[43]

Like Kierkegaard and Nietzsche, Rank celebrates what, today, is called emotional intelligence: "If I have at one time designated consciousness when it goes beyond a certain breadth or depth as destructive . . . , now while still maintaining this, I would exclude expressly intelligence, which represents exactly the factor that can realize the conscious surplus constructively if one succeeds in putting it at the service of the will."[44]

The problem of emotional experience, and willing, is not how to understand or speak about the past, which has already been interpreted over and over in memory, but how to live, consciously, in the present. In the psychic realm, the only reality is the Now, the same Now that psychoanalysts find so incomprehensible, useless, even unthinkable.[45]

In volume 3 of *Genetische Psychologie* Rank notes that in *The Trauma of Birth* he had referred to "the creation of the individual himself, not merely physically, but also [spiritually] in the sense of the 'rebirth experience,' which I understand . . . as the actual creative act of the human being." Materializing out of nothing and nowhere, a creature born from a biological mother, constructed out of two particles of cosmic dust, "the human being becomes at once creator and creature or actually moves from creature to creator, in the ideal case, creator of himself, his own personality." The evolution of consciousness and the birth of the creative self, a process of continual learning, unlearning and relearning, is never complete: "For the whole consequence of evolution from blind impulse through conscious will to self-conscious knowledge, seems still somehow to correspond to a continued result of births, rebirths and new births, which reach beyond the birth of the child from the mother, beyond the birth of the individual from the mass, to the birth of knowledge from the work."[46]

Rank disputes Freud's characterization of emotions as hysterical attacks—disguised derivatives of sexuality that need to be uprooted or drained. Because of this, Rank writes, "psychoanalysis has scarcely approached the problem of the emotional life."[47]

"The characteristic of that time," remembers Sándor Radó, who was in analysis with Karl Abraham from 1922 to 1925, "was a neglect of a human being's emotional life": "Everybody was looking for oral, pregenital, and genital components in motivation. But that some people are happy, others unhappy, some afraid, or full of anger, and some loving and affectionate—read the case histories to find how such differences between people were then absent from the literature."[48] As if he were answering the question Freud posed in 1925 to Marie Bonaparte—*Was will das Weib?*—Rank observes that, for both men and women, "the emotional tone is an index of the 'what' of the will."[49] Because Freud confounded sexuality and emotion, Rank argues that "the real I, or self with its own power, the will, is left out" of psychoanalytic theory and practice.[50]

For Rank, the act of willing is an expression of primal human energies. Willing is always relational. Tenderness, connection, and love are the quintessential emotions energizing us to unite with others; aggression, anger, and hate energize us to separate from others. Emotions are relationships.

For the patient, according to Rank, each therapeutic hour is a "moving"— back-and-forth—feeling of uniting and separating, surrendering and asserting, connecting and differentiating, holding on and letting go. Rank called this emotional dynamic the "part-whole" problem. If a patient can learn to accept his or her own will in the microcosm of therapy, without too much anxiety or guilt-feeling, then living, creating, and loving more fully outside the allotted hour may also be possible. Human development is a lifelong construction, according to Rank, requiring continual negotiation and renegotiation of the dual yearnings for individuation and connection, difference and likeness, the emotional will to separate and the emotional will to unite. Solving and continually resolving the "part-whole" problem is a never-completed process.

Willing, according to Rank, divides into two emotional currents: one toward separation and individuation, the other toward connection and union. Emotional suffering often comes from the streaming together of two anxieties, "life fear and death fear." A crisis "seems to break out at a certain age when the life fear which has restricted the ego development meets with the death fear as it increases with growth and maturity. The individual then feels himself driven forward by regret for wasted life and the desire still to retrieve it. But this forward driving fear is now death fear, the fear of dying without having lived, which, even so, is held in check by fear of life."[51]

Separating oneself from internal or external objects is traumatic because the uneasy feeling of transition reveals, once again, the primal anxiety of difference, of the "consciousness of living." Thus, the liminal meaning of the trauma of birth: "To this making real of his own ego, the individual reacts in the actual separation experience with fear which is not an original biological reaction in the sense of the death fear, but, on the contrary, is life fear, that is, fear of realizing [one's] own ego as an independent individuality. Accordingly, fear as experienced in birth, is and remains the only fear, that is fear of one's own living and experiencing."[52]

The neurotic is an *"artiste-manqué,"* a failed artist. "In spite of the predominance of death fear, [the neurotic] still stands nearer to the creative type than to the average, on account of which he can be understood only as a miscarried artist, not as an incomplete or undeveloped normal type.... Neurosis is a facing of the metaphysical problems of human existence, only [the person] faces them not in a constructive way as does the artist, philosopher or scientist, but destructively."[53]

"Fear of living" accompanies the prospect of separating and individuating; "fear of dying" the prospect of uniting and merging—the loss of individuality or identity. Separating and uniting are each a source of ambivalence, as the one correlates with the creative impulse—including self-creation—and the other the yearning for love, including dependence on persons and society. To respond narrowly—trying to separate or to merge totally—is a futile effort to deny the dynamics of living.

> The fear in birth, which we have designated as fear of life, seems to me actually the fear of having to live as an isolated individual, and not the reverse, the fear of loss of individuality (death fear). That would mean, however, that primary fear corresponds to a fear of separation from the whole therefore a fear of individuation, on account of which I would like to call it fear of life, although it may appear later as fear of the loss of this dearly bought individuality as fear of death, of being dissolved again into the whole. Between these two fear possibilities, these poles of fear, the individual is thrown back and forth all his life, which accounts for the fact that we have not been able to trace fear back to a single root, or to overcome it therapeutically.[54]

Psychotherapy cannot uproot or drain the two spiraling anxieties. They are a burden universally assumed with life, from birth. The eternal conflict between wanting and fearing both separation and union has no obvious solution. Like the "part-whole" problem, it must be solved, unsolved, and resolved throughout life, at each developmental stage, "from birth, via childhood and puberty to maturity and from there downward through old age to death." There is no final solution. "It can only be a matter of balance between the two, which, however, is not attained once and for all but must be created anew and ever anew."[55]

This life-long, rhythmic oscillation is made more bearable in a relationship with a person who accepts one's difference and allows for the emergence of the creative impulse—without too much guilt-feeling or anxiety for separating. Living fully requires "seeking at once isolation and union," finding the will and courage to bear separation and connection simultaneously.[56] Only a differentiated human being can experience a mature, loving relationship with another differentiated human being. Art, love, and creative production "originate solely in the constructive harmonization of this fundamental dualism of all life."[57]

Like angst, the creative impulse divides into two emotional currents: "Will and guilt are the two complementary sides of one and the same phenomenon." Willing and guilt-feeling define the greatness and limits of a flesh-and-blood mortal, simultaneously creator and creature, artist and worm food, whose awareness of existence is split, "wavering between his Godlikeness and nothingness, whose will is awakened to knowledge of its power [but] whose consciousness is aroused to terror before it. The heroic myth strives to justify this creative will through glorifying its deeds, while religion reminds man that he himself is but a creature dependent on cosmic forces."[58]

Willing is never "free." Although a necessary part of growth, separating and individuating have an emotional price, observes Rank: "The more we individualize ourselves—that is, remove and isolate ourselves from the other—the stronger is the formation of guilt-feeling which originates from this individualization, and which again in turn unites us emotionally with others."[59]

Not an advocate of pure "free will," Rank unwinds the helix of freedom and determinism, willing and guilt-feeling, independence and dependence in *Art and Artist*: "Man's acceptance of his dependence on nature is more honest, while freedom-ideology, beyond a certain point, presumes the negation of that dependence and is therefore, also in a deeper sense, dishonest. This fundamental dishonesty towards nature then comes out as consciousness of guilt, which we see active in every process of art. . . . The more strongly man feels his freedom and independence, the more intense on the other hand is the consciousness of guilt, which appears in the individual partly restrictive, partly creative."[60]

Guilt-feeling is not just a feeling of committing wrong against another, or a residue of sexual wishes, or fear of punishment. Like angst, guilt-feeling is existential, a given. It defines us as human beings as long as we live, grow, and create or, conversely, as long as we deny and betray ourselves by failing or refusing to live, to change, and to develop our potential, for example, by remaining embedded in the "other"—be it the safety net woven by parents, organizations, ideologies, gods, therapists, or lovers. For this reason guilt-feeling—the inescapable complement of willing—is an emotional force in the human being as powerful as the biological impulse of sexuality: "Indeed, it is even shown that in many human beings inhibitions manifesting themselves as anxiety and guilt are stronger than the drives, that these inhibitions themselves, so to say, operate 'as a driving force' although in a different way from the biological impulses. In a word, we see that the psychological has become a force at least equal to the biological and that all human conflicts are to be explained just from this fact."[61]

In its creative expression, guilt feeling is not to be condemned or analyzed away as a residue of Oedipal or pre-Oedipal complexes. It serves as a balancing factor between interlaced yearnings to separate and to unite.

> I think the guilt-feeling occupies a special position among the emotions, as a boundary phenomenon between the pronounced painful affects that separate and the more pleasurable feelings that unite. It is related to the painful separating affects of anxiety and hate. But in its relation to gratitude and devotion, which may extend to self-sacrifice, it belongs to the strongest uniting feelings we know. As the guilt-feeling occupies the boundary line between the painful and pleasurable, between the severing and uniting feelings, it is also the most important representative of the relation between inner and outer, the I and the Thou, the Self and the World.[62]

Therapy, like aesthetic experience and love, is, in Buber's famous phrase, a "healing through meeting," a process that allows therapist and patient to merge into a "greater whole" in order to reemerge, enriched and spiritually renewed by the mutual acceptance of each other's difference and individuality. "The two selves become one and the patient can now find in this enlarged self the differentiation needed for life."[63]

In the life-long, never completed, process of differentiation, we must learn to bear with courage, even affirm, the pain and suffering of human existence, including death. "My formula for greatness in a human being," said Nietzsche, "is 'amor fati' [to love one's fate]"[64] Following Nietzsche, Rank argues in Art and Artist that fate can be overcome only through "volitional affirmation of the obligatory"[65]—that is, by saying "Yes" to the "Must," accepting the need to individuate as well as the need to merge, without becoming shackled to one or other pole, or aimlessly vacillating between the two.

Rank ends *Will Therapy*: "The patient must learn to live, to live with his split, his conflict, his ambivalence, which no therapy can take away, for if it could, it would take with it the actual spring of life. The more truly the ambivalence is accepted the more life and possibilities of life will the human being have and be able to use." Neurosis is an unwillingness to accept this ambivalent condition of life, saying No to necessary suffering—"a refusal of life itself."[66]

Unlike Freud, whose gifts as a writer won him the Goethe prize for literature, Rank was no wordsmith. "I crave simplicity," he told Jessie Taft. "The other [complexity] I have myself."[67]

At one point, during a 1930 speech at the First International Congress on Mental Hygiene, Rank said: "I am no longer trying to prove that Freud was wrong and I was right."[68] Jessie Taft never heard him speak ill of Freud. Anaïs Nin recounts Rank's version of his painful break with Freud, as she heard it from him:

> Freud tried to analyze Rank, but this was a failure. . . . Like all fathers he wanted a duplicate of himself. . . . The real cleavage was achieved by the others. . . . They hoped for a fissure. Even though Rank's discoveries were dedicated to Freud, Freud could never quite forgive him for differing from his established concepts. He began to consider Rank's explorations a threat to his own work. The other disciples worked actively to point up the estrangement, to add to it. Dr. Rank was made to feel so alienated from the group that he finally went to practice in Paris. . . . He lost not only a father but a master, a world, a universe.[69]

In 1944, three years after the death of Freud and Rank, Hanns Sachs, a loyal follower of the Professor, published his memoir, *Freud: Master and Friend*. In it, he revealed publicly, for the first time, the existence of the Secret Committee. Once very close to Rank, Sachs shared Freud's own final judgment.

> [Freud] had done everything in his power to make Rank's way smooth and to bestow on him a leading part of the psychoanalytic movement. Then came a time when Rank broke away from psychoanalysis, doing it not with a clear-cut decision, but alternately renouncing all his former opinions and then again half-heartedly turning back to them. Yet, when after many ups and downs the

final rupture came, Freud did not show the soft regret that I felt at the loss of an old friend. He said, "Now after I have forgiven everything, I am through with him."[70]

"I was born beyond psychology and want to die beyond it," Rank jotted on a note dated June 1939, a few months before he died, "but first and foremost, I want to live beyond it—and formerly it has been in my way." He closes the introduction to his last book, *Beyond Psychology*: "My own life work is completed, the subjects of my former interest, the hero, the artist, the neurotic appear once more upon the stage, not only as participants in the eternal drama of life but after the curtain has gone down, unmasked, undressed, unpretentious, not as punctured illusions, but as human beings who require no interpreter."[71]

≈ ≈

Epilogue

In the thirteen years of my association with him he never discussed with me his
relations to Freud or to the others on the Committee except once in answer to
something I had said about their attachment to Freud, when he replied, "and I was in
the deepest of all"; and once painfully about Ferenczi, whom he had met in the railroad
station in New York in 1926, "He was my best friend and he refused to speak to me."
—Taft, *Otto Rank* (1958), Preface

Beginning in 1926 the American Psychoanalytic Association restricted the practice of psychoanalysis to physician members. Though a physician, Ferenczi supported nonmedical analytic candidates—as did Freud—but that provoked opposition in New York. Rank settled in Paris just as a psychoanalytic group was being formed. He mounted a large portrait of Freud over his desk, doubtless to emphasize his connection rather than the separation from his famous mentor. His patients included American visitors and expatriates. Rank sailed to the United States every year or two before settling in New York in 1935. His 22 American lectures, given from 1924 to 1938, reflect a post-Freudian approach to psychology and therapy in accessible prose. At Yale in 1929, in "The Psychological Approach to Personal Problems," he put his ideas in historical context.

I grew up, as it were, with the whole psychoanalytic movement. I first got in touch with Freud in 1905 and then began to study psychoanalysis under his guidance. Not only have I watched the whole movement from inside (from 1905 to 1925) as it were behind the curtain, but I also took an active part in it. For more than ten years I was editor of the psychoanalytic journals and secretary of the Vienna Psychoanalytic Society. For several years I was vice-president of the Society. Maybe, sometime after I have retired, I will write a history.... Personality, as I conceive of it, is dynamic. Freud's psychology, which in the beginning had the appearance of being a dynamic psychology, in my opinion is dynamic only when compared with the psychology prior to him. It is not, I think, dynamic compared with the psychology that we can see developing in the near future out of the psychoanalytic movement. With Freud the driving force, any kind of impulsion in the individual is biological. He conceives it only biologically, which means even in its highest sense, a kind of *procreative* impulse, but not a real *creative* driving force, of which I think personality consists.

The two important deviations from the Freudian school—represented by Jung and Adler—certainly went beyond this, but both Jung and Adler, each in his own way, went too far in one particular direction. Jung stressed the racial factor.... His is chiefly a psychology of types ... not sufficiently individualized to explain the personal problems that we have to deal with in neurotic or even creative types.

Adler's "individual psychology" is a social psychology; he wants to adjust the individual to circumstances, whereas Freud tries to reform the individual according to the normal, a standard that he derived from some theoretical concept of normality. But neither Freud, nor Jung, nor Adler sufficiently considers the creative part of our personality: that which is *purely individual*, not biological, racial, or social. This I consider the most important part not only for understanding personality but also for therapy and for the individual's adaptation. In 1905 my first reaction to Freud and his theory was a little book, *The Artist,* in which I pointed out the absence of a creative driving force in Freudian theory. What I called the artist in that book was something other than the man who actually paints. I meant by *artist* the creative personality; and using Freud's psychology and terminology, I tried to explain this creative type—but I found it was impossible without going beyond Freud. The chief difference already showing in my book was that, in contrast to Freud, I emphasized not the biological and external factors, but this *inner* self of the individual, something in the individual that is creative, that is impelling, that is not taken in from without but grows somehow within.... It is a kind of mental principle, contrasted with the biological principle.

I don't explain my psychology to the patient but let him develop himself, express himself. There is, especially in this country, a type of patient who already suffers from too much introspection. I don't think we can help these patients by making them more aware of their mechanisms. They need some-thing else. They need an *emotional* experience.

My approach doesn't aim at the individual's complete understanding of himself (Freudian) nor to adjust different individuals to our social situation (Adler). My aim is to enable the individual first to find himself and then to develop himself. . . . I think the neurotic type is a *failure of a creative type*. . . . If the therapist achieves a real therapeutic result the patient will not only be able to adjust himself but sometimes he *adjusts the circumstances to himself*—which means *creation*. . . . His chief job is to create himself and then to go on and cre-ate externally. Other methods of psychotherapy try to adjust the individual to a certain standard: social, biological, or normal instead of being oriented to the individual.

Psychology, understood dynamically when approaching personal problems, deals with interpretations rather than facts—interpretations of both the indi-vidual and the therapist. The individual is constantly interpreting himself, consciously or unconsciously; his whole adjustment, maladjustment, *Weltan-schauung* [world view] depends upon his interpretation of himself, upon what he thinks he is, or what he wants to be, or what other people want him to be, etc. I consider psychology to be a *science of relations* and interrelations, or a *science of relativity*. There is nothing fixed in the field of psychology, everything changes, it is constantly moving. . . . *There are no facts*. The facts are interpretations.

I found this theory insufficient and contrasted to it an inner principle, the individual's *own self-creative power* that also manifests itself ethically [as inhibi-tion, anxiety, or guilt]. We are no longer living on a purely biological principle. We are living on a moral principle.[1]

Rank had a busy practice among American psychiatrists, some of whom saw him in Paris. Among them were Bostonians George Wilbur, Martin Peck, and John Taylor (and their wives); Marion Kenworthy and Frankwood Wil-liams in New York; Frederick Allen and Edward Strecker in Philadelphia. In April 1928, Rank addressed a large Boston audience on "Beyond Psycho-analysis."

Freud's great merit was the overthrow of the medical superstition that the psy-chical is a matter of nerves, which indeed only represent the instrument on which the human life is played. His error was that in its place he wanted to put the biological sex theory. As nerves enable the instrument, so biological sex provides the material for emotional life. Thus Freud dethroned medical materialism. But we thank him for failing to set in its place the purely biological, and so brought psychology into its own as an irreducible philosophical entity. Along with the biological there is in humans an equally strong ethical principle.

The dynamic coexistence of psyche and soma is the basis of all human conflict. Just as the guilt problem can only be comprehended from the ethical side, so real understanding of the love life is to be found only beyond the sex drive in the ego, the I.

Freud used myths to name his concepts, and thought he had explained the myths. Psychological processes can be understood only in psychological—including mythical—terms. Freud himself is a myth creator in the grandest style, in Plato's sense a real philosopher.

Although called "analysis," Freud's search for the biological basis of the psyche was mainly *interpretation*. Where the psyche or soul is concerned, interpretation is almost everything. So Freud's theory is an intellectualized flight from a fact—the new relationship, beyond transference, that presents love and teaches something about it. The interpreted experience of love is ego psychology; the experience of relationship to another is Thou psychology and brings in the ethical, which is part of any relationship between two human beings. A third component of the analytic situation is a new approach to the theory of cognition: a new understanding of the relation of the I not only to other human beings but to reality in general. . . .

The two chief problems of philosophy—cognition and ethics—thus finally also represent the chief problems of psychoanalysis, of human psychology. Fundamentally they correspond to a single great problem: the contrast between I and Thou, self and world, inner and outer. . . . Psychology aims at knowledge of the internal but uses material concerning the external—reality, Thou. It is a science of relations, which easily overestimates one or the other instead of dealing with the relationship between the two.

It is a long way from the medical therapy of nervous disturbances which Freud at first wanted to heal by a kind of sexual dietetics, to the understanding of neurosis as a guilt problem. It is the fundamental difference between two opposite world views, the materialistic and the philosophic—in a more specific sense, the biological and ethical. Psychoanalysis has pushed far in both directions but has failed to see the problem in its full bearing and significance, much less to solve it. But we are grateful to psychoanalysis for bringing up this primal problem again, and for opening up new ways toward its understanding, perhaps to a better solution.[2]

Beata Rank visited Vienna often from Paris and, unlike Otto, maintained a connection with Freud. In her final visit with him in his office in 1928, she was taken aback when Freud told her she would see a man in the outer office who "gave your husband some money—at the time Otto worked for his doctorate." Freud suggested that the Ranks "return the money to this man, so he can help other people, too." Tola was shocked, not sure if the encounter was planned or spontaneous, but "I could not visit Professor Freud any more." Freud was probably aware of Rank's success—he was charging $15 per session (discounted for social workers); the Paris apartment was described by Helene Deutsch as "palatial . . . a luxurious salon frequented by many celebrated artists."[3]

In May 1930, an International Congress on Mental Hygiene took place in Washington, attracting some four thousand attendees. Anna Freud was invited by chairman Frankwood Williams but declined. Her participation would have helped the case for nonmedical practitioners that her father supported and Brill's APA opposed.

Rank was lead speaker on a panel of eight, including three psychiatrists. He spoke of the importance of human experience and emotion and criticized the attempt of science to predict and control while eliminating what is human. Jessie Taft supported him in her comments. Mary Chadwick, a British nurse and ally of Jones, castigated Rank, urging listeners not to exchange the Freudian lamp for a new one. The audience applauded. A. A. Brill scorned Rank's use of "individual will" and "human elements." He suggested that Rank had accused Freud of offering psychoanalysis as a substitute for human suffering. "Only an idiot could imagine such a thing. . . . I feel that all the stuff to which Dr. Rank treated us this morning is but an indication of his own present maladjustment." Brill referred to his long acquaintance and respect for Rank as a stalwart analyst who then underwent a conversion. "A deep conversion invariably involves deep emotional upset. My feeling about Dr. Rank is that it is this emotional upheaval that is responsible for his present confusion" [applause]. Dr. Isidor Coriat, the top Boston analyst, said, "Dr. Rank criticizes certain of the Freudian concepts, and yet he substitutes for them a metaphysical concept of the will, whereas analytically we know that the will is nothing but the wish." Franz Alexander spoke of the "interesting new theoretical ideas of Dr. Rank" but claimed they were reformulations of Freud's ideas. He was applauded, as was Rank, who concluded the session: "I take my lamp home from Washington, and leave the old lamps to everybody who wants to stick to them."

That afternoon and evening the APA held its annual meeting. On a motion by Brill, seconded by Harry Stack Sullivan, Rank was stripped of his honorary membership in the APA (Freud and Ferenczi kept theirs). Thereby Rank was disqualified as an analyst in the United States, and his analysands had to be reanalyzed or lose APA certification. That action destroyed much of Rank's referral base, which was thus redirected to American psychiatrists. Helene Deutsch, who took part in four panels in Washington, wrote her husband, Felix, "I hear a lot bad about Rank—he suffered a real calamity at the Congress, and I felt very sorry, for I see fate holding sway here, and Tola's future really worries me."[4]

Although he supported Freud's analysis in *The Incest Theme* (1912), Rank later reinterpreted Oedipus. He came to emphasize creative will and ethical relationship in human development, social evolution, and psychotherapy. He brought up the mother-role in home and society and the pre-Oedipal phase in child development. Rank valued knowledge and insight with a caveat: the need for illusion, what Ibsen called the "life lie." Rank introduced his first book with Shakespeare's "Is it possible he should know what he is and be that he is?" The question sums up fears about psychoanalysis: too much rationality, introspection, even truth, can interfere with creativity and, indeed, life itself. Jocasta's plea to stop the inquiry is a classic example. Even Freud's relentless scientific effort to explain psychological and social functioning and his contempt for religion left room for unscientific ideas like Lamarkian inheritance, telepathy, and numerology. Oedipus Rex is the quintessential self-fulfilling prophecy: belief leads to enactment. Psychoanalysis—part hermeneutic, part science—tends to validate its own presuppositions.

Rank regarded his *Psychology and the Soul* [*Seelenglaube und Psychologie*, 1930] as a definitive critique of Freudian analysis. In the book he challenges the Oedipal interpretation of *Hamlet*, arguing that "playing the fool" is "basically a refusal to perform a duty, a reluctance excused as inability, in the sense of my will-psychology. . . . [The hero] *cannot* do what he *would* not do before. [In that refusal] I see the *son's revolt against the father's right to control his life and soul.*" Rank's own professional revolt—exchanging the patriarchal Oedipus theme for a mother-child focus, came with hypomanic excitement, an ironic echo of playing the fool.

In the preface to *The Interpretation of Dreams* (2nd ed., 1909), Freud described its initial writing as "a portion of my own self-analysis, my reaction to my father's death—that is to say, to the most important event, the most poignant loss, of a man's life." This provoked a response from Rank—who suffered the presence more than the loss of his own father. He painstakingly analyzes Freud's failure to refer to Joseph Breuer, his mentor and colleague until 1896, in any published dream.

> Everyday experience, even in analysis, shows the father's death to be by no means the most important event in every man's life. . . . Why did he believe this of himself and hypothesize it to be universal? . . . Surprisingly, in the confessional that *Interpretation of Dreams* purports to be, Freud's relation to Breuer plays no role, while the banal event of a mature man losing his aged father, whom he had long since outgrown in mind and spirit, becomes all-important. There is no doubt which event in the life of the 40-year-old Freud was more important: his father's death, or his simultaneous break from Breuer, to whom he owed both the key to understanding the neurotic and the basis of his own success, and from whom he was obliged to break, as if under a compulsion, to go his own way. . . . [Psychology itself can be] a projective mechanism that comforts the self by shifting focus away from the person. . . . So we have to choose between the view that his relationship to Breuer played no role in Freud's dreams, many of which date from the period of the separation conflict, and my view that it played so large a role that Freud had to deny it and substitute the more banal relationship with his father.[5]

At a meeting of the Vienna Psychoanalytic Society in 1930, Freud criticized Rank's *Seelenglaube:*

> Rank was a highly gifted person, the ablest and most gifted of all. Then came a second phase in which he turned huckster, with only one motive: contradicting Freud. He had a new interpretation of *Hamlet*. Incest played no part in it. Hamlet is just the son who won't listen to anything his father says and refuses the son's obligation (to avenge the murder). This interpretation is trash. Hamlet's monologue makes no sense then. In his main argument Rank gets on his high horse and looks down on psychoanalysis. He uses relativity and quantum the-

ory to understand causality. What's left is soul and free will. But psychoanalysis cannot be an illusion. The new ideas may bewilder the physicists. Psychology has always suffered when other sciences are applied to it. Leave psychology in peace! Leave it to psychologists![6]

A proposed anthology based on Rank's work, mainly by his Boston colleagues, came to naught, as did Wilbur's translation of *Seelenglaube*. Ives Hendrick, a Boston Freudian, said most Rankians were "untrained women." Rank guessed that this referred to his Philadelphia colleagues Jessie Taft and Virginia Robinson, and two at Columbia, Martha Taylor and Martha Jaeger (not mentioning Caroline Newton):

> I think what gets their goat (the N.Y. analysts, I mean) is that some women whom I analyzed make (at least potentially) good analysts as women, i.e. as having accepted their femininity contrasted to most Freudian female analysts who are compensating in a masculine role (for that statement I have good real reasons). Be that as it may, they will always find fault with me! But to come back to Freud with whom it is different: his late appreciation of women enables him only now to see that they have their own makeup and are not merely "castrated" man.[7]

Rank was in Europe from mid-1930 to March 1932, when he came to the States to teach with Taft and proofread *Modern Education* and *Art and Artist*, both first published in English. Suddenly deeply depressed, he abruptly returned to France in April. He apologized by letter to Taft, saying he had worked out personal problems, had no money but no worries either, and was writing a book on humor.

A serious rift opened between Ferenczi and Freud in 1932. Freud wrote (Oct. 2): "I also knew that you didn't credit me with more insight than a little boy. (Just as Rank did, back then). . . . Each of those who were once near to me and then fell away was able to find more to reproach me with than you, of all people. (No, Rank just as little.) The traumatic effect dissipates in me, I am prepared, and used to it." Ferenczi died on May 22, 1933. That year Eitingon emigrated to Israel and Sachs to Boston.

American psychiatrist Roy Grinker quoted Freud in 1933 as having "nothing but good to say about Rank—his imagination and brilliance—but simply stated 'he was a naughty boy.'"[8] In 1934 Rank teamed up with American psychologist and future neurologist Pearce Bailey to create a summer work-shop in Paris. It was a success, but the sequel in 1935 was canceled because of political chaos in Europe due to Hitler. Rank stayed in New York; his wife emigrated to Boston, where, like Sachs, she was accepted as a lay analyst. (Daughter Helene finished college at Swarthmore and earned her doctor-ate in psychology at Stanford.) In 1936 Otto Rank's books on technique appeared as *Will Therapy* and *Truth and Reality*. He was writing a book in English for the first time: *Beyond Psychology* (1941).

In "Analysis Terminable and Interminable" (1937) Freud likened Rank's brief therapy to a fire brigade that removes an overturned lantern from a burning house instead of putting out the fire. Brief therapy was a "bold and ingenious idea" suited to profit from the haste and affluence of America. "The theory and practice of Rank's experiment are now things of the past—no less than American 'prosperity' itself." In his last work, *Moses and Monothe-ism* (1939), Freud describes a young man who grew up with a worthless father, then developed a sterling character, only to reverse that in the prime of life, "as though he had taken this same father as a model." Freud generalized: "There is always an identification with the father in early childhood. This is afterwards repudiated, and even overcompensated, but in the end establishes itself once more." Sachs, who visited Freud in England, confirmed that the passage referred to his old friend Otto.[9]

In 1939, Rank got a divorce and married his companion of four years, Estelle Buel. She was 35, a trilingual librarian born in Cleveland to Swiss immigrant parents. He applied for U.S. citizenship and they planned to move to California; On September 23, 1939, Freud died—about a year after his move to London. In late October, in New York, Rank contracted a blood-borne infection and was treated with a sulfa drug as a last resort. He died of agranulocytosis, a side-effect of the drug, on October 31.

In a 1940 obituary, Ernest Jones wrote that he opposed Rank's post–World War I "plans of unfairly using England and America for the benefit of German scientific activity." Was he making disputes about journal editing and book translations sound sinister, after Hitler went to war? In the third volume of *Freud* (1957) Jones included a long chapter on Rank, ostensibly to show that Freud tolerated dissent, but he used the story to portray Rank as crippled by "psychosis," and a failure. In the *New York Times*, literary critic Lionel Trilling, who helped abridge Jones's trilogy into one volume, wrote that Ferenczi and Rank "both fell prey to extreme mental illness and died insane." Challenged by Virginia Robinson, Trilling wrote a retraction that could hardly offset the damage done. In a belated cautionary letter to Trilling, Jones cited Rank's "very successful career" in New York, contradicting his own testimony.[10] Jessie Taft's admiring memoir *Otto Rank* (1958) drew a contemptuous review in *Time* magazine which ended, "Otto Rank was 'sick, sick, sick.'"[11] (Taft died in 1960.) There were some less prominent favorable reviews. Several hundred admirers of Rank, including analysts Martin Grotjahn and Esther Menaker, formed the Otto Rank Association in 1966 and published a journal—31 issues—over the next 16 years.

In 1981 one of us wrote to Anna Freud about Otto Rank, and she promptly replied.

20, Maresfield Gardens London NW3 5SK ¶November 6, 1981

Dear Dr. Lieberman,

Thank you for your letter of October 30th.

There are of course many people besides me who knew Otto Rank intimately and could tell you about him. Helene Deutsch in Boston is one of them, though I do not know how intact her memories are by now. All I can tell you is that Otto Rank was an indispensable help to my father for many years, at times as a liaison with the Analytic Society, at times as secretary, provider of books from libraries, etc. In that capacity, of course, he was very often in our home.

At the same time he was also a most valuable, and also quite indispensable, secretary of the Vienna Psychoanalytic Society. His books written at the time, before the birth trauma, were much appreciated and probably of permanent value. There was at that time no sign of a manic depressive illness.

Yours sincerely, Anna Freud

Anna Freud was very protective of her father's ideas and general reputation. That she responded at all to this letter is remarkable. She omits (or forgot) her trials with Rank in 1924, limiting her comment to the time before the controversy. Ambivalent toward Jones, she had criticized a draft of his chapter on Rank in the Freud biography, vol. 3: "too long" and "too unpleasant," she told her brother Ernst, in 1956.[12] Paul Roazen had two cordial interviews with her in 1965 before becoming anathema to most Freudians. Despite this he collaborated with Helene Deutsch, who had some contact with Tola Rank, a lesser light in the Boston Freudian establishment. By the time Roazen interviewed Tola, her memory was fading and she had little to offer. Her postwar exchanges with Anna are sparse and formal. Lieberman visited the Freud house in London in mid-1982; Anna Freud was too ill to meet, and she died on October 6, at 86.

A SCHEMATIC DIFFERENTIATION of Freud and Rank contrasts the two on a continuum of classical and modern; other schools may fit along the continuum in different ways. Major psychodynamic systems or schools of thought that have emerged since the founding of "depth psychology" include the object-relational (Melanie Klein, D. W. Winnicott), interpersonal (Clara Thompson, H. S. Sullivan), existential (Rollo May, Irvin Yalom), client-centered (Carl Rogers), humanistic and transpersonal (A. Maslow), Gestalt (Fritz Perls and Paul Goodman), rational-emotive (Albert Ellis), cognitive-behavioral (Aaron Beck), and dialectical behavior therapy (Marsha Linehan). In general, relational, ego-oriented, and "here-and-now" approaches have gained prominence at the expense of classical psychoanalysis and behaviorism. An early but still exemplary overview is *Schools of Psychoanalytic Thought* by Ruth L. Munroe (1955); besides Freud and Rank she includes Adler, Horney, Fromm, Sullivan, and Jung. The finest appreciation of Rank's thought is *Otto Rank: A Rediscovered Legacy* (1982), by Esther Menaker, who, along with Ernest Becker's Pulizer prize–winning *The Denial of Death* (1973), inspired a revival of interest in Rank in the last 25 years.

Science—objective, general   ≈   Art—subjective, unique

A positivist, Freud wanted to scientifically verify the intuitions of poets, artists, and philosophers. Rank, an existential humanist, embraced philosophy, paradox, and art, celebrating the unique and paradoxical without disparaging science. "For each patient I need a different theory."

The past, memories, childhood   ≈   The present, experience

Freud regarded "here-and-now" dynamics as an echo of the past: transference. Ferenczi and Rank viewed the analytic situation as a place where feeling ferments and emerges in a real relationship not to be dismissed or diluted by interpreting old family ties or assuming biological predestination.

Unconscious: Oedipus ≈ Conscious: Pre-Oedipal, Oedipal, Post-Oedipal

Freud devoted the analytic hour—his invention—to uncover that which is hidden by Oedipal repression; Rank used the relationship to tap emotions and will that the patient cannot integrate or express constructively.

Sexual wishes ≈ Creative will

Freud dismissed the will found in nineteenth-century psychology, making unconscious sexuality and aggression the focus. Including these, Rank made will the key, noting its power for action and inhibition, its ties to creativity, anxiety, and guilt. "Will therapy" is a two-person encounter: both may improvise.

Intellectual insight ≈ Emotional experience

If the unexamined life is not worth living (Freud), the uncreative life is a mixed blessing that examination may not fix (Rank). Neurotics suffer from too much self-analysis, Rank thought, while failing—due to guilt and life fear—to engage life willingly.

Transference, indifference ≈ Actual relationship, intimacy

The Freudian analyst functions as a "blank screen" for transference. For Rank real relationship is the therapeutic force in an ethical and professional context. Existence precedes essence: this experiential theme deemphasizes infantile residues, supporting emotional reality over intellectualized reconstruction.

Biology, body ≈ Psychology, mind

Freud's Oedipus complex anchors individual psychology in biology: incest wish, patricidal hostility, castration fear. Freud ignores the psychology of infanticide and adoption. Oedipus loved his actual, nonbiological parents. Jocasta gives Oedipus a Rankian warning about literal truth. According to Rank, sometimes we cannot live with the truth.

Analysis, research   ≈   Therapy, helping

Freud took the word *analysis* (Greek, "loosen up") from the vocabulary of chemistry. He cared more about research than helping. *Therapy* derives from the Greek and Latin with meanings of serving, care, and healing. Rank preferred the term *psychotherapy* to describe his work, even calling himself a philosopher of helping.

Normality   ≈   Difference

Freud allowed that psychoanalysis would only change neurotic misery to ordinary unhappiness. For Rank, however, the post-Freudian challenge is creating a person—life as an individual art work. By engaging the will, overcoming anxiety and guilt, one puts the loan of life to good use. The neurotic, a failed artist in Rank's view, tries by inhibiting life to deny death, which is repayment of the loan.

Death drive   ≈   Death fear

According to Freud, the patricidal son inhibits himself for fear of paternal punishment (castration fear), which symbolizes death. Rank sees the problem as one of individuation. Can we, unwilling, suffering newborn creatures, attain a level of consciousness that embraces our lives, affirming creative will and human responsibility without paralyzing guilt and fear? This would be psychological rebirth, evolution from creature to creator.[13]

SIGMUND FREUD CHANGED THE WAY WE THINK and feel about ourselves—mind, body, and society. He may not have found the scientific basis for the insights of poets, artists, and philosophers, but he earned his place in twentieth-century popular culture as well as in psychology, medicine, and philosophy. He invented a new form of human interaction, the analytic hour. A mental alchemist, he transformed myth into scientific theory and vice versa. As an archeologist, he liked history and digging things up. As a lover of literature and good storytelling, he made case histories into narrative works of art even while insisting he was a scientist.

Freud took on the mantle of dream-interpreter and created a new human relationship: the psychoanalytic hour, which Otto Rank called the analytic situation. An ardent atheist, Freud provided what some call the "Jewish confessional": a humane, good-humored, yet serious challenge to the religious domination of forgiveness.

Freud grew up in a century that brought scientific and engineering miracles like railroads, photography, anesthesia, x-rays, and sound recording while women struggled with long skirts and doctors plied remedies that were as likely to harm as to help. Otto Rank came of age in 1905, when Albert Einstein published his theory of relativity. Thenceforth time and space, like energy and matter, had to be considered in their dynamic relation, not as separate entities. Air travel and wireless communication made the world smaller. Weapons and wars were more destructive, but world population grew. Rank's signal myth may be the pre-Oedipal Eden, origin of birth and death. Along with consciousness came will, and with will came love, creativity, anxiety, and guilt. Solving riddles to defeat father and win mother were not so heroic compared with becoming a self that learns to bond and separate, balancing individual difference with human similarity, independence with social attachments. The remedy for the trauma of birth is not regressive sexual conquest but creative selfhood, responsible choice, and living with mortality.

Theirs was a remarkable and important mentorship. Although a stickler for loyalty, Freud proved capable of revision and innovation. He opposed requiring a medical degree for psychoanalysts (the Americans defied him). Through the 1960s, most chairmen of psychiatry departments in the United States were Freudian. Becoming a training analyst was a major goal and source of prestige for psychiatrists, like tenure in a university and publishing articles in prestigious journals. Now non-physicians are welcome in psychoanalytic training and practice, while psychiatry (soul-therapy) is dominated by neuroscience and pharmacology.

The efforts of Jones and Brill to purge Rank from the annals of psychoanalysis were effective for half a century. His ideas were kept alive in a few schools of social work and departments of psychology. Often his ideas were adopted without due credit, for political reasons or from ignorance.

One of Rank's unfinished projects was a book on humor. His favorite writer was Mark Twain, his favorite book *Huckleberry Finn*. Rank signed himself "Huck" in letters to Jessie, Anaïs (who briefly became a therapist as well as his lover), and Estelle. In Twain's chapter on freeing Nigger Jim, Huck the pragmatic idealist challenged his mentor, Tom Sawyer, who favored a complex strategy of release based on history and mythology. In the letters of Freud and Rank there is an echo of Tom and Huck struggling to release the enslaved soul. While it is important to understand how the problem came about, and what our forebears would have done, that should not interfere with finding a solution.

Where are the missing letters from Freud to Rank from 1916 to 1921? In view of Freud's eagerness to foil his biographers (he destroyed early letters, and hoped Marie Bonaparte would destroy his letters to Fliess), and Rank's mention of emotionally revealing letters from Freud during the war, we hesitantly speculate: In exchange for a promise not to publicly denounce Rank, Freud took back the wartime letters (and some others). Though disappointed and angry with him, Freud did not express the hostility and contempt toward Rank that he vented on Adler, Jung, Stekel, and others. He asked Brill not to link him to efforts to stifle Rank's career in America. He evidently gave his folders of Rank letters to Ferenczi after Rank left. All the players saved letters and probably expected that they would someday be published. While we hope that more Freud-Rank letters will be found, our expectations are low.

Acknowledgments

For grant support of translation and research materials: Robert Wallerstein, Peter Fonagy, and the International Psychoanalytical Association Research Advisory Board; Neil Elgee and the Ernest Becker Foundation; Michael Ryan, Director, Rare Book and Manuscript Library, and the Rank Fund, Columbia University, New York.

Gregory Richter, Truman State University, translated all the letters from German, expertly and patiently. We salute Ernst Falzeder for his many translations of Freud and writings on psychoanalysis and its historiography. For additional help with translation and interpretation we thank Gretl Cox, David Edminster, Elke Jordan, Kate Loewe, Paul Peucker, and Marion Wolff.

Libraries and archives: The Library of Congress: Margaret McAleer and Leonard Bruno; George Washington University: the late Cynthia Kahn; Countway Library: Scott Podolsky and Michael P. Dello Iacono; Boston Psychoanalytic Society and Institute: Sanford Gifford and Olga Umansky; Boston University, Gotlieb Research Center (Paul Roazen Papers): Adam Dixon; Gleeson Library, University of San Francisco (Anaïs Nin Papers): John Hawk; Princeton University (Caroline Newton Papers): Jens Klenner; The Washington Center for Psychoanalysis; and the late John Gach, for a generation of bibliographic support.

Others who have given valuable help along the way: Ruhama Veltfort; Judith Dupont, Alain de Mijolla, Tom Roberts, Steph Ebdon; Bertram Müller, Klaus Hölzer, Hans-Jürgen Wirth, Martin Chénard. Readers of and/or contributors to parts of the developing manuscript include Louis Breger, Jim Chapman, John Justin David, Zvi Lothane, R. Andrew Paskauskas, Hans Pols, Leonard Rosenbaum, Tommy Schmitz, Robert A. Segal, Michael Schröter, Grey Shepard, Christfried Tögel, and Gerhard Wittenberger. Close to home: Carol Lieberman, Nick Troccoli, and Betsy Hostetler.

Appendix A

Minor Letters

These letters are by F(reud) or R(ank), plus Rank to Ferenczi, cc Eitingon (Apr. 3, 1924). In the following letters, the salutation and closing have been omitted. Paragraph breaks are indicated by ⁋; computer dating numbers have been added.

June 21, 1907 F · The situation with your stipend seems secure. I will need to receive your application soon. The man will depart at the end of next week. 70621

September 22, 1907 F · Please have copies of the enclosed notice made and sent to all members so that the decisions can be returned by October 1. I am very well, and am planning to return in eight days. ⁋Greetings to you and to Dr. Adler, whom you will certainly be seeing [with enclosure of same date]. 70922

November 11, 1907 F · I am in possession of a registered letter addressed to you. 71107

April 4, 1909 F · Dr. Morris Karpas of New York has been warmly recommended by Brill (?) as a supporter 1 x [?]. Address: 26, 1 St., T. 7. He wishes to remain here for several months. He should be admitted as a guest to our Wednesday evening meetings, and indeed should be invited to the next session. A time of 8:30–9:00 should be indicated. ⁋How are things with Gartenlaube? [Karpas (1879–1918) was a guest: *Minutes*, April 7, 1909 (2:175). A founding member of the New York Psychoanalytic Society. Died in France in WWI.] 90404

October 21, 1911 F · On encouragement from Stekel, Dr. Klages of Munich will give a presentation on the "Psychology of Handwriting" next Wednesday at our meeting. Thus we will postpone the discussion of onanism. Please inform all the members of this change in the program sufficiently early. Perhaps you should add "guests welcome after registration." 111021

August 3, 1912 F · Thank you for the news of your travels. We are very well here. There is a bride in the house. I will definitely travel to England on September 10. 120803

August 11, 1912 F · Many thanks for your wishes. We will leave Karlsbad early on the 13th. Next address: Hotel Latemar, Karersee [Carezza, Italy], Tirol. ⏀It is practically certain that we—Ferenczi and I, and perhaps also Brill—will arrive in London on September 10 to meet Jones. I am wondering whether your intensive studies would prevent you from joining us for a stay of eight to ten days in London. I would invite you to be my guest; I await your decision. 120811

August 18, 1912 F · Your answer to my offer may already be on its way, but just to be certain I'll repeat it now. I invite you to make the trip with us and to stay in London beginning September 10, for eight to ten days, as my guest. You may think of this as my thanks for your recent, excellent book. ⏀The only reservation I expressed in my last letter was as to whether you are able to take off this time from studies for your examinations. However, I would not think you'd need to worry about that too much. ⏀Imago no. 3 has arrived safely. Please inform Heller (?) that he should wait for my separate article until it is completed. ⏀Cordial greetings. Awaiting your answer. 120818

January 7, 1913 R · I'm taking the liberty of submitting to you a letter from Riklin, with the request that you be so kind as to inform me (perhaps tomorrow evening!) what is to be done now, and, accordingly, how I should answer. ⏀1. Should we publish the Korrespondenzblatt in the first issue? This seems desirable to me in the interest of clarifying the relationship to the Zentralblatt. 2. Should the member lists that have been submitted thus far also be published in the first issue? This does not seem necessary to me since it would take up space and would take some time, and since the lists from Zurich and America appeared in the Zentralblatt just recently. 3. "Official Organ" will be printed in any case. 4. The fact that the membership fee has been raised 3 marks is unpleasant, but unavoidable under the circumstances. It is, in fact, not higher [than before], and the individual member will feel nothing. 5. It would certainly be simpler if subscription payments were handled by the local groups (just the changes in membership would warrant this), but I think the establishment of this mode of operation without a Congress would be more complicated than the current method of payment; the payment for the organization's account would still have to be sent to Riklin. ⏀Of course I'll come to an agreement with the chairmen of the local groups directly. ⏀The first issue is experiencing a difficult birth; printing is going slowly too. I received the philological report today; the affair has become just a bit more uncertain again, but still looks favorable for us. Forgive me for disturbing you with business details. ⏀P.S. Shouldn't I suggest in my answer to Riklin that under the title Korrespondenzblatt des Internationalen Psychoanalytischen Vereins [newsletter of the International Psychoanalytical Association] he write "edited by Dr. Freud, president of the International Psychoanalytical Association"? I think it would be desirable [for readers] to know who is making the announcement about the Zentralblatt! 130107

January 9, 1913 R · [postcard] This morning, after my letter had already been mailed, I received from Riklin the report from the local group in Zurich subscribing to the Korrespondenzblatt; he also informed me that he is in agreement with the announcement in the first issue. Despite the recent hesitation, I will write him that we will of course include the report from Zurich in the first issue. ◀In his letter today the printer promises to proceed as quickly as possible. 130109

April 12, 1913 R · I am thankfully obliged to you for so kindly sending the footnote to Ferenczi's article. I had to retain the "casuistic collection" for the next issue since I recalled that [we] still need space for the Korrespondenzblatt. I'm [...] sorry to have troubled you about this. Under these circumstances, of course, there would still have been time; please excuse the editorial overzealousness. I did insert Tausk's essay (failures). Meanwhile Tausk has submitted a new contribution [...] dream examples; representations etc.), which would perhaps be appropriate for the casuistic collection. Storfer visited me, and made a very good impression. He is a nice and extremely intelligent person. He will be here for some time, and wishes to take the liberty of visiting you as soon as he is finished with his article. I am also taking the liberty of sending you the first corrections for the Loewenfeld article, the content of which you know. 130412

February 26, 1914 R · [postcard] [...] requests, dear Professor, that you also look over Jones' text, which seems very weak to us in certain spots. Perhaps your contribution could be inserted in the middle, where dreams are discussed. 140226

June 5, 1914 R · I wrote to Abraham, Ferenczi, and Jones—also concerning the questions about the Congress. Perhaps we can discuss their votes, which I asked them for, at the meeting planned for next week. ◀The May issue appeared yesterday. I enclose the contents for the July issue. 140605

June 12, 1914 R · Herr Troedler promised [to publish] your separate contributions within 8 days; the due date at the end of June related to the composition of the entire *Jahrbuch*. (Today nearly all the missing references arrived.) *Interpretation of Dreams* requires urgent action. Herr Troedler, who will go on vacation himself at the end of the month, wants to finish everything by then. Thus the final vacation spurt has also begun with the literature. ◀Today the April issue of *Imago* appeared (the June issue will in about 8 days), as well as Jelgersma. I'll write to Regis and Hesnard about an addendum. P.S. If you have any comments about my references (Dreams and Mythology), please let me know. 140612

July 21, 1914 R · I was surprised Abraham had not reported to you on the happy event announced to you. [...] You also celebrated too early, strictly speaking. Concerning the possible announcement, I've already reached an agreement with Abraham. Yesterday I got the Congress invitation, hopefully sent only to the definite people. Otherwise it would be unclear why this should occur before the Swiss [resignation?] is announced. But it was done skillfully and practically, which was to be expected from Abraham, and which has not been noted by the Zurich members through the years. ◀Abraham's various circulars have been sent to Ferenczi, who, however, is not keeping in touch. Nor is Sachs. In connection with the [...] report, I suggested to Reik himself that one should proceed with moderation. [...] Otherwise very well and busy. It's a pity that he cannot avoid mistakes. ◀Since the articles for the *Zeitschrift* can't appear until the November issue, there is no great hurry in submitting them. Nor would I like to take charge of them in Seis [Siusi, Italy], since this seems too uncertain. If you wish to be rid of the finished manuscripts, please send them to my address in Vienna, marked "do not forward." I cannot yet provide any summer addresses, so until [...] please use the Vienna address, where my [...] and Sachs will take care of the forwarding. I will be traveling a lot, and do not know where I will settle down (in Dalmatia, if the weather permits). ◀Many thanks for your kind offer. It would of course be nice to receive funds before my departure, but I think you can wait until Deuticke's delivery. I was there yesterday to pay the postage for the five copies (K 4.55), and Herr Troedler told me that the copies arrived from the printer on Saturday (until now there were none there). I think he was just waiting for the arrival of these copies, and that you will receive the money this week. As for myself, if nothing else comes up, I'll plan to travel to the Dolomites on Tuesday or Wednesday. ◀The *Jahrbuch* has now been completely printed at the printer, and the finished product is expected next week. Herr Troedler promised that you'll get a copy before you leave Karlsbad. ◀Best regards to your wife and cordial thanks for your thoughtfulness and kindness. . . . R 140721

July 22, 1914 R · [postcard] ◀Many thanks for your letter and the materials you sent— which I accepted not because of the content, but because of the author. I'll urge Regis and Hesnard to attend. Perhaps it will be possible to speak with one of them at the Congress. ◀Today I heard from Abraham that thus far there has been no official resignation. Heller just got payment for this year's Zurich subscriptions! From July 26 to Aug. 1, Abraham's address will be Hotel Duenenhaus, Brunshaupten, Mecklenburg. Today I received a "photographic" postcard from Herr Oliver from Millstadt. Today I'll bring your sister-in-law some reading material, and will then depart. 140722

July 23, 1914 R · This is to acknowledge thankfully the receipt of the technical article. I added the heading "Further Suggestions on Psychoanalytic Technique" and labeled it No. II since the last two articles published under that main heading concerned one (continued) topic ("On the Introduction of the Treatment"). The portions marked "small" should probably be printed in (smaller) Borgis-font; that's what I've indicated. 140723

July 24, 1914 R · Herr Heller, who likes the book by Regis and Hesnard except for a few places, would like to have it translated into German and possibly edited (by me); he believes that he'd have success with it. Since I haven't seen it, and can make no decision, I'll permit myself to ask you whether you'd be favorably disposed to such a plan, and what your opinion might be. Perhaps I can tell Heller before I depart whether he should come to an agreement with Alcan and the authors. ◖Please excuse the inquiry and the disturbance. . . . R 140724

August 13, 1914 R · After receiving your letter I wrote to you yesterday in Karlsbad but I just learned from Sachs that you are already in Vienna. On the trip back from the Tirol I stayed here for a while, but I will be at home again within the next few days and hope to find you well rested. 140813

July 23, 1915 R · I'm sorry I must disturb you with something not entirely pleasant. Dr. Steiner asked me yesterday whether I knew anything officially about an increase in the subscription rate for the Zeitschrift to be charged to the members of the Association, who until now had received the publication (?) at a discount of 6 marks (for 12 marks rather than 18 marks). Heller admonished our Association quite urgently to pay the subscription fees, and simultaneously announced a reduction of 3 marks in the discount (referring to a previous letter that Dr. Steiner has, however, not received), so that now 15 marks is to be paid per member. Now I remember from our debates with Heller, among others from a discussion in his shop, that Heller mentioned this increase, but I can recall no official decision, nor even an official proposal on his part, and I've informed Steiner, who in the meantime left Heller's letter unanswered. Now I would like to ask whether you perhaps know anything about such an agreement or suggestions, and how we should act with respect to this possible reduction. Even Heller should not be treated discourteously now. ◖Issue No. 3 is still being awaited. I've managed to put together Issue No. 4 more or less. Lots of [...] from it: Tausk has made all the desired changes—except for the last footnote (small animals), where he did delete the word Angsttiere [anxiety animals, cowards] but left everything else, and extended the comments on the folktales and on the impotence (castration) meaning of the legends. I've pointed out to him that you might take exception to that passage in the second Carr. [...] since you placed so much emphasis on it specifically, and he is prepared for that. ◖You've presumably heard about Sachs' temporary return. With me things are the same as before. Hopefully you are feeling well. Do you happen to know the addresses of Spielrein and Landauer? 150723

June 25, 1916 R · I have received no news from you or from Sachs for a long time, and I'm concerned that something may not be in order. What news do you have from your family, and what are the details with Sachs' military duty. Since I've also seen nothing of the Zeitschrift or of your proof-corrections, I suspect that Heller is again acting up. From my brother, who was in Volhynia [Poland], I have heard nothing since Lemberg. Otherwise nothing very pleasant. Once again my eye problem is bothering me; at least I definitely know now that is "only" a nervous condition. Also, I'm always depressed; I'm just vegetating on. Now I'm participating (?) in various types of sport, for which I have ample opportunity here. ◖Otherwise, everything here is as before. 160625

August 13, 1916 R · My trip is nearly certain now. It's also possible I'll go to Teschen near the start of my trip, about August 22. The visit with Prochaska is already unnecessary since I got the first issue. Ferenczi, whom I'd like to visit in Budapest, is not answering my letters. What is going on with him? I spoke with Sachs by telephone the day before yesterday. He said only that you were going to Bad Aussee. Hitschmann wrote that he had an operation. What was it? I was very glad to hear of the surprise visits you got. Won't any of your sons be traveling through Krakow? I could be called from the train station, and would be very glad. My comments about Munich were not meant in that way. I merely thought you might possibly be there—quite independently of the congress. But perhaps you'll delegate me officially to report for the *Zeitschrift!* Is Abraham still in Allenstein? I'd like to come to an agreement with him. If you're in Vienna at the end of September, I hope to see you while I am traveling through, in any case. You can certainly stop writing to me. 160813

August 22, 1916 R · I had the pleasure of showing your son Oliver the beautiful sites of Krakow for two days; he was quite impressed—indeed enthralled. It's possible that we will meet again soon in Teschen if I stay there. Anyway, we discussed the possibility. However, I can't leave until September 4, when I'll go to Budapest; Ferenczi expects me. Then I'll travel on, and on the return trip be in Vienna September 23–25, where I hope to meet you. Please let me know your plans for the rest of summer, and the addresses. My colleague has been back since yesterday, and my work load has been reduced so that I can prepare a bit for the trip. 160822

February 5, 1917 R · Most sincere thanks for the letter and greetings you conveyed to me through my brother. Recently Erich Ickes was here and we spent a few pleasant hours with your son and Frau Sokolnicka. Ickes and I strongly warned Herr H., and in the future I will continue to keep an eye on the situation. You need not be concerned at all. He probably won't come to Vienna before the second half of February, but in any case, advise him by telegram of Ernst's arrival. Then things will once again be lively at your home. Please give everyone my best greetings. As for me, nothing new to report. The crisis is not yet surmounted. If he should endure it, good for him! I got galley proofs of the publications regularly, and am glad to hear that the movement is becoming somewhat active. Again, many thanks for your truly fatherly concern and your kind words, which are always a great comfort to me. 170205

February 17, 1917 R · I already feel well enough, and sufficiently removed from my winter sleep, to think about an active involvement. I'll probably be going to Romania after all, and in this connection, I'll stop in Vienna in any case. This should occur at the beginning of March. It's possible that Oli will already be there at that time, though as far as I know his departure is not yet firm. Are your two sons still in Vienna? I got the proofs from Heller quite regularly—although nothing of the Lectures for some time. I've nearly broken off all relations with Heller since I can't abide his extremely disgusting behavior. There's nothing new here. The little that there is to report you've surely learned from Ickes already. 170217

February 27, 1917 R · Many thanks for your letter. I should be in Vienna the beginning of next week, and am looking forward to breathing some analytic air again. Your
son is already planning to depart at the end of this week. I heard from him that your
youngest daughter was not well. Hopefully that was only temporary. I am anxious
to make the acquaintance of your expected grandchild, and am also hoping to meet
Ferenczi. Your comment about everyday life is really appropriate, as I'd really like to
try hard to get back into my work now. Please prepare something for me. I already
read the short book by Popper several months ago and wanted to point out to you the
nice comments on dreams, but then I lost the inclination. Prinz and Stekel have both
published new books, which I haven't read. I also saw the announcement for a critical
work by Schultz (published by Karger). ❡P.S. Heller wrote a very friendly letter in a
humane tone. My promotion to lieutenant is already underway. 170227

March 16, 1917 R · Ensign Dr. Rank, Krakow Fortress [postcard] I'd be much obliged
if you could send offprints of your work on the introduction of the virginity tabu and
on the pleasure and reality principle; I'd like to examine these two works in closer
detail and do not find them in my library. Hopefully you still have copies. Many
thanks in advance. This evening I'm traveling to Warsaw for a few days. 170316

March 26, 1917 R · Since, as I saw in Vienna, you need the typewriter more than I
do here, I'll take advantage of Dr. Praeger's temporary presence to send it to you in
Vienna. He'll bring it from the station to his home (Neulinggasse 34, Vienna III),
and I'll ask Sachs, who is of course in contact with Praeger, to get it to you so you'll
have no difficulties. The attachments that could not be packed in boxes you'll get with
this letter. Please let me know where you discuss the re-experiencing of the individual
situation in a state of mourning as a means of dealing with the same. 170326

May 3, 1917 R · Many thanks for the package. I must comment, though, that the cigars
were intended as one of those tokens of affection from the battlefield to the hinter-
land which have now become so popular. I hope to be able to repeat the gift soon
with better success. There's nothing new here. As for myself, I am slowly recovering
from some really hard blows, which, however, seem to have appeared naturally in the
course of things, and whose effects will hopefully still be integrated and dissolved
somewhere in general and other experience. I hope gradually to be able to take up the
work I'd begun. The Lectures, typeset so nicely, still haven't been printed. Otherwise,
things go well with the journals. How are your sons? I received word from Ferenczi
today. I will send him Stekel's book. 170503

May 31, 1917 R · Yesterday Dr. Praeger from Vienna was here and offered me a position as editor in a large publishing consortium he wishes to found soon in Vienna with
an entrepreneur from Berlin (whom I know well). Although I know both entrepre-
neurs well, and consider them my friends to a certain extent, and although they assure
me of extensive consideration of my personal goals and individual interests, I have not
yet accepted since I lack the actual inclination to do so. In any case, the affair is not
currently relevant for me, and if I use the enforced period of consideration until the

end of the war to decide, I will probably still have lots of time to think about it. The question as to whether the position will be held for me only if I commit myself firmly now was not discussed as Praeger knows that I would never do that. In any case, it is a chance, but one which I would grasp only if nothing else presented itself to me. It is still very uncertain how Heller would react to it, and I was already tired of the friction between our two publishers in Vienna as it is. ❡There is nothing new here. I will probably go to Karlsbad in July. And what will you do? What do you hear from Ernst, who of course must be very worn out again now? I have heard nothing from Ferenczi. Poor Sachs must really be slaving away now. For a while, Heller was bombarding me with charming notes in connection with his concert management activities—until he noticed that I have no interest. Now he is presumably displeased with me. 170531

July 20, 1917 R · I'm glad to hear that you found everything to your liking and that the visit as well as the participation of our friends made the stay pleasant for you. I wrote to you at the beginning of the month, but don't know if you got the letter. I wouldn't want you to think I was silent for such a long time. In any case, I have much to do since the principal worker here is on leave, but in a few days this torment will be at an end, though without bringing me anything better for the time being since at the moment my situation here has become extremely critical: not only my leave and the planned trip to Stockholm, but also my remaining here have become subject to doubt. Therefore, given this situation, I must decline the execution of your marvelous plan for the time being, for decisions won't be made here until around the beginning of the month. Please convey this to our friends, along with my most cordial greetings, and my sincere regret that I cannot come at the moment. I will write to you as soon as I know something more definite in one direction or the other. ❡P.S. The books must have arrived by now? 170720

July 30, 1917 R · I thankfully acknowledge your card, which I got yesterday, and I can tell you that my situation has come out well. It's true that a new difficulty has suddenly arisen again which does not concern just me alone, and which can only be resolved or intensified in the near future. Everything was already prepared for my departure this evening, and I wanted to surprise you in Csorba. But since my supervisor urgently needs to travel to Vienna today, the nice intention has been called off for the time being. Please convey this to our friends, along with my cordial greetings, and let me know how long Sachs and Ferenczi will be staying. Perhaps I'll be able to make a little hop over there at the end of the week if everything else goes well. My summer leave, too, is still uncertain. Otherwise I have nothing else to report. 170730

August 17, 1917 R · After a perfect voyage, which worthily followed after all the others—we slept stretched out until Teschen and none of us was disturbed by our bulky rucksacks—I arrived yesterday at midnight. Praeger, too, whom I left in Oderberg, also presumably arrived smoothly. Here the situation is significantly better, if still unclear. 170817

September 9, 1917 R · I arrived here with a very unpleasant catarrh which is still not better today and which, understandably, has already colored my impressions so far. But despite my diet and my lack of appetite I have noticed this much: the food here, especially in my pension, which was recommended to me by our correspondent here, is superb (better than in Csorba), although the location of the building is not the best. It's also dirt cheap. The village is situated amidst the most beautiful forests. Good air, thus everything one could wish for. In the long run, however, somewhat dull, especially if one cannot really work yet as one's head is awfully muddled from deep down. I hope soon to be able to report more, and that things will be better. 170909

September 15, 1917 R · Many thanks for the offprints by Levy, so kindly provided me by Sachs, which I shall return to you after use. My digestion is still not entirely in order, but I'm ignoring that as much as I can, and feel well in other respects. The air and food are excellent, and there are many beautiful forests. The work goes well, and faster than expected, although it takes quite an effort on my part. But perhaps that is just what was necessary. I hope to complete today, at least provisionally, the first and most difficult section. Whether I will spend the end of my leave in Hungary or in Vienna depends on how I will decide; I'm strongly inclined toward Vienna. From Krakow I have thus far received neither news nor a newspaper. 170915

September 23, 1917 R · Since in connection with Ferenczi's mixup of the letters I until today received no news from you, and since the local post office has proved not especially reliable, I'm afraid that one of your letters could have been lost—all the more since I have received absolutely nothing from you. Meanwhile Ferenczi telegraphed me that he is planning to come to Budapest, but I had to telegraph that I did not understand his telegram since I'd received no letter from him. Next week (planned for Thursday) I should be in Vienna, and will bring *The Artist* and *Mythology* in nearly complete form. I had to work quite a bit, but I also worked on my recuperation. I feel better than I have for a long time, and have gained weight. Hopefully I'll be able to tell you everything else soon in person. 170923

October 6, 1917 R · As you already know, after a three-day stay in Budapest, which was very enjoyable and also interesting, I traveled to Tatralomnicz for two days, where, thanks to the hotel secretary and your servant from Csorba, I received a room and peacetime board despite the fact that the season was almost over. I spent two gloriously beautiful days there, and thus ended my leave in as worthy a manner as would have been possible in Pest, where (for Praeger) I spent a bit too much time with writers who are considered the dregs of humanity in Budapest. Ferenczi was very kind, as usual, and is in good shape. He feels well and fit for work. He is quite busy, but hopes to get back to his literary work. ◀ Here everything is as before: the good old routine. I have not yet seen Olli. Dr. Herzfeld appeared on September 19. 171006

October 21, 1917 R · Perhaps the enclosed clipping will interest you. In a German newspaper I noticed that on October 19th Marcinowski spoke before the Sexological

Society on character and eroticism. Perhaps someone should write to him about his lecture? Nothing new with me, except that at the moment the chronic gastric catarrh has been supplanted by bronchial influenza. Heller sent a contract for the *The Artist*, 2nd ed.—the book is already being printed. However, I've not received galleys. Meanwhile I wrote the last chapter of *Mythology*, but it is something of a failure, though it could have turned out very nicely. Under these circumstances I dare not take up my work on Homer. ◀Do you have any news from your eldest son? Something should certainly be going on there again! What is Ernst doing? Olli is looking forward to his departure, though things are going very well for him here. 171021

November 19, 1917 R · Today I got from you a letter intended for Frau Sokolnicka, which I forwarded. I have good news from Oli. How are the other warriors in your family getting along? As for the news here, I will tell you in Vienna in the beginning of December. While writing down a few thoughts about the Helen myth I hit upon the idea that sole possession of the woman, so carefully observed by civilized peoples, could be a reaction to the common possession (or common disregard) which arises with totem organization. What are your thoughts on this? And doesn't this relate somehow to your tabu of virginity? 171119

December 1, 1917 R · Unfortunately I cannot come to Vienna now as planned since my colleague was suddenly sent elsewhere and there is no one else here to fill in for me. This is all the more unpleasant since the situation is threatening to become critical. I'll write today to Sachs and Heller about the literary materials I wanted to obtain in Vienna. I will try to send Olli's luggage, which I had planned to bring along. 171201

December 9, 1917 R · Today I learned from Sachs that you presented on Wednesday. I regret all the more that my trip, which was so secure that I had the official order in my pocket, came to naught. In many respects it was necessary since, once again, I am not well. Through a man I have sent Oli's luggage to my mother, who will notify you by phone. Hopefully everything will arrive in good order. I have kept a brown blanket here. Is Ernst in Vienna again? What do you hear from Martin? The new Sachs gives me of Heller is anything but encouraging. But then, what is encouraging? 171209

January 9, 1918 R · My promotion to lieutenant was successful—unofficial news! Many thanks for your kind package, which I got just as I was starting to catch up on my correspondence by writing you a few lines. Not until today have I come into balance a bit, within and without, both in my work and in my new lodgings. The work here seems quite manageable, and thus far things are going quite well, as had been my intention. I am also saving time for myself, for recuperation and for own work, which, in any case, I have not yet managed to approach. Meanwhile the first galleys of *The Artist* have arrived—after my intervention with Heller. Sachs, who is very satisfied with the introduction, kindly will bring you the galleys and I'd ask you to supply your comments in any direction since I'll wait to send back the proofs until I hear from you. In the newspaper Tuesday, Jan. 8 a supplement vividly reminds me of the poet you spoke about recently. Perhaps your daughter will be interested in the enclosed clipping. 180109

January 21,1918 R · Many thanks for the comments and corrections, which I thankfully used in order to bring a bit of light into the chaos. At any rate I am glad to have that behind me, but perhaps I will write some references to recuperate. Incidentally, a few galleys are missing from the middle; they seem to have gone astray. ¶Otherwise I'm doing quite well. The work is mechanized and narrowly delimited. The weather, especially, is now bright, sunny and warm, which is extremely good for me. I feel better than I have for a long time. Hopefully this will remain so. My promotion is still being awaited: perhaps on February 1. ¶What is the news from your warriors, and especially from Martin? ¶Is there anything new in psychoanalysis? What is going on in the Association? Tausk? ¶I hope to hear from you soon—also about your total impression of *The Artist* at this point. ¶With best regards and cordial greetings. 180121

June 27, 1918 R · *The Artist* has finally arrived, and I'm taking the liberty of sending you a copy with this mailing. I have already written to Heller that he should begin work on *Mythology*, but I don't think it will be of any use since you've written to me of the difficulties he's causing you. ¶The day before yesterday my brother was here, and we decided to bring my mother, who is convalescing from pyelitis, here for a few weeks, where she will have easy access to the foodstuffs necessary in her condition (milk and eggs). ¶Hopefully your trip to Budapest will not be adversely affected by the highly discouraging events in Budapest, which I know of through my military position, but which I cannot evaluate reliably. It would be a pity if your fine summer plans were affected. 180627

July 18, 1918 R · Your kind letter, from which I learned that you're feeling comfortable in Budapest, crossed with mine. In the meantime I have taken the liberty of sending you the latest in dream literature. I have not read the book, but Lauer certainly doesn't have a bad name, and has recently stepped forward on the side of psychoanalysis several times. My modest contributions to the new edition of *ID* aren't even worth mentioning. If you would be so good as to send me the proof corrections when convenient, that will be sufficient. ¶I enclose proofs of the Congress invitations I'm having printed here. The only problem is the addresses: I don't have the list here, and Sachs only gave me the changes. Crucially, I can't find Reutersheim's address in the journals; I need to speak to him specifically. ¶Due to Engel's absence I am really busy, and a bit overworked since I have to deal with thousands of affairs. I'm hoping to travel by car to Zakopane on Sunday; I need to take a break for a day. ¶My mother is feeling very well here and goes with open mouth and eyes—and open wallet—to the markets, where really everything is still available. We are awaiting my letter any day; then I will also discuss my chances and a possible greater fall offensive. ¶Recently I heard from Hitschmann and Jekels. I'm usually a bit removed from everything recently. I discussed the second chapter of Homer with Sachs in Vienna and benefitted in various ways from the discussion. I have now handed it over for revisions to the young woman who does our typing. ❦I hope to hear from you soon. Greetings to you and your daughter. ❦P.S. The enclosed notice will certainly interest you. 180718

July 19, 1918 R · Today I've finally found the time to ask how you are, and how Budapest suits you and Miss Anna. ❦Before my trip to Vienna I had a light case of the Spanish catarrh, and after returning I contracted a heavier case, with intestinal complications. Today is the first day I feel somewhat better. Also, Engel is on leave for four weeks, and yesterday I composed the entire newspaper from my bed, which happened to work out since I'm staying with Mama in Engel's apartment, where there is a telephone. ❦In Vienna I was very glad to see Sachs just before he left on his vacation. I needed to finish discussing things with him, which in this case meant listening to him. Judging from his comments, there seems to be hope, although he does not conceal the difficulties. For me, the arrangement was really lucky, and the position. As for me, there are no difficulties, i.e. with my transfer to Vienna, which, as you may still recall, I had planned earlier. Of course that all needs to be discussed, and I hope to have time for that in the summer so that later there will be a degree of clarity at the Congress, which I consider another brilliant idea on the part of Sachs. In a few days my brother will come here; he is also attempting to move to Vienna. ❦Heller, fortunately, was not in Vienna, and otherwise I had no time to accomplish anything else in just one day. ❦What do you hear from your family, scattered as it is through the world? Hopefully good and encouraging things from everywhere. ❦Best wishes for the summer. 180719

August 6, 1918 R · I am very worried about the absence of any news from you, since I have received no answer in response to two letters and a book I sent you in Budapest. I can only suppose that I wrote Dr. Freund's address incorrectly. This would be a pity especially because of the dream book, which was certainly not uninteresting. ❦Recently I received a letter from Ferenczi. He wrote that he will be going with you to Csorbato, and he sent me a Budapest Congress invitation, which crossed with the Vienna Congress invitation I've had printed here, and which I'm enclosing. Sachs also wrote that after a very nice stay in Rothenburg he is traveling to the Tatra, where he says I am also awaited. As I wrote you, I am really very busy now, since everyone is on leave here. At most, I could come to Csorba on a Saturday. My leave, which falls in September, I can spend only where there is an available officer's vacancy. Because of the scheduled time of year, and given the weather today and my Spanish bronchial catarrh, I would consider the South. Yesterday I received a letter from Vienna, where I am pursuing this; it opens up possibilities for Abbazia. From there I would come to Wroclaw. ❦Did you complete *ID* in Budapest, and were you satisfied with your stay there? Now that it is August, when the weather is usually constant, you will hopefully have some beautiful days in glorious Csorba. 180806

August 10, 1918 R · I'm very glad finally to hear from you, as I had received no letter from you since July 17. I'll have to assume that one letter was lost, since in today's letter you also express the hope that I already have your answer, which unfortunately is not the case. On the other hand, as the first sign of life in nearly three weeks, yesterday I already received your monthly missive, which you even had the kindness to increase. ◀It was to be expected that you would be very comfortable in Csorba. The weather, unfortunately, is miserable everywhere, but on the other hand, that's very good for the mushrooms, whose quantity at the local markets continues to amaze me. I always think of the lucky hunters and finders, whom I envy more than the eaters— which certainly means a lot. My mother feels very well here and is recovering marvelously; I'm very glad I had her come here. Your circle of companions in Csorbato is certainly ideal, especially given Ernst's presence and that of the spring guests who have become dear friends. If I possibly can, I'll come next (Saturday) Sunday. ◀Congratulations on *ID!* It's good to have such works behind one. ◀Oli already informed me of his promotion himself. ◀I am still colossally overloaded with work and can think of nothing but my military assignment, since I alone am responsible for everything. But in two weeks things will improve. ◀Good holidays to you and your family, and to our friends! Cordial thanks. ◀P.S. Sachs informs me that you will send me a letter from Pfister. 180810

August 19,1918 R · Today I arrived after a good trip, during which I missed my connection in Oderberg and therefore was not here until 10:00, having had not a bite to eat the whole way (Hungary?). The trip down here, which I completed before the rain, lasted 45 minutes, and involved colossal abbreviations which took me through swamps—but the train was equally late. ◀I hope you are once again completely well and enjoying better weather than we are; upon my arrival I was greeted by one of the storms that are so popular here. ◀I recall yesterday with joy, pride, and thanks; the day constitutes a milestone not only in the history of the psychoanalytic movement, but also in my life, and inwardly I'm hoping you'll excuse all my negative comments, of which I'm now thoroughly ashamed. ◀Please give my greetings to your dear ones and to our friends, all of whom I thank for the beautiful day, which I shall never forget. ◀P.S. Yesterday in Oderberg, while waiting for the next train, I worked through all the addenda to *ID,* and on both of my essays. 180819

August 25, 1918 R · While traveling through Vienna yesterday, after making a few corrections to my appendix, I gave The Interpretation of Dreams to Deuticke, who initially thought I was coming with a new volume written by me, and began to complain, but then was twice as glad and kind when I drew The Interpretation of Dreams from its cover. Once again, he wants to have the book printed by Prochaska. ◀Heller is expected back from Switzerland any day, where, as Sachs has of course already informed you, he wants to set up a press (competition); perhaps I'll be able to speak with him tomorrow. ◀Praeger has great plans: he wants to combine his German-Austrian theater press (Der Friede), a large daily newspaper, and (!) the psychoanalytic press into a large concern with shared printing facilities. Lots of plans for the future, but so far just complaining. ◀Here we've had tropical heat for two days. I'll be glad to get away. ◀With Sachs we've done everything that still needed to be done for the

Congress. We've sent all the announcements and have written to the boards of the local groups. ⫸Heller is behaving as usual: for Imago, which has been fully printed (he's missing a few bound sheets), there is no paper for the cover, and Sachs has heard nothing about the printing of the journal. My manuscript on *Mythology*, whose last chapter, "Myth and Folktale," I wanted to use as a Congress presentation, simply could not be located at Heller's despite the most intensive searching (also by his very nice and charming wife). My only hope rests on Heller's knowing for himself where he put it! ⫸I cannot give you my next address yet. If you wish to write, please write to Vienna, from where it will be forwarded. I will write as soon as I know more. 180825

August 29, 1918 R · Since our encounter in Csorba so much has changed that I can only write about it briefly, and must save the rest for a meeting in person. Upon my departure from Krakow my relation to Engel deteriorated so much that it is nearly impossible for me to return to Krakow, which of course will—and must—speed along the project we have in mind. On the other hand—and this will be of interest to Ernst—I've had bad luck here: my immediate acceptance at the Officers' Sanatorium will not be possible. Rather, I'll need to make another application from here and await the decision here. The freedom of movement thus gained, and which I did not have at the hospital, I'll use for a trip to Budapest in order to speak with Dr. Freund, to whom I'll also write today concerning my chances and intentions, as well as to inform him of a new idea that I hope has a chance of coming to fruition. The bad luck with the officer's vacancy is perhaps good for something: perhaps after my leave I will not have to return to Krakow, which I would like to avoid. Perhaps after the Congress I can remain here for a few weeks and await my further transfer. ⫸Here it's beautiful, just as warm as I like it, and very peaceful. I'm preparing "Myth and Folktale" as a Congress presentation, and have also brought along the second chapter of Homer to revise it. ⫸As soon as I know more about Budapest, I'll write to you immediately, perhaps from there. Please let Dr. Freund know of any change in your address. 180829

September 5, 1918 R · [to SF in Tatranska Lomnica, Slovakia] ⫸Given the changed conditions and a kind invitation from Dr. von Freund I'm traveling to Budapest on the 9th of this month to discuss things further with Dr. Freund, since, if possible, I would prefer not to return to Krakow and would like to know something halfway certain before the Congress. Before the trip to Wroclaw I may still be in Vienna, where I could perhaps meet with you, since you also need to go to Vienna before you travel to Wroclaw? 180905

October 9, 1918 R · Due to the faulty postal services, the first news from Budapest did not arrive until today, but the news was all the more encouraging, and I'm hurrying to inform you, although I must assume that you have already heard more from Dr. Levy, who is now in Vienna, than I know myself. ⫸Today I received a contract for employment with Pester Journal, which has engaged me under favorable conditions as its representative in Vienna. Dr. Freund also informed me that in Vienna today his brother-in-law Levy submitted my application for release in connection with the publication of the discussion of war neuroses. Now the application for release will probably be handled from the Pester Journal, and also, I hear, the application for transfer to Budapest. But so as to be independent of all the conceivable possibilities, I'm attempting to get a leave of several weeks starting at the end of the month, when Engel will return. During the leave it will hopefully be possible to accomplish everything—to prepare and accomplish a lot in connection with the work ahead. In any case, I hope to be in Vienna at the end of the month unless something special and unforeseen should arise. Even fewer difficulties will stand in the way of my departure as I don't think the German newspaper can carry on much longer here. ◀Concerning *Psychopathology of Everyday Life*, about the new edition of which Dr. Freund asked me today, my suggestion and wish is the following: the new press should of course definitely take it on. It will certainly be an incentive to have everything set up before the appearance of this volume so that with this first publication we'll be successful in the publishing business as well. ◀I'm looking forward to getting away from here finally and to being able to devote myself to the work I ought to be doing. I also believe that after some time to collect myself, which I will still need, I'll find my old work energy. I'm looking forward to the future, which, though perhaps not good, will certainly be pleasant for us. 180909

October 26, 1918 R · I wasn't able to answer your kind letter until today, but now I know something halfway certain—which is not easy recently. ◀Sachs wrote me that he will depart as soon as possible, and since I would certainly like to see him and speak with him before then, I will come to Vienna as soon as I can—specifically in the middle of next week, for three or four days. Then we will be able to discuss everything, since, as I hear, Dr. Freund is also planning to be in Vienna at that time. ◀Please give my regards to your family, all of whom I hope are quite well again. Please especially tell Frau Freud that I have by no means forgotten the furs, but that, given the constant decline in the price of all furs, I thought it would be better to wait a while. However, I will try to bring a selection to Vienna if possible. ◀Many thanks for the two enclosures. I'm familiar with the book on Homer, and the Lichtenberg quotation—one of the most familiar—I know by heart. 181026

October 16, 1920 R · Unfortunately I can only send today, for your signature, the Rundbrief composed yesterday; this will delay distribution a bit. Perhaps you'll be kindly deliver them to the post office. ◀I hope the little analytic joke I took the liberty of making about Jones at the end will not displease you too much. ◀Please give the courier, who comes almost every day (with galleys), the Putnam ones sent to you yesterday at your daughter's request. ◀Otherwise, there's nothing special to report. ◀With cordial greetings. 201016

August 1, 1921 R · Yesterday I received your two express letters. Many thanks! The circular is being sent out today according to schedule. I discussed it yesterday with Ferenczi. I enclose a copy; please return it when convenient. ◀Ferenczi's thorough examination by Dr. Deutsch revealed that the kidney problem, which Ferenczi supposedly had known about for many years, is indeed to be taken more seriously than before; in any case, he will have to adjust his lifestyle accordingly—which he had previously completely failed to do. The other symptoms, especially the breathing difficulties at night, which he has emphasized the most, turned out to be only minor and/or certainly associated with neurotic phenomena. I'll give you more information in person since this would be too complicated in writing. What Dr. Deutsch did not tell him, largely because it is his own personal opinion, is that he believes Ferenczi will end up with an atrophied kidney. ◀Your letter of the 28th just arrived with Jones letter enclosed. I think that in his suggestions for the new edition of your Lesser Writings one could yield to him on certain points; to the extent that you find it possible in terms of content, larger volumes could be produced (e.g. the case histories—not, of course, the first technical articles—together with the later ones; furthermore, in my opinion there is no reason not to combine metapsychology and applied psychology in one volume). ◀If you would be so kind as to send and/or return the manuscripts to me, at your convenience, that would be the simplest thing since I have other manuscripts here. ◀We will still need to discuss the Verlag in detail. I'm worried not only about money, but also about 1. finding space and personnel, which requires time and effort, and 2. the new organizational work, which will have to be done again. Also the question as to whether we should carry out production in Germany, and how we must somehow decide about this. But let us leave all that for the fall. ◀We cordially return your kind greetings—Helene almost personally—and hope everything will continue to go well for you. 210801

August 18, 1921 R · I enclose two circulars; the one from Berlin is very current, but its mainly the one from London that will be of great interest to you. ◀I also enclose a message from Pargot obviating the need for us to respond to his letter. ◀Today Harz was traveling through Vienna; I spoke with him and learned that he can only let me have the office for a short time (about two or three more months). However, he said that he would clear out some storage space for us (for book storage) and that he would investigate the availability of a suitable office. He mentioned one in Berlin (Kurfuerstenstrasse): 4 rooms, including furnishings, for 20,000 a month—which would be very cheap. I hope to learn more soon, and to make a decision about this during my trip abroad. From this perspective, the message from Harz, which of course was not unexpected, isn't really so unpleasant since it forces us to take measures immediately. ◀Since the Verlag is now at long last officially registered, by the way, it is quite appropriate that a new era is beginning. In connection with this, we'll also need to discuss who will replace poor [...], who is of course working in the Verlag as a partner; I think there is little doubt that Eitingon should be chosen. ◀Today I had to make use of your kind offer: I asked your son, Dr. Martin, for 100 francs as we have some large bills and insufficient cash; I hope this meets with your approval. ◀We're eager to learn something of your stay in the Tirol; we hope the weather has improved again, as it has here, where it's almost always hot. 210818

September 8, 1921 R · Many thanks for your comforting lines of August 31, which I will certainly take to heart. ⟨So far, of course, I have found no solution to the difficulties, nor, given the current need for haste, do I know whether anything more than a temporary remedy would be possible; even that would be difficult enough. I am thinking of handing over our local deliveries to someone in Vienna working on commission, but then the problem of office space, a pressing and difficult one, will still remain to be solved. For the last two weeks, of course, I have done nothing but look; I've found several possibilities, but cannot as yet say anything definite. I would like to get away from Harz as soon as possible since working there under these conditions is almost impossible. In fact, I also turned to Praeger, who has now closed down his own press and is working for Ullstein. He offered to provide space for us in an emergency, at least provisionally, on the premises of his old press (Fleischmarkt Square), until we have found something suitable. I will probably have no choice but to accept his offer, although I'm not enthusiastic about this. First, though, it must be insured that we can continue working undisturbed. More about that in person. ⟨Yesterday your card of the 5th arrived, reporting such good news about Brill. ⟨As for myself, of course, I long ago gave up my trip to Berlin and Leipzig since Storfer is traveling away in the middle of the month, and we cannot leave the Verlag alone for 14 days. Thus, I'll travel directly to the Congress location. Group Psychology will be sent to you tomorrow since today is a holiday. Enclosed is a discussion from the mail in which you'll see what you've gotten yourself into again (especially with me). ⟨The biggest news here is [Richard] Kola's good fortune and demise. You've probably already read the response in the Presse. Hopefully everything will go smoothly. 210908

December 19, 1921 F · [calling card] Dr. B. is planning to be analyzed by you to get training for work as an analyst in Chicago. [Lionel Blitzten, M.D. (1893–1952), became a leading analyst in Chicago.] 211219

December 29, 1921 F · I forgot to include Loewenfeld in Munich among those who are to receive the pocket edition as a gift. ⟨ [...] Please don't announce your dream book before it's ready. Shouldn't Groddeck also get it? 211229

May 20, 1922 R · Congratulations on the new Interpretation of Dreams [Freud 1922], and cordial thanks for informing me of my undeserved and ever increasing involvement in that volume. ⟨The name of the Egyptian writer clarifies for me much of the entire orientation to the topic—also the fact that I apparently mixed my ideas with his. ⟨I have not read the article in the R [?], but only leafed through it, and in so doing I observed that the originally split off, pleasurable significance reappears in the beautification of the head (the Greek ideal of beautification). The vagina dentata could certainly be relevant as well. ⟨Enclosed is Ferenczi's letter and our copy, which was not included in yesterday's mail to you. 220520

June 20, 1922 R · Enclosed is the circular from Berlin, which again includes some "Prussian" calls for order; it will certainly be easy for me to neutralize it with some Austrian charm. ⟨That also served me well elsewhere, namely in obtaining the German visas, which we'll receive, "as an exception," while on vacation, and which are valid for three months. You'll also receive "pre-approval" for Bavaria, so you need do nothing more. I enclose three passport applications since I assume your wife will apply for a visa at the same time. If you could bring the passports (and applications) Wednesday, I'll be able to obtain the visas this week. It must be done by next Wednesday (June 28) latest, since the woman in charge is going on vacation. If you still don't have the passports, then you can urge Schütz to attend to that (telephone 15141, between 2:00 and 2:30, and around 8:00 evenings). 220620

July 25, 1922 F · I enclose Jones's letter about the collection. I told him that I'd be glad to leave everything in his hands, and that it wouldn't be good to include "Transference of Drives" and "Anal Eroticism" anywhere except in the clinical section. Thus I'm sending you the letter and would ask that you express yourself to him directly about what to do. 220725

July 31, 1922 Anna Freud · ◖Dear Dr. Rank ◖Many thanks for your card. I assume that you received my brief news, which I sent to the Verlag. I just got your Seefeld address today from Papa. ◖I sent the copy of *Group Psychology and Ego-Analysis* to the Verlag on July 15. It could not be sent directly without an export permit, although I was able to show the postal officials that it was a galley. So I finally sent it to Volckmer with the request that he forward it immediately; I hope it got to Vienna some time ago. ◖The situation with Ossipow's *Tolstoy's Childhood* is: the Verlag sent me the introduction and then chapters 4 and 5. The previous chapters had been corrected by Frau Sachs. I complained, for one cannot correct or abridge what one is not completely familiar with. Now it turns out that in my portion I corrected some sections that had already been quoted and had been corrected differently by Frau Sachs. I had to ask Storfer to compare both versions. I'm sorry so much double work is resulting from this, but I don't think that I'm at fault. ◖I've seen your letter to Lou. It's such a pity that things ended up like this, but it really was everyone's opinion (including Papa's). ◖I've had a wonderful time here, and am sad to leave. On the 5th I'll be with the others in Berchtesgaden. ◖Cordial greetings to you and your wife. 220731

August 8, 1922 R · Since it suddenly occurred to me in the meantime why Reik's old affect toward me has become acute again, I have found the correct, moderate mood for responding to him (enclosed). ◖The reason is that after Frau Dr. Sachs left the Verlag in July, a replacement for her was hired, and he has also taken on the role of mediator between the central report office and the Verlag (Herr Dr. Langhammer). ◖During his first visit after my departure, Reik saw him, and reacted with all sorts of criticisms of me, which I have now understood and have largely ignored. ◖Before you answer me, I just wanted to let you know about this as well, and about the way I have dealt with the matter. ◖I would be glad to hear soon that you have arrived safely in Berchtesgaden. Cordial greetings. ◖Yours, Rank

August 22, 1906 R · I acknowledge with thanks the receipt of your mailing from Berchtesgaden, but greatly regretted that you did not include any lines about your trip and your situation there. ◀Abraham, who is coming here on the 14th, requested that I ask you whether you would approve of his suggestion to lengthen the Congress by one day (to four days); he considers the program too extensive for three days; please let me know your opinion, since Abraham clearly wants to make a decision here. ◀Enclosed are my documents re Bianchini vs. Benedicty. I'm permitting myself to appeal to your judgment, since it's your book that is involved. Otherwise, I don't think the right of the publisher of a series to publish a foreword can be disputed; at most the author or the press, but not the translator. ◀[...] informed me today that she cannot participate in the Congress. ◀Dr. Deutsch is leaving the colony today. ◀I hope you are safely reunited with your family. 220806

August 10, 1922 F · Our letters crossed. When I have your answer, I'll write in more detail, with more enclosures from Abraham [...] The extension of the Congress is not for me to decide. If he considers it necessary, he should do so. One can easily reach one's fill of presentations. 220810

August 28, 1922 F · Many thanks to you and your wife for your letter of sympathy, from which, however, I notice that our letters have once again crossed. Now I shall not write to you again until I know your new address. ◀Jones sent me the enclosed circular; I do not know whether you have also received it, though I expect that you have. The tone is not good; Flugel's defense is not successful. ◀I cannot say that my health is good, but I am writing busily so as to complete *Ego and Id* while I am still here. If possible we want to hold out [here] until the middle of the [next] month. 220828

September 8, 1922 F · We are planning to arrive in Munich on Thursday, sometime in the afternoon (after 6:00 p.m.); we'll be driven there by the Frinks. We'll stay with them at the Vier Jahreszeiten [Four Seasons Hotel], and will depart for Hamburg on Friday at 4:20 p.m. Anna is with us too. ◀Until seeing you—unless that presents difficulties for you. 220908

September 14, 1922 F · So many little details have accumulated that I needed to add this list. ◀1) The circular worked out very well this time. ◀2) Sarasin's report on Binswanger. ◀3) Mercure and an issue of the New York Evening Post for the archives. ◀4) Complaints from Reik. What is to be done? Foolishness, childishness. ◀5) On the introduction of narcissism. ◀6) So far I have one copy each of the English versions of *Beyond the Pleasure Principle* and *Group Psychology* and *Ego-Analysis*. I'll ask for more copies, and will also ask that copies be sent to Havelock Ellis and Jelliffe. ◀7) I'd like to purchase a Congress calendar. ◀8) A letter from the Spanish publisher. Please explain. ◀9) Contribution from old Spielrein. Can it be printed? Not much in itself; should be rejected, given the Russian typeface. ◀10) Eitingon writes that the French publication of *Psychopathology of Everyday Life* has been canceled in Paris. Shouldn't Payot be urged to proceed? ◀11) If the Verlag resettles, what will you do with our stocks of paper? ◀12) Mrs. Riviere, who is leaving soon, wishes to have a meeting with you to discuss the Press. Would Friday evening? Or Sunday? ◀Two points are still missing on 14). 220914

September 28, 1922 F · We are buying some necessary items, and are expecting you and Frau Beata at 1:00 for lunch here. The invitation is extended by Mrs. Bijur and Dr. Frink. 220928

March 26, 1923 R · Since Pauli was sick last week, I sent you by mail (on Thursday) the letter from Ferenczi that you wanted. Unfortunately it didn't occur to me until later that there is, of course, a strike, but I hope that in the meantime the letter has made its way into your hands. The letter seems to suggest that Dr. S. is involved— whom our colleague Reich thought he was so sure of. ◀Just as a precaution, I'll take this opportunity to repeat that the meeting of April 4 has been postponed, although the numerous analysts I met yesterday outside Vienna still didn't know anything about this (presumably as a consequence of the postal strike). ◀Perhaps, dear Professor, you'll let me know, through Pauli, whether you expect me on Wednesday, and whether you've heard from Ferenczi, since my plans for Easter would be affected accordingly. 230326

December 5, 1923 R · Mr. Money-Kyrle asked me to pass on a request to you since it's so difficult for him to make himself understood on the phone. ◀Given the recent pregnancy of his wife—who incidentally has left for England to visit a sick relative— he'd like to know when he could continue with his analysis and how long it might last, since the child is expected in July and the delivery is in England. ◀Perhaps you could answer him directly (Hotel Regina) and invite him for a brief discussion, which would be very beneficial for him now. ◀I enclose an article on "Mignon"*; based on the title I ordered it for you! ◀*Goethe poem (involves father-daughter relationship). 231205

April 3, 1924 R to Ferenczi and Eitingon · I acknowledge with thanks your detailed letter of the 30th, as well as the enclosures, which I return with this letter. ◀Yesterday evening the Professor announced to me that upon the urging of his family he has decided to remain far from the strains of the Congress and to take a long recuperative vacation in the Easter period since he hasn't fully recovered from his last cold. I didn't even try to dissuade the Professor from this decision—on the one hand since I could not oppose the firm will of his family (including Hollitscher), and on the other hand because I honestly had to admit that the vacation would suit him better than the Congress. ◀In any case, I did not conceal the fact that this would absolutely devalue the Congress for the participants this year, or might even make it impossible. Then we discussed the extent to which this already given situation would simplify the problems that have been occupying us so much recently, whereupon the Professor openly confessed to me that that was an additional motive leading him to agree to his family's plan, already formed weeks ago. ◀For us, the situation seems to be: if the Congress is canceled, which is not impossible, all the problems disappear for the time being. By Fall, they could well have developed in various directions—differently, and in a way more favorable to resolution, hopefully. If, however, the Congress is held, then the discussion of the former Committee announced by Abraham will certainly be canceled; after all, it was intended mainly for the Professor. I definitely support holding the scientific discussion on the first day of the Congress: your idea of canceling it does not strike me as especially fortunate, and also seems impracticable since the Professor is also opposed to it. Concerning the election of the president, the arguments of Max (to whom I am simultaneously sending a copy of this letter) have not completely convinced me, but in conjunction with a certain change in mood they led me to tell the Professor yesterday that I would not publicly protest against the Abraham election. An important factor was Max's friendly offer to take over for me the position of secretary so that I would not be compelled to work together with Abraham. I shall accept this friendly offer—all the more since my absence from Europe for several months could in any case make it difficult for me to carry out my duties as secretary. In compensation for this, the Professor has offered me the presidency of the Vienna group. In any case, I have had to serve as president pro tempore almost continuously this year; the Professor no longer wishes to serve as president. About this decision, too, he seems firmly decided, but he does not wish to announce it officially before informing the two of you, as former Committee members and current friends. Anyway.... ◀In conclusion, I would add that there is only one point concerning which I am willing to make no concessions whatsoever: the non-existence of the Committee. I am convinced—as is the Professor too, by the way—that it has brought about its own demise and is no longer worthy of support. Having said this, I think I've said everything essential; I don't see much occasion or material for any further preliminary discussions between us. It will be a question of acknowledging our agreement, as it were—which, hopefully, has been restored to the greatest possible degree. The Professor also seems to place great value on this; today he wrote to Max that he should try to arrive in Vienna somewhat earlier than planned, since the Professor himself plans to depart by the 17th. The Professor also hopes that you, dear Sandor, will be here by then so you'll be able to speak with him. Of course I'd be glad to see you in Vienna if the Congress is canceled, to say farewell before my departure for America, about which the Professor again expressed his strong personal agreement yesterday. 240403

April 9, 1924 R · Once again I have a bad cold, and before the trip I can't risk going out at night. Therefore at today's meeting Federn will take on the position of president pro tempore. ◀If you begin your weekend this Friday, which hopefully was beneficial to you last time as well, I won't know whether I'll be able to see you this week, though I would like to see you once more before the beginning of the official wave of visitors—next week. Eitingon telegraphed that he'll arrive early on the 16th; the Ferenczis are arriving on the 15th. ◀I enclose the letters that arrived in the meantime. The one from Ferenczi, which arrived today, is a surprise for me, but a pleasant one, since he's prepared for the situation—and this was necessary. I'm glad that Sandor has done this so tactfully, yet decisively. ◀As soon as I am able to go out, and as soon as I know that you are in Vienna, I'll ask you by phone when I can see you. 240409

August 14, 1924 R [from NY] · Dr. Wechsler, who left a few days ago for a brief trip to Palestine, would like to pay you a visit during his journey, and asked me to recommend him to you. ◀Dr. Wechsler is a member of the local (N.Y.) psychoanalytic group; although he is a neurologist, he is interested in psychoanalysis, which he supports here. 240814

October 21, 1924 R · Since we arrive in Vienna on Sunday, October 26, and the general meeting, as Federn informed me, is scheduled for Wednesday the 29th, please let me know in Vienna when I might speak with you prior to the meeting; Sunday afternoon would be fine if you would prefer that. 241021

August 26, 1925 R · Sincere thanks for your kind invitation. I'll take the liberty of telling you that I'll arrive in Semmering on Saturday the 29th of this month at 4:11, so I'll be able to visit you at 4:30. 250826

October 1, 1925 R · For various reasons, I've delayed my departure, but now I must go: I'll leave Sunday evening at 11:00. I'd be very glad if you could spare a quarter hour before then to see me so that I can bid you farewell. May I ask you to let me know by phone perhaps whether and when this would be possible? 251001

Appendix B

A Precocious Dream Analysis

In 1905 Rank produced three essays based on his reading of Freud: an essay on the artist that was reworked with Freud and published in 1907, the dream analysis presented here, and a paper, "The Essence of Judaism."

We insert the Frau Doni dream from The Interpretation of Dreams (1900). *Rank used quotation marks to imply Freud's unspoken reaction to the material. Rank refers, of course, to page numbers in the first edition of the book. At the end of the analysis, we add comments written by two scholars, recognizing that even psychoanalysts differ on interpretation.*

Introduction

In October last year, when I was engaged in a brief study of child psychology, Dr. Adler made me aware of your book, *The Interpretation of Dreams.* I then read it through, really enthused. I understood it for the most part—of course, only to the extent that I found the particular topics of interest.

It wasn't until April this year that the wish arose to study the work again thoroughly, going into all the sections. However, unable to get the book right away, I meanwhile read *Studies on Hysteria* (1895) and several of your essays in various journals. Toward the end of April, Dr. Adler was kind enough to provide me with *The Interpretation of Dreams.* My knowledge of the "psyche" had meanwhile grown somewhat deeper, and a numerical analysis I conducted myself (22) opened my eyes completely.

Then, in reading your book again, I came across the dream labeled "III," which I undertake to analyze now.

This is all I know about you, your circumstances, and your works. (I was unfortunately unable to obtain your other books.)

[The Frau Doni dream: "I was going to the hospital with P. Through a district in which there were houses and gardens. At the same time I had a notion that I had often seen this district before in dreams. I did not know my way about very well. He showed me a road

315

that led round the corner to a restaurant (indoors, not a garden). There I asked for Frau Doni and was told that she lived at the back in a small room with three children. I went towards it, but before I got there met an indistinct figure with my two little girls; I took them with me after I had stood with them for a little while. Some sort of reproach against my wife, for having left them there." *S.E.*, 4:483]

Analysis

"I was going to the hospital with P. Through a district in which there were houses and gardens." With P you have "come a way in life on the same path." The houses therefore aren't close together, as in city streets, but "in the area." Thus there is open space. The opposite, for example, would be narrow, small, tight circumstances (from which you yourself came?). Houses, gardens, and space: this surely brings to mind "villa." If your parents had been wealthy, if they had possessed a villa with a garden (opulent circumstances), things would have been different for me. (The villa is also found in a dream on page 217 ["Villa Secerno," 352]. There, "the first word is vague, perhaps Via, or Villa . . . or even Casa. The second word [Secerno] . . . expresses my anger that he kept his address secret from me for so long.") (Was the friend in Italy perhaps P? [It was Fliess: see 352n1].) In Dream III, in front of the "Villa," you keep your humble origins a secret, as it were; instead of that, you [...] expression. To dream of houses and gardens in an area. Casa, by the way, immediately suggests house; Italy suggests garden (Earthly Paradise). Via is associated with Frau Dona A——y, and leads back to villa. Dona brought to your mind Donna (with double "n"); via sounds like a child's pronunciation of villa, and Frau A——y corresponds: you convert the "y" to "i"; you keep the "a"; the double "n" reminded you of double "l" (Villa). For a long time, your passion was Rome (city, as opposed to villa), Italy, a villa. Rome: city. Not in the city ([...] narrow rooms, chambers), but in the town (villa): area of houses and gardens. Wish. But now you go through the area. Thus, you were not permitted to awaken in a villa (nor later to live in one). You enter the hospital: in any case, as a child you could certainly have slept in the same room with your parents (narrow circumstances; few rooms). It was at this time that you probably developed the germ of the neurosis: you enter the hospital. (I believe I can conclude from the "Sparrow-Hawk Dream" that you slept in the same room with your parents. There you say: "I awoke crying and screaming, and disturbed my sleeping parents.")

"At the same time I had a notion that I had often seen this district before in dreams."

In your dreams and in the analyses there are frequent occurrences of the fear that you could die before leading your children beyond puberty. (You have seen the area numerous times.) The point of this worry is that you wish to spare your children what you yourself were not spared in childhood. You probably still do not possess a villa (though you may have a large home). The fear as to whether your home was large enough (with individual children's rooms), or whether the children would have to sleep in the "bedroom." Would they too have to go to the hospital now? You must also have had frequent doubts as to whether you had thus far preserved your children from everything. You parry: "this worry is of course only an idea, only a dream."

"I did not know my way about very well."

In fact, you do not know whether you have spared your children or not.

"He showed me a road that led round the corner to a restaurant (indoors, not a garden)."

P shows you what you should have done to proceed right through all your doubts (conflict), without being touched by them, into a cheap restaurant (around the corner: with your [...] and your children you are standing at a corner, as it were). Unmarried men are often childless men. Married couples usually dine in more elegant restaurants. Thus, either you should have wished to remain unmarried or you should have wished to have no children in your marriage. Then you would not have these worries. "Large room, not garden." (The large room is the opposite of "Frau Doni's" little room, and of the "narrow room" you slept in as a child?) It was one room, not a garden (villa). If you had no children, you wouldn't wish for a "villa." Then you could sleep with your wife in one room (chamber), unconcerned.

"There I asked for Frau Doni and was told that she lives at the back in a small room, with three children. I went towards it, but before I got there met an indistinct person with my two little girls. I now take them with me after I had stood with them for a little while."

On the day before the dream you had read in the newspaper the obituary of Frau Dona A——y, who died in childbirth. You heard from your wife that the dead woman had been attended by the same midwife "as she herself with our two youngest."

Thinking about your children apparently brings your wife to mind (whom you presumably love less than you love your children). You tell yourself: "Even if I really 'asked about' the woman, i.e. even if I really stopped, even if I really wanted to go into her room, it would not have been appropriate: 'first, I come across an indistinct person.'" (Your wife also came from small, narrow circumstances: in the context of another dream you mention that you informed your father of your engagement, undertaken against his will (due to the poverty of the bride?).) "I could have had regular sexual relations" (as perhaps you previously had, in fact) "without marriage, with an indistinct person" (by switching the "circumstances," by taking another woman and forgetting the first one (unthinkable); ambiguous ladies).

You identify Frau Dona with your wife, and now you can shift some of your self-accusations to your wife: If our children were not "spared," it's the fault of my wife: she was the one who came from narrow circumstances (for I didn't go all the way into the room). She habitually slept in her parents' bedroom, and it was she who took our children in: Frau Doni, of course, lives with her children in her room. Your wife came from narrow circumstances. In the context of another dream you state that you had to wait four or five years before you could marry. What happened with you, in terms of sex, also relates to this dream. Your wife is at fault for everything. But since you married her, after all, it would certainly have been better, you tell yourself, if she had died in childbirth (like Frau Dona) rather than bringing the children into the world and ruining them. Frau Doni (your wife) lives in the background (narrow circumstances), and now you live together with her. (Your wife (the eternal feminine) has dragged you down, as it were, like these circumstances.)

P has passed you by: he lives in the foreground, he is childless. (He does not lead you into the "garden" usually found behind a cheap restaurant, but into the large room, which is in front, along the street.) People with children always live in the background, for they must use their energies to produce and feed their families, while the childless can use their extra energies "for culture." He has passed you by. But if I had wanted to have children, there should have been fewer of them. At the time you were writing the book, as I learned from the book itself, you had six children. Frau Doni has three. Thus, your wife is also at fault for that. If there had been fewer children, you could have spared them better. First, you come across an indistinct person with your two little girls. If you had wanted to have children, it should have been with an indistinct "person," about whose children you wouldn't have concerned yourself. Then you would not have entered the room (indeed, you do not enter the room in the dream) where this person had lived with her little ones. You simply would not have concerned yourself with them. "With my two little girls." The girls represent the accusations you make against your wife. The little girls: indeed, you wanted to have fewer children. The little girls (the last two: Frau Doni's midwife) should have died in your wife's childbed (thus remaining indistinct). You further declare that if everything you wished out of existence must remain a fact, it should at least be only the girls who are not "spared" (apparently you love the boys more, especially the eldest; you're very proud of him)—the girls, since it cannot harm them as much, but also due to the blame you place exclusively on your wife (both of these children are female): women are at fault for everything. "I now take them along with me after standing with them for a while." For a while you stood there and quietly watched your wife bring the children into the bedroom (but perhaps she did this behind your back, or not at all; you shift to your wife the responsibility for the possible damage your children may have suffered), until you finally took them along with you (before you discovered the etiology of the neuroses, you probably paid no attention to this): as for them, whatever has been redeemed is your own achievement.

"Some sort of reproach toward my wife" for leaving you there.

You have now dampened the strict accusations you aimed at your wife in the course of the dream to "a sort of reproach." (This is reminiscent of the situation in which a husband on the way home decides to have it out with his wife over some fault, to scold her severely, even to become crude, yet when he actually stands before her he brings forth only a timid objection.) Some of the comments you now associate with the dream strike me as still belonging to the dream content, such as your "satisfaction"—hence my analysis thereof.

"Upon awakening I feel great satisfaction, which I motivate with the thought that I shall now discover from analysis what it signifies. I have already dreamed about this." (Comment below: "a topic about which an extensive discussion has been spun out in the latest volumes of the Revue philosophique.") "But analysis teaches me nothing about this. It only shows me that my satisfaction belongs to the latent dream content, and not to any judgment upon it. It is the satisfaction that in my marriage I have had children."

In the course of the dream it is quite clear that there occurs a dampening of the initially postulated ruthless, ego-centered wishes. You make more and more concessions. I shouldn't have married; but if I married, I should have had no children; but if I had many children, it should have been with an indistinct person; but if I had to have them with my wife, they should all have been "spared"; but if they could not all be spared, at least the boys should have been; and if not all the boys, then at least the eldest (the fact that the date of the dream was the eve of your son's birthday allows one to surmise this last step). The result of all these dampenings—the manner of your reproach toward your wife in lieu of highly forceful accusations—was not solid enough for this compromise-forming court of appeals (which found itself dealing with an experienced dream interpreter, and used all its wits, as it were, to deceive you): it finally converted the affect (satisfaction) into its opposite. In the latent dream content you feel satisfaction that you have no children (the first thought of the dream: you are walking with P!), whereas you later believe the opposite. On the same page as the dream being analyzed (p. 258), is a dream designated as "II," in which the patient, upon waking, immediately says: "I'll have to tell the doctor about that." The analysis provides hints about a relationship he had planned to tell you nothing about. Here, you have a similar reversal. The dream work can deal with the affects of the dream thoughts in other ways than merely admitting them or repressing them to the null point: it can convert them to their opposite (p. 277). Since this clever "court of appeals" knows that you know about the possibility of the conversion of "affects into their opposite," it grasps you to prevent you from discovering this reversal here, in your ambition. You motivate your happiness upon awakening with the thought that you will now discover from analysis what it means: "I have already dreamed about this." The court of appeals flatters you with the idea that you will now solve the problem about which the extensive discussion has been spun out in the latest volumes of the Revue philosophique (it thus grasps you with astounding acuity precisely where it fears you the most: in the realm of "scientific dream interpretation"). The fact that precisely in this case the analysis could teach you nothing about paramnesia is very clear. Indeed you did not dream that you "already dreamed about this." Rather, the idea is already present that you have already seen this area several times in dreams. The other details were only a mirage intended to mislead you; when you were brought before the court of appeals, it did not grant you, as it were, what had been promised. You did not find the solution to the problem (which of course does not exclude the possibility that you could have solved the problem in another way).

Conclusion

I shall explain the "wish fulfillment" as follows: above, I already deduced the final step in the sequence of concessions—that if nothing else goes according to wish, then at least your eldest son should be "spared"—from the comment that you had the dream the night before your son's birthday. Through the sequence: Frau Dona A . . . y— Doni (your wife)—Dona from the English novel, which proceeds from your poetically talented son, you arrive at everything else. Your son is the core of this dream. The fact that he does not even appear in the dream—that, precisely, is the wish fulfillment. He has had nothing to do with these matters; he shall know nothing about your doubts, nothing about your reproach toward your wife, and thus nothing about your marital secrets (he shall not have been in the bedroom); he shall know nothing about the hospital, nothing about the childbed and midwives, and nothing about indistinct (ambiguous) women with little girls. He shall have remained far from all these things. Indeed he has remained far from them: he doesn't even appear in the dream (just as Wotan, the "hero" of Götterdämmerung, does not appear there; this expresses the highest negation of Wotan: he acts no more). You have converted your wish to fact. Your son stands above all those things: he is a poet, and in the end "for us, having children is not the only path to immortality" (p. 285). Thus you avenge yourself after all, as it were, upon the court of appeals. If you could not explain paramnesia, if you do not become immortal through your children, you are nevertheless immortal. The wish (like women) must always have the last word.

Now I believe I have also discovered that in this interpretation (by no means flawless and complete) lies the core of the entire book. The book is a defense, playing itself out in the unconscious, against the fear that you may be a neurotic. The book says: I am not a neurotic, but rather a "dreamer," i.e. a "quite normal person"; nor is my son a neurotic, but rather a poet—a superior person. All of you may consider me a neurotic, and this can be easily excused, for "When we deduce their driving forces from phenomena themselves, we recognize that the mental mechanism utilized by neurosis is not created by a pathological disturbance of inner life; rather it already lies ready in the normal structure of mental apparatus." (that is your defense).

Illness—at least the sort correctly designated as functional—does not aim for the destruction of this apparatus or the distortion of new splits within it. This illness must be explained dynamically, through the effects and weakening of the components in the interplay of forces—an interplay by which so many effects are hidden during normal function. Elsewhere, one might also demonstrate how the bringing together of the apparatuses before the two courts of appeal "also permits a refinement of normal achievement that could not be effected by one court alone" (p. 362). That is the special defense of your son (refinement: poet).

The wish fulfillment of the book is this: "my dream theory is true. It is correct. It has scientific value. Consequently I really am not a neurotic, and my son is a poet."

(Indeed, for unprejudiced persons, I would like to say that the truth of the theory is guaranteed precisely by the fact that your book is an auto-apology. Thus, you really are not a neurotic—but something close to it—and your doubts and fears have left you no peace.) Thus, the book is your therapy, and the motto you place before the entire text—"Flectere si nequeo superos, Acheronta movebo" [If I cannot bend the gods, then I shall move Acheron]—I would freely translate back into Freudian language more or less as follows: "If I cannot convince people of the correctness of my theory, I can at least tame my 'unconscious' (Acheron)."

The apparent contradiction between the first dream thought ("I have no children") and the wish fulfillment of the dream (my eldest son is spared), is explained by the origin of the dream, which I imagine approximately as follows.

You must often (consciously or unconsciously) be plagued by doubts as to whether you have protected your eldest son from childhood sexual experiences, given how dangerous these are. When you are awake, you pacify these doubts: This is only an "idea" of mine, a "dream." Now during sleep, stimulated by the experiences of the day (your son's birthday, obituary of Frau Dona A——y) and supported by them—with their approval, as it were—resistance has presented itself and has teased its opponent, the pacifying court of appeals: "Your son is really not spared, the court is correct," etc. Yet the other court of appeals wishes to deal swiftly with the teaser, and declares: I have no children at all (I go with P [into the cheap restaurant]). Period. And now I want to sleep. Accordingly, due only to your opinion (wish) that your son should be spared, you go so far as to deny his existence completely: better dead than ruined.

Even in a dream, though, it would probably never have occurred to you to feel satisfaction at the naked fact that you have no children. Rather, you feel satisfaction because you have so thoroughly dealt with your resistance, have so completely given it the lie, have so thoroughly destroyed it in its very foundations. (Indeed, you have no children!) Still, your resistance is not destroyed, as you believed (in the dream); it arises again, and the entire following portion of the dream is a compromise between the two forces, until your resistance manages to turn your satisfaction—initially opposed to your resistance—to the advantage of your resistance itself: you feel satisfaction that you have children. (From this, your resistance might conclude that it is possible, after all, that your children were not spared.) Thus the thought (wish) that you should have no children (like P), is first of all a lie in the dream—a lie used by one court of appeals to destroy the other. Secondly, the completion of the thought lies concealed therein—the thought which later surfaces: "I have no children who could have had anything to do with these matters." (Your son does not appear in the dream.)

In the context of another dream, you remark that you had always felt timidity about publishing anything, and that "Old Brücke" (or someone else?) had to order you to publish your first scientific discovery. Unconsciously, the fear was always present within you that through your scientific clothing someone might see your own naked body. (I believe you would never have discovered the etiology of the neuroses had you not come from the experience "with a black eye" yourself.) You also had this fear with the "Dream book". For a long time you let the manuscript lie unpublished, but finally you had to publish it: it was really too marvelous (said in your conscious mind). In your unconscious was the wish to see your theory recognized, and if not, at least "Flectere si nequeo . . ."

I could also explain to you why I had to be the one to "discover" all of this, but—! Anyway, perhaps you'll guess the reason yourself.

Otto Rosenfeld II Rote Kreuzgasse ◀March 12, 1905

Two Contemporary Comments

Rank's analysis is daring, and amazingly insightful into the lingering effects of Freud's poverty, the crowded family circumstances of his childhood, his disdain for his wife, and the way his interpretations both reveal and cover all this up. His son Martin was a bit of a poet, and wrote a novel, though it was not published.

Rank figures out Freud's fear of poverty and his wish to protect his children from it: "I know from my youth that once the wild horses of the pampas have been lassoed, they retain a certain anxiousness for life. Thus, I came to know the helplessness of poverty and continually fear it" (*The Complete Letters of Sigmund to Wilhelm Fliess, 1887–1904*, ed. Jeffrey Moussaieff Masson [Cambridge, MA: Harvard University Press, 1985], 374). And: "The expectation of eternal fame was so beautiful, as was that of certain wealth, complete independence, travels, and lifting the children above the severe worries that robbed me of my youth. Everything depended upon whether or not hysteria would come out right" (266).

Rank found out Freud's dislike of his wife (Erich Fromm, *Sigmund Freud's Mission* [New York: Harper & Bros., 1959], 36) and the way the whole of *The Interpretation of Dreams* is both creative and a defense against Freud's own neurosis. Rank shows himself a master of interpretation of symbols, better than Freud himself, who is always trying to reveal and conceal at the same time. To send this to Freud when he was so young, and unknown, shows such daring.

—Louis Breger, Ph.D., psychoanalyst; author, *Freud: Darkness in the Midst of Vision* (2000) and *A Dream of Undying Fame: How Freud Betrayed His Mentor and Invented Psychoanalysis* (2009)

In reading Freud's Frau Doni dream, Freud's interpretation of it, and Rank's reinterpretation, I remain convinced that Rank is implicated in the same practice that he accuses Freud of exercising. Freud, he claims, used interpretation as the final stage of wish fulfillment, and so does Rank. The key here is Rank's state of mind at the time he discovered Freud and this dream in 1904–5. He is expressing a profound loneliness and the need of a son for protection. As a result, he responds especially strongly to Freud's reference to his son in Freud's interpretation of the dream: it is Freud's son, who doesn't appear in the dream, who is exempt from Freud's worries and even despair. It is he that Freud yearns for in contrast to the bleakness in Freud's dream of his little girls living with their mother in dark poverty. For Rank, Freud's reference to his son with poetic gifts makes a special impression, for it is he, Otto Rosenfeld, who will shortly become Otto Rank, who aspires to poetic achievement. In the dream Rank believes he has discovered Freud's wish for a son like him—a belief that constitutes a perfect example of psychological projection. He's that object of Freud's desperate wish fulfillment and, if nothing else, he can believe that he has found a worthy and plausible source of protection.

Rank's reinterpretation is extraordinary and shows his special gifts. He is compelling in showing Freud's search for a way out of predicaments that burdened him considerably. Freud's Rome dreams in his *Interpretation of Dreams* indicate a strong desire, indeed, an ambition, for significant accomplishment. In his Frau Doni dream, Rank is right in showing the dramatic light and dark contrast that characterized it: Freud's preferred association with P in the "gardens" on the one hand and, on the other, his descent to the back rooms of the restaurant. His begins the dream among "villas," or, as Rank notes, his "via," an interpretation that is consistent with the dream book's salient narrative—an expression of triumph over rivals and obstacles. But beyond that, Rank is overinterpreting, and this is especially notable in his assertion that Freud's son's absence is the most significant part of the dream: Rank argues that Freud's son is exempted from the onus that Freud's little girls represent. But Freud's reference to his son in his interpretation and the fact that Freud's attributed to him poetic promise may just as easily be interpreted as an example of Freud's assertion of satisfaction with his children and not a commentary on his eldest son alone.

What I like about Rank's analysis of Freud's Frau Doni Dream and his interpretation of it is the love-hate ambivalence it expresses for Freud and psychoanalysis. It makes clear Rank's germinating attachments to a father figure and his worldview. But is also shows simultaneously a precipitous defection or, seen differently, a creative spark that I believe could have taken place only as a result of an acquired self-confidence and sense of security that he believed Freud and his movement could provide him. Indeed, he needed a mentor not just for protection and context but also for energizing his own quest for accomplishment.

—Dennis B. Klein, Ph.D., historian; author,
Jewish Origins of the Psychoanalytic Movement (1981)

Appendix C

Major Figures in the Freud-Rank Correspondence

Abraham, Karl (1877–1925). German physician, cofounder and president of the Berlin Psychoanalytic Society, developer of the "classical" model of psychoanalytic training, and member of the Committee. Married his cousin Hedwig Bürgner in 1906; they had two children, one of whom, Hilda Abraham, later became a psychoanalyst. Studied psychiatry under Jung at the Burghölzli. Analyzed Edward and James Glover, Ella Sharpe, Melanie Klein, Helene Deutsch, Theodor Reik, and Sándor Radó.

Adler, Alfred (1870–1937). Viennese physician, original member of the Wednesday Society; president of the Vienna Psychoanalytic Society in 1910. Left Freud in 1911 with nine of the 35 members of the VPS; founded the Society for Individual Psychology. Unlike Freud, who emphasized infantile sexuality, he and his followers focused on aggression, inferiority, sibling rivalry, and social feeling.

Alexander, Franz (1891–1964). Hungarian physician, first graduate of the psychoanalytic training program in Berlin. Moved to the U.S. in 1930, founded the Chicago Institute of Psychoanalysis, and later worked in Los Angeles. A major figure in psychosomatic medicine and American psychoanalysis, he formulated the "corrective emotional experience," derived from Ferenczi and Rank.

Bernays, Minna (1865–1941). Sister of Martha Freud. "Tante [Aunt] Minna" moved into Berggasse 19 in 1896, where she lived with the Freud family until her death. She frequently accompanied Sigmund Freud on trips and summer vacations.

Binswanger, Ludwig (1881–1966). Swiss physician and first president of the Zurich branch society of the International Psychoanalytical Association. Cordial friend of Freud, pioneer in existential psychiatry, he was influenced by the writings of Martin Heidegger, Edmund Husserl, and Martin Buber.

Bleuler, Eugen (1857–1939). Swiss director of the Burghölzli, formally known as the Cantonal Sanatorium and Psychiatric University Clinic in Zurich. Along with Carl Jung, opened psychiatry to the ideas of psychoanalysis. Many psychiatrists came to psychoanalysis through Bleuler or Jung, including Karl Abraham, Roberto Assagioli, Ludwig Binswanger, A. A. Brill, Max Eitingon, Sándor Ferenczi, Smith Ely Jellife, and Ernest Jones. Coined the terms *ambivalence, autism,* and *schizophrenia* (formerly called *dementia præcox*).

Brill, Abraham Arden (1874–1948). Austrian, came to the United States as an adolescent. First practicing psychoanalyst in the U.S. and earliest translator of Freud's work into English. Founded the New York Psychoanalytic Society in 1911 and served during 1919–20 as president of the American Psychoanalytic Association and again from 1929–35. President of the New York Psychoanalytic Society from 1911 to 1913 and, again, from 1925 to 1936. Opposing Freud, who advocated lay analysis, he insisted that only medical doctors could practice psychoanalysis in the United States.

Deutsch, Helene Rosenbach (1884–1982). Psychiatrist, wife of Felix Deutsch (1884–1964), physician, internist, and analyst. Studied in Munich with Emil Kraeplin and served as assistant to Julius Wagner-Jauregg during World War I. Analyzed by Freud and Abraham. In 1924, became first director of the Vienna Psychoanalytic Training Institute. Helene and Felix were close friends of the Ranks. She wrote two volumes on the psychology of women.

Eitingon, Max (1881–1943). Russian physician and first Burghölzli staff member to meet Freud, in 1907; from 1908 to 1909 underwent the first training analysis by Freud and became a lifelong trusted confidant. Married Mirra Jacvoleina Raigorodsky, a Russian actress, in 1913. Founded the Berlin Psychoanalytic Training Institute in 1920, along with Karl Abraham and Ernst Simmel. Replaced Anton von Freund on the Committee in 1920. A wealthy man, he financed the Berlin Polyclinic. President of the IPA (1927–33) and founder of the International Training Committee (1925–43). After settling in Palestine, he organized the Palestine Psychoanalytic Society (1934). Although fluent in six languages, a slight speech defect made him reluctant to speak in public.

Ferenczi, Sándor (1873–1933). Hungarian physician and psychoanalyst. Met Freud in 1907 and corresponded extensively with him. Committee member, author of many papers, he developed Active Therapy. Analyzed Ernest Jones, Anton von Freund, and Clara Thompson. Practiced briefly in New York. Rank's closest ally, he stayed with Freud but was alienated from him near the end of his life, as revealed in his *Clinical Diary.*

Groddeck, Georg W. (1866–1934). German physician, pioneer of psychosomatic medicine, director of the Baden-Baden clinic, and self-described "wild analyst." Close friend of Ferenczi, with whom he conducted a mutual analysis. Supported by Freud and Rank, and in 1921 the Verlag published his Rabelaisian novel *Der Seelensucher* (The Soulseeker) and in 1923, *Das Buch vom Es* (*The Book of the It*), a collection of thirty-three "Psychoanalytic Letters to a Friend." His "It," the power that makes a human being act, think, grow, become sick or sound, found an echo in Freud's "Id."

Jones, Ernest (1879–1958). Welsh-born psychiatrist, worked in Canada and was an early organizer of psychoanalysis in the U.S. Headed the movement in England; first suggested the Committee in 1913. Wrote the most influential Freud biography, in three large volumes, 1953–57. Had two children with third wife, Katherine. Founded the International Psycho-Analytical Press, an English branch of the Verlag, which published the *International Journal of Psycho-Analysis,* books in the International Psycho-Analytical Library, and James Strachey's translations of Freud.

Newton, Caroline (1893–1975). American social worker. Analyzed by Freud and Rank. Fluent in German and worked with Thomas Mann. Member of the Vienna Psychoanalytic Society, 1924–38. Translated *The Development of Psychoanalysis* (1925) by Ferenczi and Rank. Stirred controversy by practicing psychoanalysis in New York.

Radó, Sándor (1890–1972). Hungarian lawyer and medical doctor. Replaced Rank as chief editor of the *Zeitschrift* in 1924. Analyzed Wilhelm Reich, Heinz Hartmann, and Otto Fenichel. Moved to New York in early 1930s and founded the first training institute of the New York Psychoanalytic Society and, later, the Psychoanalytic Clinic at Columbia University's medical school.

Rank, Beata ("Tola"), née Mincer or Munzer (1886–1961). Polish wife of Otto, member of the Vienna Psychoanalytic Society, and, after her emigration, a child psychoanalyst in Boston. Their only child, Helene (1919–99), became a clinical psychologist, practiced in San Francisco, had two children. In 1923, Tola translated Freud's *Über Träume (On Dreams)* into Polish. Cofounded the James Jackson Putnam Children's Center in 1943 and served for decades as a training analyst at the Boston Psychoanalytic Institute. The Ranks divorced in 1939.

Riviere, Joan H. (1883–1962). A founding member, with Jones, of the British Psychoanalytic Society in 1919. English translator of Freud and translation editor of the *International Journal of Psychoanalysis* (1920–37). Analyzed by Ernest Jones and by Freud. A proponent of Melanie Klein's ideas, in conflict with Anna Freud. Analyzed John Bowlby and Donald Winnicott.

Sachs, Hanns (1881–1947). Austrian lawyer, lay analyst, and member of the Committee. With Rank, coauthor of *The Significance of Psychoanalysis for the Mental Sciences* (1913) and co-editor of the journal *Imago,* created in 1912. Training analyst at the Berlin Psychoanlytic Institute, trained Franz Alexander, Michael Balint, Erich Fromm, Rudolf Löwenstein, and Karen Horney. After moving to Boston in 1932, taught at the Harvard Medical School. In 1944, published *Freud: Master and Friend,* the first book to reveal the existence of the Committee.

Stekel, Wilhelm (1868–1940). Austrian physician, early associate of Freud. Prolific author and active contributor to meetings of the Vienna Psychoanalytic Society, he opposed Freud's views on the harmfulness of masturbation and the existence of the actual neuroses. In 1912, split with Freud over his role as editor of *Zentralblatt für Psychoanalyse.* Pioneered in short-term therapy. He committed suicide in London in 1940.

Taft, Jessie (1882–1960). American psychologist and social worker. Studied at the University of Chicago with George H. Mead and completed a doctorate in 1913 with "The Woman's Movement from the Point of View of Social Consciousness." Heard Rank in June 1924 at the annual meeting of the American Psychoanalytic Association, became his patient in 1926, and thereafter, a friend and Rank's American translator (*Will Therapy* and *Truth and Reality*) and biographer (*Otto Rank*, 1958). She and her life partner Virginia Robinson taught at the University of Pennsylvania School of Social Work. Robinson cofounded the Otto Rank Association in 1966.

Williams, Frankwood E. (1883–1936). American physician and psychiatrist. From 1916 to 1931, a prominent member and chair of the National Committee for Mental Hygiene, founded by Clifford Beers and Adolf Meyer. Underwent analysis in Vienna with Rank in 1925. Traveled to Russia to study the Communist system.

Appendix D

Family Chart of Sigmund Freud in 1905

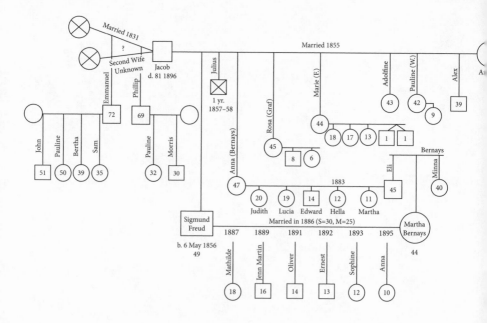

Freud's father, Jacob, had two prior marriages. Sigmund had two half-brothers his mother's age. Emmanuel's son John, though a nephew, was two years older than Sigmund, his childhood companion. Freud had five sisters and a brother, 12 full and six half nieces and nephews. Martha and Sigmund had six children, all younger than Otto Rank, who was then 21. Martha's unmarried sister Minna lived in the Freud household; their brother Eli married Freud's sister Anna. [Circle indicates female; square indicates male. Individual ages as of 1905.]

Appendix E

Otto Rank Family Tree

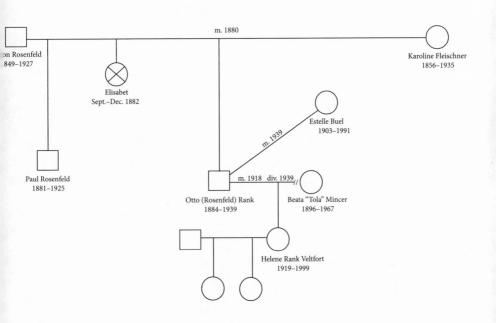

m. 1880

on Rosenfeld
849–1927

Karoline Fleischner
1856–1935

Elisabet
Sept.–Dec. 1882

Estelle Buel
1903–1991

m. 1939

Paul Rosenfeld
1881–1925

Otto (Rosenfeld) Rank
1884–1939

m. 1918   div. 1939

Beata "Tola" Mincer
1896–1967

Helene Rank Veltfort
1919–1999

Notes

Abbreviations

Brief excerpts from letters usually do not carry notes, since date, sender, and recipient are evident. The minor Freud-Rank letters appear in full in Appendix A. Notes indicate sender with * before initial: *F-Fer or F-*Fer. The notes use the letter dates and numbers given in the primary sources (not page numbers, which vary in different editions).

AoW	Lieberman, *Acts of Will* (1985)
BPS	Archives, British Psychoanalytical Society, London
F-Ab	Freud-Abraham, *Complete Correspondence* (2002)
F-Anth	Freud, *Letters* (1960)
F-Eit	Freud-Eitingon, *Correspondence*, vols. 1–2 (2004)
F-Fer	Freud-Ferenczi, *Correspondence*, vols. 1–3 (1993–2000)
F-Jo	Freud-Jones, *Complete Correspondence* (1993)
F-Jung	Freud-Jung *Letters* (1974)
GP	Rank, *Genetsiche Psychologie*, 3 vols. (1927–29)
ID	*Interpretation of Dreams*
IJP	*International Journal of Psychoanalysis*
J	Jones, *Sigmund Freud: Life and Work*, 3 vols. (1953–57)
LoC	Freud (and others) papers, Library of Congress, Washington, DC
Minutes	Nunberg and Federn, *Minutes*, Vienna Psychoanalytic Society, 4 vols. (1962–75)
OR	Otto Rank papers, Rare Books and Manuscript Library, Columbia University
PoD	Rank, *Psychology of Difference* (1924–38) 1996
Rbr	Wittenberger and Tögel, *Die Rundbriefe*, 4 vols. (1999–2006)
S.E.	Freud, *Standard Edition* (1953–74)
ToB	Rank, *Trauma of Birth* (1929 [1924])
TR	Rank, *Truth and Reality* (1936 [1929])
WT	Rank, *Will Therapy* (1936 [1929–31])

Preface

1. Falzeder 2007.

2. Martin Freud, *Glory Reflected: Sigmund Freud as Man and Father* (London: Angus and Robertson, 1957), 17, 107, 121.

3. Ibid., 26–27, 32–33.

4. Taft 1958, xvi.

Introduction

1. The original and translated diary (unpublished) are in OR; excerpts in *AoW*, 1–43.

Chapter 1. The Vienna Psychoanalytic Society, 1906–1910

1. *Minutes*, 1:75, Dec. 5, 1906.

2. *Minutes*, 1:60, Nov. 21, 1906.

3. *F-Jung 8F, Dec. 6, 1906.

4. *F-Jung 11F, Jan. 1, 1907.

5. Rank 1907, 38. *AoW*, 81.

6. F-*Jung, 17J, Mar. 31, 1907.

7. *F-Jo, 18F, Apr. 7, 1907.

8. *Minutes*, vol. 1, Jan. 23, 1907.

9. *The Interpretation of Dreams*, 2nd ed., 1909, *S.E.*, 4:135.

10. *F-Jung 92F, May 10, 1908.

11. J. Keith Davies and Gerhard Fichtner, *Freud's Library: A Comprehensive Catalogue* (London: Freud Museum, 2006). The item referred to is #2885 (we used the CD version).

12. F-*Jo 18, Oct. 17, 1909.

13. *Minutes*, vol. 2, Oct. 8, 1909.

14. "A Dream That Interprets Itself," *Jahrbuch*, vol. 2, 1910; *Psychoanalytic Review* 5 (1918): 230–34.

15. F-*Jo 51, Feb. 8, 1911.

16. *F-Fer 130, Apr. 24, 1910.

17. E. Hitschmann, 1911: E. Mühlleitner, *Bibliographisches Lexikon der Psychoanalyse* (Tübingen: Diskord, 1992), 150; *F-Fer 130, Apr. 24, 1910.

18. *F-Jung 218F, Nov. 30, 1910.

Chapter 2. Alfred Adler Departs, 1911

1. *Minutes*, vol. 3, Feb. 22, 1911.

2. *F-Jo 54, Feb. 26, 1911.

3. *F-Jung 238F, Mar. 1, 1911.

4. *F-Fer 204, Mar. 12, 1911.

5. *Minutes*, vol. 3, May 3, 1911.

6. *F-Fer 223, May 28; 230n2, June 20, 1911.

7. Heinrich Leuthold, *Gedichte* (Zurich, 1879); trans. E. James Lieberman.

8. *Die Sache:* The "cause," "matter," thing. Freud often used the term as shorthand for psychoanalysis. See Kramer, 1997.

9. J2:85.

10. *F-Ab 117F, Nov. 2, 1911.

11. *Minutes,* vol. 3, Dec. 20, 1911; Vienna Psychoanalytic Society, Diskussion der Wiener Psychoanalytische Verein, *Die Onanie* (Wiesbaden: Bergmann, 1912).

12. Rank, *Jahrbuch* 3, 1911. Havelock Ellis, *Psychology of Sex* (London, 1933), 134–35.

Chapter 3. Judging Jung, 1912–1913

1. Freud, *Psychopathology of Everyday Life* (*S.E., 6*) 68, and *Introductory Lectures* 33 (ch. 2, "Parapraxes").

2. Original in Zurich Zentral Bibliotek, O Pfister Nachlasse 3.30; copy in OR and LoC.

3. *F-Fer 316, Jul. 28, 1912.   4. F-*Fer, 317 Aug. 6, 1912.

5. F-*Fer 331, Oct. 25, 1912.

6. *F-Fer 332, Oct. 27; *F-Jo 99, Nov. 8, 1912.

7. F-*Jung 323J, Nov. 11, 1912.   8. F-*Jung 338J, Dec. 18, 1912.

9. *F-Fer 359, Dec. 23, 1912.   10. *F-Jung 342F, Jan. 3, 1913.

11. *F-Fer 353, Dec. 9, 1912.

12. *Z. Pathopsychologie,* no. 1, 1911, critical of psychoanalysis, Jung wrote from Germany.

Chapter 4. The Committee, 1913–1914

1. J2:154. Jones said they ranked as follows in Freud's esteem: Ferenczi "easily first," Abraham, Jones, Rank, Sachs.

2. F-*Jo 114, Jan. 30, 1913.   3. *F-Jo 115, Feb. 10, 1913.

4. F-*Jo 121, Apr. 25, 1913.   5. *F-Ab 159F, June 1, 1913.

6. F-*Fer 391, May 3, *F-Fer 392, May 4, 1913.

7. *F-Jung 145F, June 24, 1909.

8. J. Laplanche and J.-B. Pontalis, *The Language of Psycho-Analysis*, trans. Donald Nicholson-Smith (New York: W. W. Norton, 1973), 92.

9. F-Fer, 2:xiv.   10. F-*Jo 122, June 3, 1913.

11. *F-Jo 123, June 8, 1913.   12. F-Fer, vols. 1 and 2 Intros.; F-Jo, Intro.

13. J2:99; Ellenberger 1970, 817–19; F-*Jo 133 and 139: Aug. 8 and 22, 1913.

14. J2:149.

15. J2:387. Evidence that Freud and Minna B. registered as husband and wife in a Swiss hotel in 1898 came to light in 2001. Documentation and discussion in Burston 2008.

16. *F-Fer 424, Oct. 12; 432, Nov. 9; 435, Nov. 13, 1913.

17. Editions 4–7, 1914–22; Marinelli and Mayer 2003 includes Rank's two chapters.

18. *F-Ab 184F, Nov. 9, 1913.

19. *F-Fer 470, Apr. 24; 480, June 22, 1914.   20. J2:106.

Chapter 5. War, 1914

1. F-*Jo 191, May 25, 1914.

2. *F-Jo 192, June 2, 1914.

3. *Zentralblatt* 4 (1914): 293–95; English translation in Kiell 1998, 392–96.

4. Some of these articles were reprinted in *Mythenforschung* 1919 and 1922 and in *Künstler* 1925.

5. F-*Fer 469, Apr. 18, and *F-Fer 470, Apr. 24, 1914.

6. Breger 2000, 236.

7. Freud and Andreas-Salomé 1972: *F-Lou, June 29, 1914.

8. *F-Ab 228F, July 15, 1914.

9. *F-Anna Freud, Freud Papers, LoC. *F-Jo 200, July 22; Young-Bruehl 2008, 66–68. *F-Fer 488, July 17, 1914.

10. F-Anth 167: *F-Herbert and Loe Jones (undated: Aug./Sept. 1914).

11. *F-Ab 244F, Aug. 25, 246F, Sept. 3, 1914.

12. *F-Fer 519, Nov. 25; *F-Fer 521, Dec. 2; *F-Fer 524, Dec. 15; *F-Ab 260F, Dec. 21, 1914.

13. Ernest Jones papers, BPS. Cited in F-*Jo 435, Sept. 29, 1924, n4.

Chapter 6. Limbo, 1915–1916

1. Freud and Binswanger 2003: *F-Bin 104F, Jan. 10, 1915.

2. Sigmund Freud, "Thoughts for the Times on War and Death," 1915, *S.E.*, 14: 273–300.

3. Freud and Binswanger 2003: *F-Bin 105F, Apr. 1, 1915, *F-Fer 542, Apr. 8, 1915, and *F-Fer 544, Apr. 23, 1915.

4. *F-Fer 557, July 27, 1915, from Karlsbad.   5. *F-Fer 550, July 10, 1915.

6. J2:185.

7. Sigmund Freud, *An Autobiographical Study*, 1925, *S.E.*, 20:1–76.

8. F-Anth: *F-Putnam, 169, July 8, 1915, translation modified; *AoW*, 62.

9. *F-Fer 573, Oct. 31, 1915. Published 1916–17, *The Introductory Lectures* is Freud's most translated and widely read work.

10. J2:187, 333, and 160.

11. *F-Fer 583, Dec. 17, 1915; 573n6: Galicia, population about 8 million, Polish-speaking 54 percent, Ruthenian (Ukrainian) 43 percent, German 3 percent.

12. F-*Fer 586 and n1, Dec. 26, 1915.

13. *F-Fer 589, Jan. 6; 591, Jan. 18, 1916.

14. Philologist U. v. Wilamowitz-Moellendorff (1848–1931) on Kaspar Hauser (1812–33), noted for his claim that he grew up with minimal human contact.

15. *F-Fer 607, Apr. 29, 1916.

16. *F-Fer 611, June 1, 1916.

17. *Zeitschrift* 2 (1914): 50–58; *Der Künstler und andere Beiträge*, 4th ed, 1925, 158–70. "On Conquering Cities," trans. David Winter, *Political Psychology* 31.1 (2010): 6–19.

18. German *Ubw.* ("ucs."), elaborated in Sigmund Freud, "Das Unbewusste," *Zeitschrift* 3.4 (1915): 189–203, and ibid. 3.5 (1915): 257–69; *S.E.*, 14 (1914–16).

Chapter 7. Krakow, 1916–1918

1. See Introduction by Andre Haynal to vol. 1 and Axel Hoffer to vol. 2 of F-Fer.

2. *R-F Aug. 22, 1916, app. 1.

3. *F-Fer 629, Nov. 16; 631, Nov. 26, 1916.

4. *Der Vertriebene* [The Refugee], 1917, F-*Fer 646, Jan. 28, 1917.

5. F-*Jo 219, Feb. 20, 1917. Morfydd Owen died Sept. 7, 1918, of appendicitis. F-*Jo 221, Oct. 4, 1918.

6. F-*Fer 660, Apr. 25, 1917.

7. *F-Ab 319F, July 13, 1917; see Breger 2000, ch. 17, "The First World War."

8. F-*Fer 700, Aug. 18, 1917.

9. *F-Fer 706, Sept. 17, and 798, Sept. 24, 1917.

10. *F-Fer 713, Nov. 6, 1917.

11. *F-Fer 717, Dec. 16, 1917.

Chapter 8. Active Therapy and Armistice, 1918

1. *F-Ab, 332F, Jan. 19, 1918.

2. *F-Ab, 334F and *F-Fer 729; F-*Ab 344A, 27 Oct. 27, 1918.

3. Beata Rank, interviews by K. R. Eissler (LoC; *AoW*, 169).

4. *F-Fer 742, May 9, 1918; notable mention of active therapy; also A. Haynal, "Ferenczi and the Origins of Psychoanalytic Technique," in *The Legacy of Sándor Ferenczi,* ed. Lewis Aron and Adrienne Harris (New York: Analytic Press, 1993), 53–74.

5. *Zeitschrift* 5 (1919): 34–40. Paper 15 in Ferenczi's *Further Contributions to the Theory and Technique of Psychoanalysis* [1926] (London: Hogarth Press, 1969), 189–97.

6. Duration, 1910–14; published in 1918: "From the History of an Infantile Neurosis."

7. *R-F 29 Aug.; *F-Ab 342F, Aug. 27, 1918.

8. F-*Fer 754, Sept. 10, 1918.

9. Young-Bruehl 2008, 79–81; Paul Roazen, *Meeting Freud's Family* (Amherst: University of Massachusetts Press, 1993), 109. Freud's analysis of Anna came to light in *Brother Animal,* by Paul Roazen (1969); Freud had revealed the fact to Edoardo Weiss in a letter.

10. *Minutes,* I:xxii; *AoW,* 154.

11. *F-Fer 765, Oct. 22, n2: Anna's analysis: Oct. 1918 to spring 1922; May 1924 to mid-1925.

12. F-*Ab 344A, Allenstein, Oct. 27, 1918.

13. *F-Fer 772, Nov. 17, 1918.

14. F-*Fer 774, Nov. 24 and *F-Fer 775, Nov. 27, 1918. (In 776, Dec. 3, Rank is mistakenly cited as author of Reik's paper.)

Chapter 9. Eros Meets Thanatos, 1919 and 1920

1. *Rank-Toni von Freund, Oct. 18, 1918, OR file, LoC, folder 1.

2. *F-Fer 787, Jan. 24, 1919.

3. *F-Fer 788, Feb. 3, 1919.

4. *F-Fer 790, Feb. 13, 1919. On the Swiss event: 787n5.

5. *F-Fer 794, Mar. 17, 1919. Rank's travel dates: 793 and 805. Young-Bruehl 2008, 104ff.

6. F-*Jo 234, Mar. 17, 1919; J2:160, J3:12–13.

7. F-*Lou, Aug. 25, 1919.

8. Sigmund Freud, "Analytic Therapy," *The Complete Introductory Lectures on Psychoanalysis* (1916–17), trans. James Strachey (New York: W. W. Norton, 1965), 462.

9. Sigmund Freud, *Beyond the Pleasure Principle,* ed. Todd Dufresne, trans. Gregory C. Richter (Peterborough, ON: Broadview, 2011). This new English edition, with background history and 25 commentaries, includes a significant essay by Richter on translating Freud; Breger 2000, 264–68, describes the context of Freud's work on this idea.

10. Otto Rank, *The Incest Theme in Literature and Legend: Fundamentals of a Psychology of Literary Creation* [1912], trans. Gregory C. Richter (Baltimore: Johns Hopkins University Press, 1991), 34 (ch. 2).

11. Lili Peller, *Development and Education of Young Children* (New York: Philosophical Library, 1978), 312.

12. F-*Fer 819 Aug. 28; *F-Fer 825, Dec. 11, 1919.

13. F-*Fer 823, Nov. 18, n4; On Reik: *F-Fer 824, Dec. 3, 1919.

14. *F-Jo 256, Dec. 11; sent prior to receiving 255 of Dec. 8, 1919.

15. F-*Jo 255, Dec. 8; *F-Jo 257, Dec. 23, 1919.

16. *F-Jo 267, Feb. 12, 1920. In fact, Freud was 40.

17. *F-Jo 267, Feb. 12, 1920; Havelock Ellis, *The Philosophy of Conflict* (Boston: Houghton Mifflin, 1919).

18. *F-Jo 275 and n7, May 13, 1920; Rank's (monthly) salary of 48,000 crowns appears in *F-Eit 178F, May 27. The crown was dropping in value steadily.

19. J3:31.

20. *F-Fer 837, Mar. 15, 1920 (F-Fer, vol. 3).

21. *AoW,* 169; Beata Rank, interview by K. R. Eissler, 195.

22. *F-Fer 852n2, Aug. 20, 1920.

23. *F-Fer 857, Nov. 28, and F-*Fer 859, Dec. 21, 1920. Martin had a son in April 1921.

24. *Rbr,* 1:72: Jones, Oct. 7; Rank, Oct. 15, 87ff.

Chapter 10. Rising Tension, 1921

1. R to Committee, Oct. 28, 1920.

2. *Wiener Allgemeine Zeitung,* mid March 1921. January rate in *F-Eit 1:232, 194F, Jan. 23.

3. *F-Jo 296n4, Jan. 24, 1921.   4. *F-Jo 306, Apr. 12, 1921.

5. J3:79; $1 = 4.2 marks.

6. Medical and humanitarian prizes, respectively. F-*Fer 872, June 6, 1921.

7. *Vom Vater habe ich die Statur / Des Lebens ernstes Führen / Vom Mütterchen die Frohnatur / Und Lust zum Fabulieren.* Zahme Xenien 6 (1796).

8. *F-Fer 882n6, Aug. 18, 1921. The *Journal of Nervous and Mental Disease* published Rank's *Myth of the Birth of the Hero* in 1913 and as a monograph in 1914.

9. Intro to F-Fer, 3:xx, by Judith Dupont.

10. J3:81 and F-*Fer 889 Sept. 9, 1921. Both mention climbing the highest mountain, Brocken.

11. F-*Jo 324, Sept. 6, 1921. The author was Albert Polon (n3).

12. Oberndorf 1953, 136; Kardiner, in Nelson 1958, 48–49; *F-Jo 330, Dec. 9; *F-Fer 895, Dec. 15, 1921.

13. *F-Fer 870, May 8, 1921.

14. F-Anth 194: *F-Ernst and Lucie, Dec. 20, 1921, translation modified; F-*Jones 334, Dec. 26, 1921.

Chapter 11. Favorite Son, January to July 1922

1. OR: *Massenpsychologie* is better translated as "crowd" or "mass" psychology.

2. *Rbr,* Dec. 11, 1921, and Jan. 22, 1922; cited in *AoW* 432n25.

3. J3:52ff (ch. 2, "Disunion").

4. *S.E.,* 19:107–22, 1923 (quoted from 112–13).

5. See epigraph. Rank, "Don Juan-Gestalt," *Imago* 8 (1922): 142, tr. 1975, 121–23; and "Literary Autobiography," *Journal of the Otto Rank Association* 16 (1981): 16.

Chapter 12. Fratricide, August to December 1922

1. F-*Fer 909, Aug. 17, 1922.

2. J3:86: Maus was pregnant; Rosa, widowed in 1908, lost her other child, Hermann, in the war.

3. Beata Rank, interview by K. R. Eissler, Mar. 30, 1953, 12, LoC. Mrs. Bijur became Frink's second wife.

4. Rank, "Perversion and Neurosis," *IJP* 4.3 (1923): 287.

5. *Rbr,* 3:238–39.

Chapter 13. Birth of the Mother, January to June 1923

1. *Jo-Ab Jan. 1; Abraham papers, LoC.; *AoW,* 212; *F-Fer 917, Jan. 25; F-*Fer 916, Jan. 22, 1923.

2. Gay 1988, 420.

3. F-*Fer 951, Mar. 24, 1924.

4. *F-Fer, Jan. 10, 1910; Weiss 1970, 37.

5. "Recommendations to Physicians," *S.E.,* 12 (1912), 115 and 118.

6. Ferenczi and Rank 1925, 33 and 34; Freud 1926, vol. 1.

7. Ferenczi and Rank 1925, 54, 34, and 31.

8. Ibid., 25–26 (ch. 2).   9. Ibid., 38–43.

10. J3:58.

11. *Minutes,* 1:71–72, Nov. 28 1908; *S.E.,* 5:400–401.

12. *ToB,* 9.

13. *ToB,* 44, 87n2, 90, 155, and 215. Ferenczi's undated note was found in Rank's proof copy of *ToB,* OR.

14. *ToB,* 199.   15. *ToB,* 207.

16. *ToB*, 201, 203, and 207.   17. Kenworthy 1928 (1966), 178–200.

18. Thomas Mann, *Freud und Zukunft*, 1936; quoted in Ellenberger 1970, 209.

Chapter 14. Under the Knife, June to December 1923

1. Schur 1972, 359; Gay 1988, 422; J3:92; F-Anth 203: *F-L. and K. Levy, June 11, 1923.

2. Rank 1924, 119 and 197. Not translated into English.

3. Ernest Jones papers, BPS; Jones to Brill, Apr. 9, 1923, Brill papers, LoC, re Jones to Katherine Jones.

4. F-*Jo 406n2, Sept. 12; Jones papers, BPS; *AoW* 189. Gay 1988, 424; F-*Fer re: Abraham, 951, Mar. 18, 1924.

5. J3:55.

6. Jones papers, BPS; Jones-Brill, Apr. 9, 1923, Brill papers, LoC.

7. Schur 1972, 364 and 365. Re Anna: J3:96.

8. Gay 1988, 426.

9. Grosskurth 1991, 136: Abraham's *Rbr*, Nov. 7, 1923.

10. Schur 1972, 363.

11. Version 1: Freud papers, LoC; 2: Rank letters, Dupont.

12. *D.h. im Traume tut es L.G. an Ihrer Stelle, noch dazu indem er gegen einen Ihrer Grundsätze verstößt, nämlich die Analyse im Dienste der Politik missbraucht. Das heißt wohl: "Es ist doch höchste Zeit, dass ich wieder in die Arbeit gehe, spreche, denn die anderen *verstehen mich* ja doch *nicht*, 'übersetzen,' d.h. interpretieren mich schlecht (the I and the it) und missbrauchen die Psychoanalyse für ihre persönlichen Interessen. Die andern *verstehen nichts* (nothing) oder noch weniger als nichts (over-nothing)." (Erinnert an die Steigerung: nix, nix, aber gar nix!) Dabei ist zu beachten, dass das "Wortspiel" sich aber aufs Deutsche bezieht: Das *Ich* und das N-Ich-T, was wohl den Zweifel bedeutet: Werde *ich englisch* sprechen können oder *nicht*; werden *mich* die andern "verstehen" oder nicht? Im Traum ist diese Frage von Seiten des *Ich* gelöst, welches das *will*; aber noch nicht von Seiten des *Es* (des Organischen!), das unerörtert bleibt. (Der ganze Traum geht ja auch, mit seinem gedanklichen Charakter, mehr vom Ich bzw. Über-Ich aus.)

13. Wittels, 1924, 133.

Chapter 15. Crisis, January to April 1924

1. F-*Fer 946, Jan. 30; J3:57: "10 pages"; F-*Fer 948.

2. F-*Eit 290E, Jan. 31, 1924.   3. F-*Eit 291F, Feb. 7, 1924.

4. F-*Fer 948, Feb. 14, 1924.

5. Rundbrief first published as F-Ab, 429ff. We translate *Trieb* as "drive" rather than "instinct."

6. The Wolf Man case, 1918. "Under the inexorable pressure of this fixed limit, his resistance and his fixation to the illness gave way, and now in a disproportionately short time the analysis produced all the material that made it possible to clear up his inhibitions and remove his symptoms. All the information, too, which enabled me to

understand his infantile neurosis is derived from this last period of the work" (*S.E.,* 17:11). Sometime during the end-setting, "the patient lamented his flight from the world in a typical womb-phantasy and viewed his recovery as a typically conceived re-birth" (*S.E.,* 7:102). See ch. 19 for Rank's pre-Oedipal interpretation of this case.

7. *Rbr,* Jan. 4, 1924; the patient was Cavendish Moxon, therapist and author.

8. *Fer-Rank, Mar. 30, 1924; published as 953 in F-Fer.

9. Hanns Sachs, but not Eitingon. The letter was first published in *AoW,* 223–24.

Chapter 16. New York, May to October 1924

1. Rank's of Aug. 9 and Freud's of Aug. 27 are quoted in F-*Fer 972 nn2 and 3, Aug. 27, 1924.

2. *Eine Neurosenanalyse in Traümen.* F-*Fer 974, Sept. 1, and *F-Fer 976, Sept. 4, 1924.

3. F-Eit 306F, Sept. 27. F-*R Sept. 16, thought to be lost, was in the Dupont archive.

4. On Frink, *AoW,* 182. Beata Rank, interview by K. R. Eissler, 1953, 12, Freud papers, LoC. Lavinia Edmunds, "His Master's Choice," *Johns Hopkins Magazine,* Apr. 1988, 40–49, reprinted as *Unauthorized Freud: Doubters Confront a Legend,* ed. Frederic C. Crews (New York: Viking, 1998); Daniel Goleman, "As a Therapist, Freud Fell Short," *New York Times,* Mar. 6, 1990.

5. Paper read at the American Psychoanalytic Association. *PR* (1924) 11: 241–45. In *PoD,* lecture 3.

Chapter 17. About-face, October to December 1924

1. Taft 1958, x.

2. Sept. 16, 1924. Anna Freud papers, LoC; some in Young-Bruehl 2008, 148ff.

3. F-*Fer 949, Mar. 18, 1924.

4. *F-Jo 438, Nov. 5; F-*Jones 440, Nov. 11, 1924.

5. F-*Brill, Nov. 17; Brill papers, LoC; partly quoted in Lieberman 1997; (*AoW*).

6. F-*Eit 317F, Nov. 19; F-*Fer 989–92: Nov. 28, Dec. 2, 4, 7, 13. No information found about Otto and Paul.

7. Young-Bruehl 2008, 151.   8. *Rbr,* F-*Ab 467F, Dec. 15, 1924.

9. F-*Fer 996, Dec. 25, 1924.   10. Taft 1958, 113n51.

11. Kay Redfield Jamison, *Touched with Fire: Manic-Depressive Illness and the Artistic Temperament* (New York: Free Press, 1993).

Chapter 18. Reunion and Ending, 1925–1926

1. F-*Eit 324F, Dec. 29, 1924. Only 25 hours per week for 25 weeks earns $12,500.

2. Cited in part F-*Fer 998n4.

3. Brill papers, LoC.

4. A. Kardiner: oral history, 1963, Psychoanalytic Movement Project, Butler Library, Columbia University.

5. Celia Bertin, *Marie Bonaparte: A Life* (New York: Harcourt, 1982), 145. *Rbr,* 4: 233–37.

6. Sachs, review of *ToB, Zeitschrift* 11 (1925): 106–13.

7. F-*Fer 1009, Apr. 12. *F-Fer 1010, Apr. 14, 1925. *Reproduce* includes *reexperience, reenact, act out.* Franz G. Alexander and Sheldon T. Selesnick, *The History of Psychiatry: An Evaluation of Psychiatric Thought and Practice from Prehistoric Times to the Present* (New York: Harper & Row, 1966), 249.

8. *Rbr,* 4, Mar. 3 and Apr. 13, 1925. Jones, 20.4.1925/L[ondon]. Summary: F-*Fer 1011, n2.

9. *F-Eit 336F, May 13, n3: Marina Leitner, *Freud, Rank und die Folgen: Ein Schlusselkon-flikt fur die Psychoanalyse* (Vienna: Turia + Kant, 1998), 137, supposes a marital problem was involved.

10. J3:111. A tribute to Blitzten (1893–1952) appeared in 1961 (International Universities Press, privately printed). He was a leading teacher in the Midwest after Alexander moved to California.

11. *F-Fer 1021, Aug. 14, n4, and P. Ries, "Popularize or Be Damned," *IJP* 76 (1995): 759–91.

12. F-*Ab 495A, Sept. 8. F-*J 464, Sept. 19, 1925. J3:75: Jones had the Abraham and Ferenczi letters.

13. F-*Fer 1036, Nov. 28; *F-Fer 1037, Dec. 1, 1925.

14. Martin Freud, *Glory Reflected: Sigmund Freud as Man and Father* (London: Angus and Robertson, 1957), 193. Walter was a war hero for Britain against Hitler.

15. *F-Eit 368F, Jan. 28, 1926. *Rbr,* 4:299, Feb. 18, 1926/W[ein], n2.

16. *F-Fer 1052 and 1054, Feb. 27 and Mar. 3, 1926.

17. *F-Jo, 489, Aug. 30; F-*Jo, 490, Sept. 23; *F-Jo, 491, Sept. 27, 1926.

18. J3:77.

Chapter 19. Willing, Feeling, Living, 1926–1939

1. Fall 1926 lecture, New York, *PoD,* 116–27; *GP,* 1:24–40; *Mental Hygiene* 11 (1927): 176–88.

2. *ToB,* 199, 205, and 115.

3. *New Introductory Lectures* (1933). In a footnote here, J. Strachey reports equivalent statements by Freud idealizing the mother-son relationship in *Introductory Lectures* (1916–17), *Group Psychology* (1921), and *Civilization* (1930). Freud never idealized the mother-daughter relationship.

4. "*Was will das Weib?*": Dec. 8, 1925, J2:468; "*dark continent*": *S.E.,* 20:212; italics in the original.

5. Jessie Taft translated volumes 2 and 3 of *Technik* (1929 and 1931) as *Will Therapy: An Analysis of the Therapeutic Process in Terms of Relationship* (1936). With Rank's agreement, she composed the subtitle to differentiate his "two-person" relational therapy from Freud's "one-person" intrapsychic approach. The terms *will therapy* and *relationship therapy* were synonymous for Rank and Taft. Willing is always relational, according to Rank.

6. Rank 1926, 3–4. Although Freud introduced the word *pre-genital* in the sexual sense, Rank coined the word *pre-Oedipal* and was the first to employ it in the modern relational sense: "The only real new viewpoint in [my] contribution [is] the concept of the pre-Oedipus level," he said in January 1925 to the New York Psychoanalytic

Society. The phrase "pre-Oedipal development" (*präödipalen Entwicklung*) appears in "The Genesis of Genitality," presented at the Bad Homburg Congress, September 1925. Rank's typescript contains the phrase, as does *GP*, 1:71 (OR).

7. Rank 1926, 7 and 9. Rank combines "now" and "here": "jetzt (hier)"—his parentheses.

8. Rank, 1926, 14.

9. Rank, 1926, 39. A patient said, "Not free love, but loving freely." *AoW*, 270.

10. Ibid., 23 and 6.   11. Ibid., 16–17.

12. In therapy his entire life, Pankejeff (1887–1979), who called himself *Wolfsmann*, never achieved psychological separation from Freud (Mahony 1984). "According to Freud," Pankejeff stated "remembering is enough. But to remember something isn't enough. The element of experience is lacking" (Obholzer 1982, 148). He faulted the absence of will in psychoanalytic theory and practice: "There is no such concept as 'will' in Freud. For Freud, will is drive. But actually, it is the opposite, it is the capacity to repress the drive and to do what one considers rational. Which would mean that drive does not equal will" (94).

13. Rank 1926, 153.   14. Ibid., 152.

15. F-*Fer 1060, May 30, 1926.   16. *F-Fer 1061, June 6, 1926.

17. *F-Eit 387F, June 18, 1926.

18. Ferenczi, *IJP* 8 (1927): 97–100. In his 1932 *Clinical Diary*, Ferenczi reopens the debate over the priority of mother over father: "The question arises whether the primal trauma is not always to be sought in the primal relationship with the mother" (Ferenczi 1988, 83). In a letter to Freud in 1930, Ferenczi regrets that "you did not comprehend and bring to abreaction [my] negative feelings" (F-*Fer 1179, Jan. 17). Shortly before his death, Ferenczi lamented in the *Clinical Diary* his ambivalence about separating from Freud: "Not yet being born is *the danger* ... I had never really become 'grown up.' ... Is the only possibility for my continued existence the renunciation of the largest part of one's own self, in order to carry out the will of that higher power [Freud] to the end (as if it were my own)? ... Must I (if I can) create a new basis for my personality, if I have to abandon as false and untrustworthy the one I have had up to now? Is the choice here between dying and 'rearranging myself'—and this at the age of fifty-nine? On the other hand, is it worth it always to live only the life (the will) of another person—is such a life not almost death?" (Ferenczi 1988, 212).

Expressing his will was critical for Ferenczi in 1932, as it was for Rank in 1926. Strikingly, Ferenczi uses the term *will* in his *Clinical Diary*: "imposition of an alien will" (16); "the harmful superego (alien will) ... penetrates the other person with all its tendencies, while a piece of the person's own spontaneity is forcibly driven out" (77); "adults forcibly inject their will ... into the childish personality" (81). According to Dupont, Ferenczi considered Freud "incapable of making his patients (and first and foremost his pupils) independent of himself" (F-Fer, 3:xxiii), which echoes the Wolf Man's reminiscences (Obholzer 1982, 172–73).

19. *F-Fer 1079, Sept. 19, 1926.

20. Nin 1992, 294, 297, 299, and 394, Nov. 1933–Oct. 1934. The unexpurgated

diary. She reports wearing the ring in *Fire* (41). It came back to Rank, and eventually to his daughter.

21. *GP*, vol. 2; some chapters became the American Lectures: *Psychology of Difference.* Volume 3 of *GP* became *Truth and Reality: The Human History of the Will.*

22. *GP*, 1:iii–iv.

23. See Freud's 1925 essay, "Some Psychical Consequences of the Anatomical Distinction between the Sexes": "[Women's] super-ego is never so inexorable, so independent of its emotional origins as we require in men" (*S.E.*, 19:257).

24. *PoD*, 101–2. In "Literary Autobiography" Rank identifies analyst Charles Odier, who cites him in 1926 regarding "the primal source of the super-ego in the pre-Oedipal (maternal) inhibitions. The pre-Oedipal super-ego has since been overemphasized by Melanie Klein without any reference to me" (Rank 1930a, 37).

25. *GP*, 1:113–14. Gay 1988: "There is no evidence that Freud's systematic self-scrutiny touched on this weightiest of attachments, or that he ever explored, and tried to exorcise, his mother's power over him" (505).

Freud's unwillingness to analyze his mother's power over him may account for Ferenczi's remark in 1932 to Brill that "he couldn't credit Freud with any more insight than a small boy; this happened to be the very phrase that Rank had used in his time—a memory that could but heighten Freud's forebodings" (J3:172). In one of Freud's last letters to Ferenczi, Freud wrote: "I also know from [Brill] that you don't credit me with more insight than a little boy. [Just as Rank did back then.]" (*F-Fer 1238, Oct. 2, 1932; brackets in the original). See Kramer 2003 for discussion of this letter.

26. In 1929, Freud wrote to Frankwood Williams, "R[ank] has ceased to be an analyst. If you have not undergone a thorough transformation since then, I would have to dispute also your right to this name" (Gay 1988, 484). See Rudnytsky 1991 for Rank as the first object-relations theorist.

27. *GP*, 1:42, 110, 111, and 122.

28. *F-Eit 435F, June 20, 1927; *F-Eit 439F, July 2, 1927.

29. *GP*, 2:75, and *PoD*, 153. Beata said of Rank, "He was a very tender person, always wrapped up in his deep feelings. He was close to Professor and his family, very appreciative of Mrs. Freud and, I think Anna was very close to him" (*AoW*, 201).

30. *GP*, 2:76 and *PoD*, 154. Only through mutual recognition is healing—or becoming "whole"—possible. Freud nowhere writes of "I-Thou." Instead, he speaks of "I-It" to advocate the "draining" of the patient's emotions in analysis: "Where It was there I shall be," he urges. "It is a work of culture, not unlike the draining of the Zuyder Zee" (*S.E.*, 22:80). In his post-Freudian writings Rank argues for a deepening of the life of feelings. In *Modern Education* (1932b), feeling, "as I have already mentioned [*GP* 2], consists of the union of the I with the Thou, of the individual with his fellow men, in the broadest sense, with the community" (80). In *Beyond Psychology* (1958): "The [I] needs the Thou in order to become a Self" (290).

31. "Means of healing," *WT*, 1; "Philosophy," *WT*, 2; "Learn to will," *WT*, 9; "Feeling of experience," *WT*, 5. See Kramer 1995 for what Carl Rogers learned from his 1936 meeting with Rank.

32. "Actual feeling experience": *WT*, 37. "But to eliminate the will altogether, to suspend each and every affect, supposing we were capable of this—what would that mean but to *castrate* the intellect?" (Nietzsche 1989 [1887], 119; italics in the original). Willing, for Rank as for Nietzsche, is an expression of the intelligence of the emotions. Rational decision-making is impossible without the judgment provided by feelings. Unwilling to "*castrate* the intellect," Nietzsche infuses emotions into all of his thinking, reflecting a conviction that feelings are non-rational but intelligent, not irrational. For Nietzsche, the passions contain a high degree of intelligence. Strong emotions are constitutive of "the will to power" or its correlative, "the will to life" (79).

33. Alexander 1925, 487.   34. Thompson, 1924, 234.

35. *WT*, 8, 13, and 6.

36. *WT*, 37 and 39. Rank's first use of "here and now."

37. *WT*, 27, 28, and 65.

38. *WT*, 49 and 41.

39. *TR*, 25. By shifting his attention to consciousness, Rank is following in the tradition of William James, whose work he studied as a Ph.D. student at the University of Vienna (Karpf 1953, 55n). Today, consciousness is at the forefront of neuroscientific research (Taylor 2009, 315–38). See Wallace 2000 for a history of the neglect of consciousness by Western science.

40. In *Art and Artist* (1932), Rank writes: "For if one is not prepared to interpret the unconscious in the rationalistic sense of psychoanalysis as [a container for] the repressed impulse, it remains but a pseudo-scientific metaphor for the inconceivable, the divine" (xxvi).

41. *WT*, 55.

42. *WT* resonates strongly with the thought of Kierkegaard (Becker 1973; Schneider and May 1995). Rank does not cite him here, but he quotes Kierkegaard in his adolescent *Daybooks* (Jan. 1, 1905, OR) and in *Art and Artist* (413).

43. *WT*, 53 and 55.

44. *WT*, 177. "I sense an intelligence rendered clairvoyant by feeling," remembers Nin of her experience in therapy with Rank. "I sense an artist" (Nin 1966, 286).

45. Rank 1930b, 127.

46. "Creator and creature" and "Births, rebirths and new births": *TR*, 11–12.

47. *TR*, 8. In *Inhibitions, Symptoms and Anxiety*, Freud argues that emotions are "reproductions of very early, perhaps even pre-individual, experiences of vital importance" that correspond to "hysterical attacks" (*S.E.*, 20:133). Unruly feelings were seen by Freud as a cause of mental disorder, with "unpleasure" defined as an increase in emotion and "pleasure" as a reduction in emotion. Classical analysts declared that patients used "emotional experience" for sexual gratification, not insight or transformation. Understood through Freud's hydraulic metaphor, emotions were to be drained.

In *Will Therapy*, Rank criticizes Freud for reducing emotional experience merely to a derivative of sexuality: "The emotional life develops from the sexual sphere; therefore [Freud's] sexualization, in reality, means emotionalization" (165). The confusion between sexuality and emotion continued for decades among Freud's followers. "Emotions have long been seen as less than fully real, as mere epiphenomena, as derivative from those essential motivators, the instinctual drives," according to Donna Orange (1995). "Since emotion signified trouble, a psychoanalytic cure meant reducing or eliminating emotion. Making the unconscious conscious, full of cognitive insight, should render emotional signals from the unconscious almost unnecessary" (89). Since 1939, the year of Freud's death, many articles in the official psychoanalytic journals lament the absence of a psychoanalytic theory of emotions (Weinstein 2000, 15–51). The chorus includes such distinguished Freudians as Marjorie Brierly, David Rapaport, Bertram Lewin, Ernst Kris, Charles Brenner, Jacob Arlow, John Gedo, Leo Rangell, Edith Jacobson, Arnold Modell, Frank Lachmann, Robert Stolorow, Michael Franz Basch, Ethel Spector Person, John Munder Ross, and Adrian Applegarth (193–94). "Fifty years after Brierly's statement [in 1937], William Meissner noted that the psychoanalytic psychology of affective experience remains to be written, and such comments persisted throughout the 1990s" (40).

Writing in 1932 in his *Clinical Diary*, Ferenczi identified the "personal causes for the erroneous development of psychoanalysis" (1988, 184): "One learned from [Freud] and from his kind of technique various things that made one's life and work more comfortable: the calm, unemotional reserve; the unruffled assurance that one knows better; and the theories, the seeking and finding of the causes of failure in the patient instead of partly in ourselves . . . and finally the pessimistic view, shared only with a few, that neurotics are a rabble [*Gesindel*], good only to support us financially and to allow us to learn from their cases: psychoanalysis as a therapy may be worthless" (185–86).

48. Roazen and Swerdloff 1995, 82–83.

49. *TR*, 24.   50. *WT*, 113.

51. *WT*, 188–89.   52. *WT*, 82.

53. "*Artiste-manqué*": Rank 1932a, 25; "metaphysical problems": *WT*, 127.

54. *WT*, 124.   55. *WT*, 134 and 91.

56. Rank 1932a, 86.   57. ibid., xi.

58. *TR*, 31.   59. *GP*, 2:15.

60. Rank 1932a, 328–29.   61. *GP*, 2:4.

62. *GP*, 2:82.   63. *WT*, 176.

64. Nietzsche 1989 [1908], 258.

65. Rank 1932a 64. German: "*willensmäßige Bejahung des Gemußten*." Nietzsche's "*amor fati*," in *TR*, 18.

66. "Actual spring of life": *WT*, 206, and "refusal of life": 108.

67. Taft 1958, 183.

68. "I am no longer trying to prove . . . ," *PoD*, 222.

69. Nin 1966, 279. This does not appear in the unexpurgated *Incest* (1992), which "complements" the earlier version. In his preface to *Incest*, Rupert Pole alleges—falsely—that Anaïs was encouraged to seduce her father by her "psychiatrist" Otto

Rank (she was then supposed to abandon her father to punish him for abandoning her). After publication, Pole retracted his allegation.

70. Sachs 1946, 149.

71. "I was born beyond psychology": OR; Rank 1958, 16. Written in English, *Beyond Psychology* was published posthumously.

Epilogue

1. In *PoD*, 240–48.

2. *Psychoanalytic Review* 16.1 (1929); reprinted as Lecture 18 in *PoD*, 228–39.

3. Beata Rank, interview by K. R. Eissler, 1953, 9–13, LoC. Helene Deutsch, *Confrontations with Myself* (New York: W. W. Norton, 1973), 146.

4. Williams, F. *Proceedings of the First International Congress on Mental Hygiene* (New York: International Committee for Mental Hygiene, 1932), 2:142–49; *IJP* 9 (1930):513 (APA ruling). Deutsch: May 13, 1930 "calamity" in Paul Roazen, *Helene Deutsch: A Psychoanalyst's Life* (Garden City, NY: Doubleday/Anchor Books, 1985), 275.

5. Rank (1930b) 1998, 86–89.

6. Richard F. Sterba, *Reminiscences of a Viennese Psychoanalyst* (Detroit: Wayne State University Press, 1982), 116; later ed. in German: *Erinnerungen eines Wiener Psychoanalytikers* (Frankfurt: Fischer 1985), 119–20. The quotation combines the two slightly different texts.

7. Rank to Wilbur, Jan. 14, 1932; EJL, "Rank-Wilbur Correspondence," *Journal of the Otto Rank Association* 14.1 (1980): 15–16.

8. Roy Grinker, "Reminiscence," *American Journal of Orthopsychiatry* 10 (1940): 850–55, 1940; rpt. Ruitenbeck, *Freud as we Knew Him*, 1973.

9. "Analysis Intermindable," *S.E.* 23: 216; *Moses, S.E.* 23: 125; Sachs, 1946, 115; George Wilbur in Roazen 1975, 589n39.

10. See Jones to Trilling, Oct. 11, Lionel Trilling papers, Butler Library, Columbia University, and *New York Times Book Review*, Nov. 17, 1957.

11. *Time* magazine, June 23, 1958, by Gilbert Cant, *Time* medicine editor. His similar review appeared in the *New York Post*.

12. Jones to Anna Freud, Feb. 7, 1956. AF papers, LoC.

13. Earlier versions: "Trennung und Selbstschaffung: Leben und Werk von Otto Rank," *Psychoanalyse im Widerspruch* 5 (1994): 56–64. EJL, "The Evolution of Psychotherapy since Freud," in *Creative Dissent: Psychoanalysis in Evolution*, ed. Alan Roland, Ann Ulanov, and Claude Barbre (Westport, CT: Praeger, 2003).

Bibliography

Alexander, Franz. 1925. Review of *The Development of Psychoanalysis*. *International Journal of Psychoanalysis* 6: 484–96.

Becker, Ernest. 1973. *The Denial of Death*. New York: Free Press.

Breger, Louis. 2000. *Freud: Darkness in the Midst of Vision*. New York: Wiley.

Burston, Daniel. 2008. "A Very Freudian Affair." *Psychoanalysis and History* 10: 115–30.

Ellenberger, Henri F. 1970. *The Discovery of the Unconscious*. New York: Basic Books.

Falzeder, Ernst. 2007. "Is There Still an Unknown Freud?" *Psychoanalysis and History* 9: 201–31.

Ferenczi, Sándor. 1927. Review of *Technik der Psychoanalyse*. *IJP* 8: 97–100.

———. *The Clinical Diary of Sándor Ferenczi*. 1988. Edited by Judith Dupont. Translated by Michael Balint and Nicola Zarsay Jackson. Cambridge, MA: Harvard University Press.

Ferenczi, Sándor, and Otto Rank. 1925. *The Development of Psychoanalysis*. Translated by Caroline Newton. New York: Nervous and Mental Disease Publishing.

Freud, Sigmund. (1953) 1967. *The Interpretation of Dreams*. Translated by James Strachey. New York: Avon Books.

———.1953–74. *The Standard Edition (S.E.) of the Complete Psychological Works* of *Sigmund Freud*. Edited and translated by James Strachey et al. 24 vols. London: Hogarth Press and the Institute of Psychoanalysis.

———. 1960. *Letters, 1873–1939*. Edited by Ernst Freud. New York: Basic Books.

———. 1992. *The Diary of Sigmund Freud, 1929–1939: A Record of the Final Decade*. Edited and translated by Michael Molnar. New York: Charles Scribner's Sons.

———. 2002. *Unser Herz zeigt nach dem Süden: Reisebriefe, 1895–1923*. Edited by Christfried Tögel. 2nd ed. Berlin: Aufbau-Verlag.

———. 2010. *Unterdess Halten Wir Zusammen: Briefe an Die Kinder*. Edited by Michael Schröter. Berlin: Aufbau-Verlag.

Freud, Sigmund, and Karl Abraham. 2002. *The Complete Correspondence of Sigmund Freud and Karl Abraham, 1907–1925: Completed Edition*. Edited by Ernst Falzeder. London: Karnac.

Freud, Sigmund, and Lou Andreas-Salomé. 1972. *Letters*. Edited by Ernst Pfeiffer. Translated by William and Elaine Robson-Scott. New York: Harcourt, Brace.

Freud, Sigmund, and Martha Bernays. 2011. *Sei mein, wie ich mir's denke. Die Brautbriefe*. Edited by Gerhard Fichtner, Ilse Grubrich-Simitis, and Albrecht Hirschmüller. Vol. 1. Frankfurt am Main: S. Fischer.

Freud, Sigmund, and Ludwig Binswanger. 2003. *Freud-Binswanger Correspondence, 1908–1938*. Edited by Gerhard Fichtner. Translated by Arnold J. Pomerans. New York: Other Press.

Freud, Sigmund, and Max Eitingon. 2004. *Briefwechsel, 1906–1939*. Edited by Michael Schröter. 2 vols. Tübingen: Edition Diskord.

Freud, Sigmund, and Sándor Ferenczi. 1993, 1996, 2000. *The Correspondence*. Edited by Eva Brabant-Gero, Ernst Falzeder, and Patrizia Giampieri-Deutsch. Translated by Peter T. Hoffer. Vol. 1, *1908–1914*; vol. 2, *1914–1919*; vol. 3, *1920–1933*. Cambridge, MA: Belknap Press of Harvard University Press.

Freud, Sigmund, and Ernest Jones. 1993. *The Complete Correspondence of Sigmund Freud and Ernest Jones, 1908–1939*. Edited by R. Andrew Paskauskas. Cambridge, MA: Belknap Press of Harvard University Press.

Freud, Sigmund, and C. G. Jung. 1974. *The Freud/Jung Letters: The Correspondence between Sigmund Freud and C. G. Jung*. Edited by William McGuire. Translated by Ralph Manheim and R. F. C. Hull. Princeton: Princeton University Press.

Gay, Peter. 1988. *Freud: A Life for Our Time*. New York: Norton.

Grosskurth, Phyllis. 1991. *The Secret Ring*. Reading, MA: Addison-Wesley.

Karpf, Fay B. 1953. *The Psychology and Psychotherapy of Otto Rank: An Historical and Comparative Introduction*. New York: Philosophical Library.

Kenworthy, Marion. (1928) 1966. "The Prenatal and Early Postnatal Phenomena of Consciousness." In *The Unconscious: A Symposium*, intro. Ethel S. Dummer. Freeport, NY: Books for Libraries Press.

Kiell, Norman. 1988. *Freud without Hindsight: Reviews of His Work, 1893–1939*. Madison, CT: International Universities Press.

Kramer, Robert. 1995. "The Birth of Client-Centered Therapy: Carl Rogers, Otto Rank, and the Beyond." *Journal of Humanistic Psychology* 35: 54–110.

———. 1997. "Otto Rank and the 'Cause.'" In *Freud Under Analysis: Essays in Honor of Paul Roazen*, 221–47. Edited by Todd Dufresne. New Jersey: Jason Aronson.

———. 2003. "Why Did Ferenczi and Rank Conclude That Freud Had No More Emotional Intelligence Than a Pre-Oedipal Child?" In *Creative Dissent: Psychoanalysis in Evolution*, 23–36. Edited by Claude Barbre, Barry Ulanov, and Alan Roland. New York: Praeger Publishers.

Lieberman, E. James. 1979. "The Rank-Wilbur Correspondence." *Journal of the Otto Rank Association* 14: 7–26.

———. 1985. *Acts of Will: The Life and Work of Otto Rank*. New York: Free Press. Published in French in 1991: *La volonté en Act: La vie et l'œvre d'Otto Rank*. Paris: PUF, and in German in 1997: *Leben und Werk*. Gießen: PsychoSozial.

Mahony, Patrick J. 1984. *Cries of the Wolf Man.* New York: International Universities Press.

Marinelli, Lydia, and Andreas Mayer. 2003. *Dreaming by the Book: Freud's "The Interpretation of Dreams" and the History of the Psychoanalytic Movement.* Translated by Susan Fairfield. New York: Other Press. Includes Rank's chapters in editions 4–7 (1914–1922) of *The Interpretation of Dreams.*

Nelson, Benjamin, ed. 1958. *Freud and the Twentieth Century.* London: Allen & Unwin.

Nietzsche, Friedrich. (1887) 1989. *On the Genealogy of Morals.* Translated by Walter Kaufman and R. J. Hollingdale. *Ecco Homo* (1908). Translated by Walter Kaufman. New York: Vintage Books [combined edition].

Nin, Anaïs. 1966. *The Diary of Anaïs Nin.* Vol. 1, *1931–1934.* Edited by Gunther Stuhlmann. New York: Harcourt, Brace & World.

———. 1992. *Incest: From "A Journal of Love," 1932–1934.* New York: Harcourt Brace Jovanovich.

———. 1995. *Fire: From "A Journal of Love," 1934–1937.* New York: Harcourt, Brace.

Nunberg, Herman, and Ernst Federn, eds. 1962–1975. *Minutes of the Vienna Psychoanalytic Society.* Vols. 1–4. New York: International Universities Press.

Oberndorf, Clarence P. 1953. *A History of Psychoanalysis in America.* New York: Harper.

Obholzer, Karin. 1982. *The Wolfman: Conversations with Freud's Patient.* Translated by Michael Shaw. New York: Continuum.

Orange, Donna M. 1995. *Emotional Understanding: Studies in Psychoanalytic Epistemology.* New York: Guilford Press.

Rank, Otto. 1907. *Der Künstler.* Vienna: Heller. Translated by Eva Salomon as *The Artist, Journal of the Otto Rank Association* 15.1 (1980).

———. (1922) 2004. *The Myth of the Birth of the Hero: A Psychological Exploration of Myth.* 2nd ed. Translated by Gregory C. Richter and E. James Lieberman. Baltimore: Johns Hopkins University Press, 2004. Originally published, 1909.

———. 1924. *Eine Neurosenanalyse in Träumen.* Leipzig: Internationaler Psychoanaltischer Verlag.

———. (1924) 1975. *The Don Juan Legend.* Translated and edited by David G. Winter. Princeton: Princeton University Press.

———. (1924–38) 1996. *A Psychology of Difference: The American Lectures.* Edited by Robert Kramer. Princeton: Princeton University Press.

———. 1926. *Technik der Psychoanalyse: Die Analytische Situation.* Vol. 1. Leipzig: Franz Deuticke.

———. 1927. *Genetische Psychologie: Grundzüge einer Genetischen Psychologie auf Grund der Psychoanalyse der Ich-Struktur.* Vol. 1. Leipzig: Franz Deuticke.

———. 1928. *Genetische Psychologie: Gestaltung und Ausdruck der Persönlichkeit.* Vol. 2. Leipzig: Franz Deuticke.

———. 1929a. *Genetische Psychologie: Wahrheit und Wirklichkeit.* Vol. 3. Leipzig: Franz Deuticke.

———. 1929b. *Technik der Psychoanalyse: Die analytische Reaktion in ihren konstruktiven Elementen.* Vol. 2. Leipzig: Franz Deuticke.

——. (1929c) 1993. *The Trauma of Birth*. New York: Dover. German ed., 1924.

——. (1930a) 1981. "Literary Autobiography." *Journal of the Otto Rank Association* 16: 3–38.

——. (1930b) 1998. *Psychology and the Soul: A Study of the Origin, Conceptual Evolution, and Nature of the Soul*. Translated by Gregory C. Richter and E. James Lieberman. Baltimore: Johns Hopkins University Press.

——. 1931. *Technik der Psychoanalyse: Die analyse des Analytikers und seiner Rolle in der Gesamtsituation*. Vol. 3. Leipzig: Franz Deuticke.

——. 1932a. *Art and Artist: Creative Urge and Personality Development*. Translated by Charles Francis Atkinson. New York: Knopf.

——. 1932b. *Modern Education*. Translated by Mabel Moxon. New York: Knopf.

——. (1936) 1945. *"Will Therapy" and "Truth and Reality."* Translated by Jessie Taft. New York: W. W. Norton & Company, 1978.

——. (1941) 1958. *Beyond Psychology*. New York Dover.

Roazen, Paul. 1975. *Freud and His Followers*. New York: Knopf.

Roazen, Paul, and Bluma Swerdloff, eds. 1995. *Heresy: Sándor Radó and the Psychoanalytic Movement*. Northvale, NJ: Jason Aronson.

Rudnytsky, Peter. 1991. *The Psychoanalytic Vocation: Rank, Winnicott, and the Legacy of Freud*. New Haven: Yale University Press.

Ruitenbeek, Hendrik M. 1973. *Freud as We Knew Him*. Detroit: Wayne State University Press.

Sachs, Hanns. 1946. *Freud: Master and Friend*. Cambridge, MA: Harvard University Press.

Schneider, Kirk, and Rollo May. 1995. *The Psychology of Existence: An Integrative, Clinical Perspective*. New York: McGraw Hill.

Schur, Max. 1972. *Freud: Living and Dying*. New York: International Universities Press.

Taft, Jessie. 1958. *Otto Rank*. New York: Julian Press.

Taylor, Eugene. 2009. *The Mystery of Personality: A History of Psychodynamic Theories*. New York: Springer.

Thompson, Clara. 1964. *Interpersonal Psychoanalysis*. Edited by Martin G. Green. New York: Basic Books.

Wallace, Alan B. 2000. *The Taboo of Subjectivity: Toward a New Science of Consciousness*. New York: Oxford University Press.

Weinstein, Fred. 2001. *Freud, Psychoanalysis, Social Theory: The Unfulfilled Promise*. Albany: State University of New York Press.

Weiss, Edoardo. 1970. *Sigmund Freud as a Consultant: Recollections of a Pioneer in Psychoanalysis*. New York: Intercontinental Medical Book.

Wittels, Fritz. 1924. *Sigmund Freud*. London: George Allen & Unwin.

Wittenberger, Gerhard. 1995. *Das "Geheime Komitee" Sigmund Freuds*. Tübingen: Edition Diskord. 1995.

Wittenberger, Gerhard, and Christfried Tögel, eds. 1999–2006. *Die Rundbriefe Des "Geheimen Komitees."* Vol. 1–4. Tübingen: Edition Diskord.

Young-Bruehl, Elisabeth. 2008. *Anna Freud: A Biography*. 2nd ed. New Haven, CT: Yale University Press.

Index